An Introduction to

Manish K. Sethi • William H. Frist

Editors

An Introduction to Health Policy

A Primer for Physicians
and Medical Students

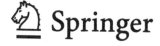 Springer

Editors
Manish K. Sethi, MD
Director of the Vanderbilt Orthopaedic
 Institute Center for Health Policy
Assistant Professor of Orthopaedic
 Trauma Surgery
Department of Orthopaedic Surgery
 and Rehabilitation
Vanderbilt University School of Medicine
Nashville, TN, USA

Senator William H. Frist, MD
Department of Cardiac Surgery
Vanderbilt University School
 of Medicine
Nashville, TN, USA

ISBN 978-1-4614-7734-1   ISBN 978-1-4614-7735-8 (eBook)
DOI 10.1007/978-1-4614-7735-8
Springer New York Heidelberg Dordrecht London

Library of Congress Control Number: 2013941871

Printed on acid-free paper

Springer is part of Springer Science+Business Media (www.springer.com)

We dedicate this book to our patients—may we continue to pursue an American health-care system that provides them the best care in the world.

Manish K. Sethi, MD
William H. Frist, MD

Preface

As the United States finds itself strapped with $16 trillion of debt, future generations of America's physicians can no longer enter their practices and clinics without a sound understanding of health care. In 2012, the total national health-care spending was $2.9 trillion, and it is expected to continue to increase at similar levels, potentially reaching 20 % of the GDP by 2016. Young doctors and medical students are likely to see a dramatic transformation of the manner in which America offers medical care to its citizens over the course of their careers.

But today, most physicians leave medical school without a sound comprehension of the key issues facing American health care; doctors understand the medicine, but not the policy. It is crucial that those on the front lines of medicine develop a sense of health care's evolution and understand potential directions of change.

An Introduction to Health Policy: A Primer for Medical Students and Physicians is the first of its kind, authored by physician leaders in health policy at major academic policy centers across the United States. This book allows busy physicians and medical students to quickly develop an understanding of the key issues facing American health care. It seeks to efficiently and effectively educate physicians and medical students on the past, present, and potential future issues in health-care policy.

This book is comprised of four sections. In Parts I and II, the reader will be introduced to the basic elements of health care and will become comfortable with essential concepts. Part III focuses on further developing these basic concepts into a "health-care system"—how all of the moving parts come together. Finally, the concluding section focuses on the manner in which health-care policy is created at both the state and federal levels.

Our ultimate goal is for a reader to leave with a balanced understanding of health care in America and the critical importance of health-care policy: physicians equipped to deliver the best possible care to their patients in a changing environment.

Nashville, TN, USA

Manish K. Sethi, MD
William H. Frist, MD

Contents

Contributors

Jordan C. Apfeld, BA Vanderbilt Orthopedic Institute Center for Health Policy, Vanderbilt University Medical School, Nashville, TN, USA

Elaine Besancon, MD Department of Internal Medicine, Brigham and Women's Hospital, Boston, MA, USA

Kevin J. Bozic, MD, MBA Department of Orthopedic Surgery, University of California, San Francisco, CA, USA

Phillip A. Choi, BS University of Pittsburgh School of Medicine, Pittsburgh, PA, USA

Perrin T. Considine, BS Vanderbilt University School of Medicine, Nashville, TN, USA

Alexander Ding, MD, MS Department of Radiology, Massachusetts General Hospital/Harvard Medical School, Boston, MA, USA

Walid F. Gellad, MD, MPH Center for Health Equity Research and Promotion, VA Pittsburgh Healthcare System and University of Pittsburgh, Pittsburgh, PA, USA

Daniel Guss, MD Department of Orthopedic Surgery, Massachusetts General Hospital, Boston, MA, USA

Bruce Lee Hall, MD, PhD, MBA Washington University in St. Louis—Barnes Jewish Hospital and BJC Healthcare, St. Louis, MO, USA

Andrew Han Department of Orthopedic Trauma, Vanderbilt University Medical Center, Nashville, TN, USA

Michael Hochman, MD AltaMed Health Services, Los Angeles, CA, USA

Benjamin S. Hooe, BS, BA Vanderbilt University School of Medicine, Nashville, TN, USA

Neil M. Issar, BS Vanderbilt University Medical Center, Vanderbilt University School of Medicine, Nashville, TN, USA

A. Alex Jahangir, MD Department of Orthopedic Surgery, Vanderbilt University Medical Center, Nashville, TN, USA

Sachin H. Jain, MD, MBA Boston VA Medical Center , Harvard Medical School, and Merck and Company, Boston, MA, USA

Rishin J. Kadakia, BS Vanderbilt University School of Medicine, Vanderbilt University Medical Center, Nashville, TN, USA

Jason D. Keune, MD, MBA Department of Surgery, Barnes-Jewish Hospital, St. Louis, MO, USA

Richard Latuska, BS Vanderbilt University School of Medicine, Nashville, TN, USA

Emily R. Maxson, MD Department of Internal Medicine, Brigham and Women's Hospital and Harvard Medical School, Boston, MA, USA

Danny McCormick, MD, MPH Chief of Social and Community Medicine, Cambridge Health Alliance, Harvard University Medical School, Boston, MA, USA

Samir Mehta, MD Department of Orthopedic Surgery, Hospital of the University of Pennsylvania, Philadelphia, PA, USA

Hassan R. Mir, MD Department of Orthopedic Surgery, Vanderbilt University Medical Center, Nashville, TN, USA

Cesar S. Molina, MD Department of Orthopedic Trauma, Vanderbilt University Medical Center, Nashville, TN, USA

Benedict U. Nwachukwu, BA Harvard Medical School, Oliver Wendell Holmes Society, Boston, MA, USA

Alexandra Obremskey University of Southern California, Los Angeles, CA, USA

Ilisa Halpern Paul, MPP Government and Regulatory Affairs Practice Group, Drinker Biddle & Reath LLP, Washington, DC, USA

David Polakoff, MD, MSc Commonwealth Medicine, University of Massachusetts Medical School, Shrewsbury, MA, USA

David A. Rosman, MD, MBA Department of Abdominal Imaging, Massachusetts General Hospital, Boston, MA, USA

Vasanth Sathiyakumar, BA Department of Orthopedic Trauma, Vanderbilt University Medical Center, Nashville, TN, USA

Manish K. Sethi, MD Director of the Vanderbilt Orthopaedic Institute Center for Health Policy, Assistant Professor of Orthopaedic Trauma Surgery, Department of Orthopaedic Surgery and Rehabilitation, Vanderbilt University School of Medicine, Nashville, TN, USA

Roshan P. Shah, MD, JD Department of Orthopedic Surgery, Hospital of the University of Pennsylvania, Philadelphia, PA, USA

Heather A. Smith, MD, MPH Department of Obstetrics and Gynecology, Yale University, New Haven, CT, USA

Audrey Smolkin, MPP Commonwealth Medicine, University of Massachusetts Medical School, Shrewsbury, MA, USA

Daniel J. Stinner, MD Vanderbilt Orthopedic Institute, Vanderbilt University Medical Center, Nashville, TN, USA

Amy L. Walker, BA Government and Regulatory Affairs Practice Group, Drinker Biddle & Reath LLP, Washington, DC, USA

Eleby R. Washington IV, BA Meharry Medical College, Nashville, TN, USA

Part I

Understanding the Basics I

The History of Health Care in the United States Pre-1965

1

Alexander Ding

Learning Objectives

After completing this chapter, the reader should be able to answer the following questions:
- Understand the history and causes contributing to the rise of the medical profession as an institution and authority.
- Understand the historical context in which health care evolved in the twentieth century, prior to the establishment of Medicare and Medicaid.
- Recognize why health care is becoming of increasing political and public interest.
- Comprehend the development of health insurance as an entity and the private/public struggles associated therewith.

Introduction

The close relationship between health care and politics and policy is not always appreciated by physicians or their patients. In fact, many medical students and resident physicians eschew the notion that the two apparently detached institutions are indeed deeply and intimately related in our society. Like it or not, health policy directly influences the practice of medicine at the clinical level.

As the health system in the United States shifts away from the doctor as the individual practitioner to systems and organizations with teams of practitioners, physicians must recognize the leadership role they must take to ensure that patient care remains the paramount priority. Understanding health policy and the history of our health system should be a critical piece in medical education because it informs us how to impact the dynamics and institutions that define our practices. The importance of the voice of physicians and medical students in health policy and politics should not be lost on the reader because our clinical perspective and ethical obligation to our patients must be present to guide policymakers and politicians.

This chapter will discuss the history of health care in the United States from the beginning of the twentieth century through the establishment

A. Ding, M.D., M.S. (✉)
Department of Radiology, Massachusetts
General Hospital/Harvard Medical School,
Boston, MA 02114, USA
e-mail: alexding@gmail.com

M.K. Sethi and W.H. Frist (eds.), *An Introduction to Health Policy: A Primer for Physicians and Medical Students*, 3
DOI 10.1007/978-1-4614-7735-8_1, © Springer Science+Business Media New York 2013

of Medicare and Medicaid in 1965. Further discussion of Medicare and Medicaid and the evolution of these programs and health care under these programs will be covered in Chaps. 2 and 3, respectively. Despite the existence of physicians and the profession of medicine since the beginning of our colonial history, it was not until the early twentieth century that medicine became more intertwined with politics. The consolidation of authority as a profession along with new medical discoveries and treatments paved the way for the view that medicine and health care were essential, leading to their politicization. The story of health-care politics and policy focuses around provision of coverage and health insurance.

Pre-Twentieth Century: The Rise of a Profession

The profession of medicine in the United States prior to the twentieth century consisted of inconsistent training and licensure, practice by a multitude of practitioners including lay folk remedies, and lack of public recognition. Physicians aspired to attain a privileged status for the practice of medicine, comparable to the status the profession had in Europe. However, this attempt at a distinct status was met with resistance from the public in the early days of our country.

By the time the American colonies were established, medicine was a regarded profession in Europe, particularly in England. In the early years of the United States, however, the structure and culture of our newfound country set up barriers to achieving this same status. In an expansive and primarily agrarian society, dependence on a medical professional was not practical, and most of the care of the sick was considered the role of the wife [1]. Understanding of disease was also limited, with lack of effective diagnosis and treatment options. Jacob Bigelow of Harvard Medical School and the Massachusetts General Hospital noted the dearth of therapeutics in medicine at the time: "the amount of death and disaster in the world would be less, if all disease were left to itself" [2].

There was perhaps nothing greater to counter the push by physicians to become a proper profession than our democratic culture [3]. Professions by their nature are inegalitarian institutions, granting special rights and privileges to their members. American democratic culture espoused equality and shunned special status, particularly royalty and nobility. As a result of these various factors, medicine carried little in the collective consciousness of the public sphere.

Physicians sought to draw boundaries around their profession and to instill credibility and authority. They faced fierce competition for the healing arts with other practitioners, including apothecaries, midwives, botanists, and lay healers. Lax credentials within the profession itself eroded their attempts for a standard of care. Efforts were made for state licensure "to distinguish between the honest and ingenious physician and the quack or empirical pretender" [4]; these attempts were rejected on multiple occasions. In 1760, New York City was the first to pass licensure, but it could be considered an honorific title at best, as the act was unenforced [5]. Authority for licensure was passed to the medical societies, but their attempts remained toothless as there remained no standard for education or skill and no enforcement or penalty for practice without a license [6].

Medical societies were organized to further attempt to isolate "quacks" from learned physicians and to provide a means for establishing a floor of qualification of its physician members. The oldest continuously operating state medical society, the Massachusetts Medical Society, was incorporated in 1781 so "that a just discrimination should be made between such as are duly educated, and properly qualified for the duties of their profession, and those who may ignorantly and wickedly administer medicine" [7].

Considered prestigious for universities, medical schools proliferated without added expense, as all costs were borne by matriculants through tuition fees. Lacking standards or accreditation, medical schools had disparate curricula and variation in pedagogy, if any at all. Schools were also reluctant to fail any students due to loss of tuition fees [4].

Attempts to create boundaries in the late eighteenth and early nineteenth centuries in order to define the profession took on multiple faces, including licensed versus unlicensed, medical school diploma versus none, and medical society member versus nonmember, none of these exclusive. The proliferation of easy and quick medical school degrees and lack of barriers to practice saw the proliferation of physicians grow from 5,000 to 40,000 from 1790 to 1850 [8]. However, these attempts were largely unsuccessful until decades later when a medical school diploma was needed to earn a license to practice and medical society membership was granted once an individual was practicing in good standing [3].

In 1877, a watershed Illinois law established that the state board of medical examiners could reject diplomas from disreputable medical schools, a first attempt at establishing a minimum standard and limiting the proliferation of diploma mills [9]. Licensure was further legitimized by the Supreme Court in 1888 in the case of *Dent v. West Virginia.* The Court upheld a law requiring physicians to hold a degree from a reputable medical college and pass an examination to practice, stating that the State could protect society by imposing conditions for the exercise of that right, as long as they were imposed on everyone and were reasonably related to the occupation in question [10]. There continued a gradual extension of authority to credential physician through state board examinations and licensing authorities such that by 1901 all states had a licensing statute of some sort, all of which were enforced [11].

While the American Medical Association (AMA) was founded in 1847, its influence was limited as was its membership. However, in 1901 the organization revised its Constitution, forming the House of Delegates, and became a federation and umbrella organization of state medical societies. In the process, the AMA gained legitimacy and membership. Membership rose from 8,000 in 1900 to over 70,000 by 1910, and by 1920 included over 60 % of physicians in the US [12]. After its reorganization, it declared medical education reform its top priority, and in 1904 formed the Council on Medical Education, charged with elevating standards and requirements of medical education.

The AMA commissioned the Carnegie Foundation, which selected Abraham Flexner to report on and make recommendations for the state of medical schools in the country. Flexner and the Secretary of the AMA Council personally visited every medical school in the country and reported on medical schools not meeting standards, leading to the closure of many substandard schools. Subsequently, organized medicine set up the Federation of State Medical Boards as a voluntary association of medical boards in 1912, and the AMA Council on Medical Education began to accredit all American medical schools and medical internships [3]. This self-regulation lent legitimacy and authority to the profession.

With higher educational standards, the caliber of students increased but the number of matriculants decreased. In order to remain financially secure, medical schools had to become more interconnected with universities, whereas previously they had only been nominally affiliated. This led to the development of full-time academic positions in clinical medicine, and the training and education shifted from apprenticeships with private practitioners to internships and residencies with faculty at academic hospitals. This fundamental shift in training led doctors to be trained according to the scientific method and with deeper foundations in basic science [3].

One of the problems with early medicine was that the practice was reliant more on mysticism and dogma from preceptors and was less scientifically rigorous. This inevitably was associated with limited diagnostic accuracy and an inadequacy of therapeutics, ranging from the ineffective to the toxic and lethal, including what was known as "heroic therapy" consisting of bloodletting and administering heavy doses of mercury [3]. With the elemental shift of training to a focus on science and the development of the clinician-researcher, the advances in medical technology at the turn of the century paved the way for medicine to elucidate its effectiveness and ultimately its essential nature [3]. At the turn of the century, diagnostics were improved with the development of the microscope, X-ray, and EKG. Bacteriology made scientific leaps with the isolation of tuberculosis, syphilis, diphtheria, and typhoid, and the practice of antisepsis in surgery.

During this period, hospitals rose in parallel to the profession, and the two became more interdependent. In the early nineteenth century, hospitals were considered sick houses for the poor and destitute, while patients of means preferred to be taken care of at home. However, at the beginning of the twentieth century, hospitals, aided by advances in the nursing profession and antisepsis, had become complex organizations that provided much of the technical, capital, and supportive corporate embodiment for the medical profession [3]. The integration of the hospital and medical practice became so important, and remains so today, that the number of hospitals in this country grew from 200 in 1873 to 6,000 by 1920 [13].

From the early colonial days to the turn of the twentieth century, the profession of medicine established itself as the authority in health care. It faced significant challenges in our burgeoning nation, but through the development of licensure, educational standards, and self-regulation, it established itself as the health-care provider of the nation. This authority in conjunction with the advances in diagnosis and therapeutics led to increased public demand for medical care, which, with erected barriers to entry to the profession, led to higher costs. When the middle class began to struggle with costs, proposed solutions were brought forth in the political arena.

The Progressive Era: 1900–1920

As medicine and health care became more scientifically advanced and effective at diagnosing and treating disease, the view of medicine as a vital necessity became more adopted. While the democratic view in our early nation had been that every man can be his own healer, the democratic view had evolved in that the services of physicians should see wider distribution to the population at large [14]. The history and politics of health care in the twentieth century centered

around health insurance, first becoming a political issue in the run up to World War I.

Demand for health insurance started due to the changing economic realities associated with industrialization. As families became more dependent on wages for their income, sickness could interrupt cash flow and family resources in a significant way. The initial impetus for the creation of so-called health insurance was actually disability insurance and replacement of income during sickness. And while families became more reliant on doctors and hospitals for medical treatment, insurance coverage of medical expenses was only a secondary feature of sickness insurance policies [3].

Europe was significantly ahead of the United States in the adoption of social insurance, in particular compulsory sickness insurance. Health insurance was first implemented by Kaiser Wilhelm in Germany in 1888. These efforts in Europe were more widely accepted and easier to adopt due to differences in governance structure and social culture, and in many cases was implemented to palliate social unrest and dissatisfaction. The United States, however, was more reluctant and disinterested. At this time, the government played a minimal role in social welfare and particularly in health, and most of the population agreed with this limited governmental role. The fundamental notion of a social insurance went against the founding American ideals of individualism and self-reliance.

Health insurance for the working population was first endorsed by the Socialist Party in 1904. The movement was then carried by a largely academic group of social Progressives who founded the American Association for Labor Legislation (AALL) in 1906. This group played a prominent role in the push for workers' compensation legislation, which was successfully passed in 1910. AALL saw this as a public desire for further social and labor insurance and believed sickness insurance would be the next logical path forward [15].

During the early part of the twentieth century, the Progressive movement was becoming more successful and considered social insurance an important part of its agenda. When Republican President William McKinley was assassinated in 1901, Teddy Roosevelt, his Vice President, ascended to the presidency. Roosevelt was considered a reformist in the Republican Party, and he pushed forward with a Progressive agenda. As a Progressive, Roosevelt supported social insurance, including health insurance. The Progressive movement reached its peak in 1912, when Roosevelt ran for the presidency as a third-party candidate from the Progressive Bull Moose Party, after a break with the GOP and President Taft, a fellow republican. Despite what many see as the decline of the Progressive agenda with an electoral defeat to Woodrow Wilson in 1912, Wilson's Commission on Industrial Relations still recommended health insurance for labor in its report.

In December 1912, shortly after the election, the AALL formed a committee on social insurance and organized a national conference in June 1913. It called for health insurance for the working class consisting of four main benefits to include: coverage of medical expenses, sick pay, maternity benefits, and a death benefit. Their message, rather than appealing to the traditional arguments for socialism of redistribution, focused on stabilizing incomes, preventing poverty during illness, and improving worker productivity. During this time, the AALL worked very closely with the AMA in pushing for health insurance. In fact, the two organizations had a joint office in New York.

However, the health insurance advocates faced opposition on many fronts, including unlikely partners in labor and business. The American Federation of Labor (AFL) and its spokesman Samuel Gompers strongly disagreed with the notion that the government should play a role in raising the worker's standard of living and represented the position that this was the role of unions [16]. He strongly held the view that government involvement would weaken the unions' role to provide social benefits for its members. Business interests were also opposed. They believed that health insurance would raise their costs and did not believe that their companies would see any of the benefits directly. On the issue of health insurance, labor and capital were united in opposition. They wanted no competition from the government to provide services that they believed would undermine their worker's loyalties to them,

respectively [17]. Additionally, the inclusion of a death benefit led to opposition from insurance companies which at the time were predominantly large insurance companies such as Prudential and MetLife; most of their business was life insurance, which provided death benefits.

The year 1917 saw the defeat of the Progressive's push for health insurance. They faced strong united opposition from labor, business, and insurers. At the time, they were aligned with the AMA, who in June 1917 at its House of Delegates meeting approved a report supporting health insurance. However, the AMA faced a groundswell of opposition in unhappy doctors from the local and county medical societies and had to make an about-face in order to avoid a mutiny [18].

However, perhaps the biggest factor leading to the push for health insurance to be stopped in its tracks happened in April 1917, with the entrance of the US into World War I. Doctors went into the service, the national debate was suspended, and, because the German's had pioneered social insurance, anti-insurance propaganda made it un-American to support such measures [18]. Health insurance failed in multiple states including those taken up by the legislature and those voted on by public referendum.

Rising Medical Costs and the New Deal: The Roaring Twenties and the Great Depression

After World War I and the Progressives' attempts, much of the political and public appetite for compulsory health insurance was lost during the prosperous and politically apathetic 1920s. However, at the end of the decade, there were growing concerns over the costs of medical care. The focus, in fact, pivoted from insurance covering lost wages to that of covering medical care. More and more the notion of insurance for catastrophic medical needs shifted to that of a system for financing medical care in total. This was due in large part to the rising costs of health care.

At the end of the decade, medical costs were 85 % higher compared with the lost wages incurred by a typical middle class family. Not only were the economics such that medical care was more important than income protection, but because medicine had become so effective in treating disease, it was also considered a more important commodity than just having cash [19]. During this time, meeting the rising medical costs was the most common concern and grievance amongst the middle class [20].

Health-care costs at the time were primarily rising due to the technological developments from scientific advances. Hospitals became more costly as they transformed from lowly caretaking homes to technologically advanced, professional organizations. Physician services also increased in price as quality improved with better education, and the prestige of the profession rose as the AMA's influence grew. The first reliable estimate of medical care costs in the United States was published in 1929 and consisted entirely of private costs, as the government was not yet playing a role in financing or providing health care. The country, at the time, spent $3.7 billion a year or 4 % of the gross national product on health care.

The Great Depression occurred on Black Tuesday with the stock market crash in October 1929, greatly changing the political and social landscape. With the election of Franklin D. Roosevelt, a Democrat, the idea of social insurance was again revived. The priorities of social insurance, however, changed. In the previous generation, health insurance was the priority after the implementation of workman's compensation. Now, however, unemployment insurance and elderly pensions were of primary concern due to exceptionally high unemployment [21].

In 1934, President Roosevelt appointed a Committee on Economic Security charged to work on old-age and unemployment insurance, but with an additional charge to include health insurance in its consideration. Many, including members of the committee and even advocates of the social security movement, expressed concern that pursuing health insurance would be politically unrealistic and reinvigorate prior opposition. There was real concern that its inclusion could jeopardize and defeat the entire bill. In 1935, the Social Security Act was passed as a cornerstone to FDR's New Deal with the omission of health insurance, but with coverage of unemployment and elderly pension.

During the Great Depression, increased government financing of medical services did start to take hold, despite the lack of any clear legislation passed intently addressing this. Because of falling incomes, people were using less medical care and were simply not paying their medical bills. As a result, doctors and hospitals also fell upon hard times. But, beginning in 1930, medical care became recognized as an "essential relief need," thereby allowing for the use of public and welfare funds to pay for medical services for those who were unable to afford them [22]. With the passage of the Social Security Act, the pensions that the elderly received were also a means to indirectly pay for care. While these two practices were meant to be temporary during the Depression era, the practice remained popular well thereafter.

In the late 1930s, FDR softly pushed for a new effort for health insurance. In 1937, multiple departments within the federal government were coordinated to form a Technical Committee on Medical Care. This committee's report favored federal subsidies to the states to implement health insurance programs rather than a reliance on a national system. Furthermore, the committee recommended the expansion of public health and maternal and child health services, aid to hospitals and doctors for patients who could not pay, and a federal disability program, all supported by taxes or insurance. This report was presented at a National Health Conference in summer of 1938 [23].

Unfortunately for this effort, the 1938 elections brought a conservative resurgence. Republicans and southern Democrats resisted the passage of any further social policies of the New Deal through Congress. Additionally, Roosevelt never pressed that hard on this issue because he was not feeling strong pressure for health insurance from the general public or advocacy groups as he had for unemployment insurance and old-age pensions. Just as with the prior effort, timing ultimately became a significant barrier as the United States entered World War II and turned its focus from a domestic social agenda to a wartime effort and foreign attention.

The Blues: A Response to Public Insurance

Much of the medical establishment at the time was opposed to government-sponsored health insurance, but they did feel the pressure exerted by its proponents. As a result, a push for private insurance plans as the counter solution was propagated in the 1930s. Private plans, in particular, the Blue Cross/Blue Shield entities, started and grew significantly in this decade.

Blue Cross began at Baylor Medical Center in late 1929 as a prepaid plan for group hospital services. The plan covered 1,500 local Texas school teachers and provided up to 21 days of hospital care for $6 per person [24]. Soon other hospitals recognized this business strategy as a good and reliable revenue generator and started their own competing plans. These plans were issued by individual hospitals and spawned fierce competition amongst hospitals in the same locality. The logical next step would be to eliminate this competition and cooperate to produce hospital services contracts for employed groups to a community-wide or city-wide range of hospitals. Eventually, these plans came to be known as the "free choice" plans, and, with the endorsement of the American Hospital Association, they became the dominant form of private hospital insurance [24].

During the Great Depression, particularly as hospitals' unpaid care grew as people were less able to pay their bills, these plans would become a business stop-loss and promotion of these plans became more widespread. From virtually a nonexistent market at the beginning of 1930, just 10 years later by 1940, Blue Cross claimed more than six million members, and other competing private hospital insurers had 3.7 million members [25].

The Blue Cross programs covered hospital services only, as physician services were and are considered separate and therefore not covered. However, physicians were a residual beneficiary from hospital insurance, particularly during the Great Depression. Because hospital stays were covered, patients had more money left over, thereby making it more likely that they could pay for the physician services incurred [26].

Some attempts were made by hospital plans to hire physicians to provide care or to prepay for care; however, generally speaking, they were not largely successful. The first true insurance coverage of physician services came in 1939. Again, in an effort to counter government attempts at health insurance, the California Medical Association started the California Physician Service [27]. Because of its success, Blue Shield plans were formed to cover physician services and served as partners to Blue Cross. By 1945, Blue Shield covered more than two million members [28].

World War II and the Rise of the Cold War

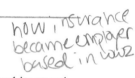
how insurance became employer based in war

Even though the government turned its attention from domestic issues to international and military problems during World War II, medicine and health insurance continued to forge their own paths, which had a profound impact on our country's health system decades into the future. The provision of health insurance through labor unions or employers made labor union members or company workers more loyal to the unions and employers, respectively. Employers increasingly favored providing health insurance as a fringe benefit to attract workers or encourage retention. The current American health insurance system, which is predominantly private and employer-sponsored, is the by-product of this time period.

During World War II, strict wage controls were imposed by the federal government as part of a larger price control scheme that were intended to be anti-inflationary during the wartime period. However, the National War Labor Board in 1942 declared that fringe benefits, such as health insurance, were not considered wages. As a result of what some considered a loophole, employers dramatically started to increase their offering of health insurance to attract and retain workers. Employers during the war were finding labor particularly scarce, given the deployment of so many men of working age to the European and Pacific theaters. In the years spanning World War II, the number of hospital insurance plan subscribers increased from under 7 million to over 26 million in a relatively short period of time [29].

Scarce labor + wage freezes = side benefits growth

During this time, unions began to increase their power due to their important role in collective bargaining with employers for health benefits. And in 1945, the Internal Revenue Service confirmed that health benefits provided by employers would be tax-exempt or paid with pre-tax earnings, thereby giving health benefits a massive implicit government subsidy and further increasing their desirability to employers and employees alike.

In 1943, just as the tide was turning in favor of the Allies, the Wagner-Murray-Dingell Bill was introduced and picked up the debate on national health insurance [30]. This Bill would extend Social Security benefits to include health insurance. Furthermore, in his 1944 campaign, FDR called for an "economic bill of rights" that included a right to medical care and insurance against sickness and accident. While it was unclear that Congress or the President would move forward on these issues during wartime, it was a signal that national health insurance would be a priority in the postwar period.

Despite FDR's death, his successor President Truman was just as enthusiastic about national health insurance. Only 3 months after the war concluded, President Truman called upon Congress to pass national health insurance as part of his "Fair Deal" program [31]. While this was yet another presidential attempt to pass national health insurance, the focus of the program was radically different. Prior proposals were focused on covering the needy people in American society, but Truman pressed for all Americans to be covered, regardless of income or wealth. The AMA opposed this proposal and instead called for expansion of voluntary insurance and public services only for the indigent [30]. Given the new focus on coverage for all instead of only the relatively needy or working class and juxtaposed to the rise of the Cold War, Truman's "socialized medicine" became a political and symbolic issue in America's fight against the Communist influence; this scenario contributed largely to the demise of Truman's plan.

Postwar Prosperity and the Vast Expansion of Health Care

Post–World War II United States saw a rapid increase in its wealth and economic status both as a country and for individual Americans, even as Europe was picking up the pieces and rebuilding. During this time, the United States engaged in its first proxy fight of the Cold War on the Korean peninsula. Once again, war would turn the country and politicians' attention from domestic issues such as health insurance externally toward war efforts.

American postwar prosperity, however, would lead to huge growth in medicine largely funded by research and discovery from unprecedented economic growth. From 1950 to 1970, the healthcare workforce expanded from 1.2 million to nearly 4 million people. Health expenditures rose from $3 billion in 1940 to $12.7 billion in 1950, and then to $71.6 billion in 1970. This represented 4.5–7.3 % of American GNP from 1950 to 1970 [32].

Medical research expenditures from all sponsors swelled from $18 million in 1941 to over ten times that amount a mere decade later in 1951 at $181 million [33]. During this period of prosperity, government investment in the sciences exploded. The National Institutes of Health budget inflated from $81 million in 1955 to over $400 million in 1960 [34]. The economic model of science laboratories changed dramatically from one predominantly funded by private monies to government-run laboratories to, as is presently the case, academic labs funded by government extramural grants. And, as this was immediately after World War II, pains were taken to eschew the German model of political priorities dictating research endeavors. As a result, the government funds did not come with an attached dictum, and academic and scholarly freedom to decide was a major victory for scientists.

Virtually everything within the realm of health care was expanding during this time period.

The construction of hospitals was rapidly ramped up, thanks to the Hill-Burton Act, also known as the 1946 Hospital Survey and Construction Act. $75 million a year for 5 years was provided to aid in the building of local hospitals. Since two-thirds of the funding was to be paid by the community itself and the remainder one-third from federal funds, most of the local community hospitals erected at this time went to middle-income neighborhoods [35].

Medical schools and medical education saw their own unprecedented expansion in the 1940s and 1950s. Faculty positions at teaching hospitals increased 51 % from 1940 to 1950 [36]. Medical school income exploded from $500,000 per school in the 1940s to $15 million per school by 1960 [37].

As more medical staff practiced in centralized hospital settings, specialization accelerated, especially as research had led to an exponential growth in medical knowledge. In 1940, 24 % of physicians were specialists compared with 55 % in 1960 [38]. Medical education with internship and residency positions grew from 5,000 spots nationally in 1940 to over 25,000 in 1955 as a result of government subsidies and the relatively cheap labor cost of internships and residencies to hospitals [39]. In 1959, a government report detailed the shortage of health-care workers, particularly doctors and nurses. In response, Congress adopted legislation to aid and expand medical education in 1963; the government remains the primary payer of medical training in this country [40].

The United States earned a new global confidence, and Americans believed that future success in the world and leadership during the Cold War could be won with scientific progress. We saw firsthand during World War II the power of the atomic bomb and the lifesaving power of antibiotics. During this time, the combination of effective and widespread antibiotic use coupled with prosperity shifted the health concerns of the day from primarily infectious diseases to chronic diseases, such as diabetes, heart problems, and cancer. The expansion of health care at the time was seen as a greater good and as a sign of prowess and success.

The Prelude to Medicare and Medicaid

During the tumultuous 1960s, the good feelings from the 1950s quickly subsided and gave way to a time of rebellion and turmoil in the era of the Vietnam War. Once again, the issue of national health insurance, now a longtime holy grail for the Democratic Party, was pressed. Some politicians believed that perhaps the implementation of social policies would pacify some of the public's discontent.

Due to the failings from the Truman proposal for universal nationalized health insurance, a more modest plan was proposed. In 1958, Representative Aime Forand of Rhode Island proposed legislation covering hospital expenses for the elderly on Social Security. By this time, this plan was starting to attract more traction because of its limited scope and also because care had continued to increase in cost, particularly for the retired population. Hospital care had doubled in the 1950s, and, of those aged 65 and older, almost 20 % needed hospital care and tended to stay twice as long compared with younger patients.

In 1960, two very powerful members of Congress, Senators Robert Kerr and Representative Wilbur Mills, put forward a competing proposal. Theirs proposed expanding welfare to cover medical costs for the poor by subsidized state programs already in effect. At the time, the Democrats had opposed this legislation because they opposed means testing [41].

Despite President Kennedy's support, Medicare legislation remained short of the needed votes to enact. It was not until a Democratic sweep in 1964 that President Johnson, riding off of the post-assassination goodwill, made health coverage again a top domestic priority under his Great Society Program.

The Republicans countered with a plan to expand voluntary health insurance for retirees; this plan would be subsidized according to a sliding scale on par with the Social Security benefits the individual received. Interestingly, while hospital services had been a proposed benefit, physician services were not included largely because of prior AMA opposition and the fear that including physician fees would be controversial and put the legislation at increased jeopardy. The AMA reacted by stating that physician fees should also be included under the voluntary private health insurance for the elderly, called Eldercare.

In a grand omnibus and compromise bill, a three-pronged plan was offered. The federal government would start Medicare with two parts: Part A to cover hospital expenses and Part B to cover physicians' bills; then Medicaid would cover the indigent through the expansion of the states' existing welfare programs. It is because of this political compromise of competing resolutions that we have these various parts of Medicare and Medicaid as they are structured today. Since then, various amendments have been made, including adding a Part C for a managed care option and Part D to cover drug costs. Medicare and Medicaid passed Congress in a bipartisan manner and were signed by President Johnson in 1965.

Conclusion

Medicine and health care in the history of the United States present an interesting narrative about the rise of a profession and the scientific advancement of medicine. Studying this history also provides insight into the evolution of politics in health care, the multiple struggles to increase access to care, and the factors leading to the organic growth of a health industry, presenting an explanation of why our health system is structured as it is presently.

Through the colonial times and the history of our nascent nation, the medical profession and physicians sought to establish and consolidate medical authority and fight for legitimacy and arguably, supremacy over other healing practitioners. Because of the professions stringent adherence to the scientific method, remarkable medical progress and health improvements have been achieved in just the last century. Life expectancy in 1900 was 47 years for the average American. By the time Medicare and Medicaid were enacted in 1965, life expectancy was 70 years. Certainly, medicine alone does not explain the remarkable progress made. However, it is impressive to think that in approximately three generations, life expectancy increased nearly 50 %.

With improvements in medical technology and care, however, medical services, which were once a relative luxury that provided more comfort and less healing, became a necessity and, to many, a human right. Such a shift in medicine in conjunction with its continuing increasing costs put the issue of medicine on the list of political priorities. In the twentieth century, no fewer than six American Presidents, from Teddy Roosevelt to Barack Obama, have pushed for efforts to expand national health insurance.

While this chapter ends with the passage of Medicare and Medicaid, the story of health care and the complexities involved continues in the subsequent chapters of this book. At the time of this writing, President Obama's Patient Protection and Affordable Care Act had withstood a Supreme Court challenge, the American Medical Association had made an about-face and supported national health reform, Accountable Care Organizations were introduced with much fanfare and concern, and a new national focus on implementation of electronic health record systems and medical quality and patient safety programs was being ushered into practice. We encourage all readers of this book to remain engaged in their clinical practices while keeping an eye on how health systems, governments, academia, and professional organizations are addressing some of the greatest challenges facing health care today. We strongly encourage you to take a proactive and leadership role in these efforts, as the importance of a patient-centric and clinical perspective cannot be emphasized enough.

References

1. Risee GB, Numbers RL, Leavitt J, editors. Medicine without doctors: home health care in American history. New York: Science History Publications; 1977. p. 11–30.
2. Bigelow J. Modern Inquiries: classical, professional and miscellaneous. Boston: Little, Brown; 1867. p. 230–311.
3. Starr P. The social transformation of American medicine. Cambridge, MA: Basic Books; 1982. p. 30–59.
4. Rothstein W. American physicians of the nineteenth century. Baltimore: Johns Hopkins Press; 1972. p. 73.
5. Duffy J. A history of public health in New York City, 1625–1866. New York: Russell Sage Foundation; 1968. p. 65–6.
6. Kett J. The formation of the American medical profession: the role of institutions, 1780–1860. New Haven: Yale University Press; 1968. p. 14–30.
7. Fitz RF. The rise and fall of the licensed physician in Massachusetts, 1781–1860. Trans Assoc Am Physicians. 1894;9:1–18.
8. U.S. Bureau of the Census. Historical statistics of the United States, colonial times to 1970. Washington, DC: Department of Commerce; 1975. p. 76.
9. Bonner TN. Medicine in Chicago, 1850–1950. Madison: American Historical Research Center; 1957. p. 208.
10. DeLancy FP. The licensing of professions in West Virginia. Chicago: Foundation Press; 1938.
11. Laws regulating the practice of medicine in the various states and territories of the United States. JAMA: American Medical Association; 1901;37:1318.
12. Burrow JG. AMA: voice of American medicine. Baltimore: Johns Hopkins Press; 1963. p. 49–51.
13. Tomer JM. Statistics of regular medical associations and hospitals of the United States. Trans Am Med Assoc. 1873;24:314–33.
14. Ohio Health and Old Age Insurance Commission. Health, health insurance, old age pensions. Columbus: F.J. Heer Printing; 1919. p. 136.
15. Rubinov IM. Public and private interests in social insurance. Am Labor Legis Rev. 1931;21:181–91.
16. Karson M. American labor unions and politics, 1900–1918. Carbondale: Southern Illinois University Press; 1958.
17. Tishler HS. Self-reliance and social security, 1870–1917. Port Washington: Kennikat Press; 1971. p. 179–89.
18. Numbers RL. Almost persuaded: American physicians and compulsory health insurance. Baltimore: Johns Hopkins University Press; 1978. p. 67–77.
19. Davis MM. Preface to Millis HA, sickness and insurance. Chicago: University of Chicago Press; 1937.
20. Davis MM. The American approach to health insurance. Milbank Memorial Fund Q. 1934;12:214.
21. Flora P, Heidenheimer AJ, editors. The development of welfare states in Europe and America. New Brunswick: Little, Brown; 1976. p. 22.
22. Goldmann F. Public medical care. New York: Columbia University Press; 1945.
23. Interdepartmental Committee to Coordinate Health and Welfare Activities. A national health program: report of the technical committee on medical care. In: Proceedings of the National Health Conference; 1938 July 18–20; Washington, DC. Washington, DC: US Government Printing Office; 1938. p. 29–63.
24. Rorem CR. Blue cross hospital service plans. Chicago: Hospital Service Plan Commission; 1944.
25. Somers HN, Somers AR. Doctors, Patients and health insurance. Washington, DC: The Brookings Institute; 1961. p. 548.
26. Dunstan EM, Alexander JC. Group hospitalization plan: survey of local organized medical opinion on the Baylor University Hospital. Hospitals. 1936;10:75–81.
27. Garbarino JW. Health plans and collective bargaining. Berkeley: University of California Press; 1960. p. 89–106.
28. Anderson OW. Blue Cross since 1929: accountability and the public trust. Cambridge, MA: Ballinger; 1975. p. 75.
29. Applebaum L. The development of voluntary health insurance in the United States. J Risk Insur. 1961; 9:15–23.
30. Poen MM, Harry S. Truman versus the medical lobby. Columbia: University of Missouri Press; 1979. p. 31–6.
31. Truman HS. A National Health Program: message from the President. Social Security Bulletin. Washington, DC: US Government Printing Office; Dec 1945.
32. US Public Health Service, Office of Research, Statistics and Technology. Health: United States 1981. Hyattsville: US Dept. of Health, Education and Welfare; 1970. p. 4.
33. Endicott KM, Allen EM. The growth of medical research 1941–1953 and the role of the public health service research grants. Science. 1953;118:337.
34. Congressional Quarterly Service. Congress and the Nation, 1945-64: A Review of Government and Politics in the Post War Years. Washington, DC: Congressional Quarterly Service; 1965. p1132.
35. US Department of Health, Education and Welfare. Facts about the Hill-Burton Program, July 1, 1947–June 30, 1971. Washington, DC: US Government Printing Office; 1972.
36. Detrick JE, Berson RC. Medical schools in the United States at mid-century. New York: McGraw-Hill; 1953. p. 195.
37. Stevens R. American medicine and the public interest. Berkeley: University of California Press; 1998. p. 350–1.
38. Coombs RH, Vincent RH, editors. Medical specialization: trends and contributing factors in psychosocial aspects of medical training. Springfield: CC Thomas; 1971. p. 460.
39. Curran JA. Internships and residencies: historical backgrounds and current trends. J Med Educ. 1959; 34:873–4.
40. Surgeon General's Consultant Group on Medical Education. Physicians for a growing America. Washington, DC: US Government Printing Office; 1959.
41. Marmor TR. The politics of medicare. 2nd ed. Hawthorne: Aldine De Gruyter; 2000. p. 35–8.

Medicare and Its Evolution to 2011

Kevin J. Bozic and Benedict U. Nwachukwu

Learning Objectives

After completing this chapter, the reader should be able to answer the following questions:
- What is Medicare and who qualifies for it?
- What are the origins of the Medicare Program?
- What benefits were originally available under Medicare?
- How has Medicare changed up to 2011?
- What are the major challenges facing Medicare beyond 2011?

Introduction

In 1965, the United States Congress created Medicare under Title XVIII of the Social Security Act. The aim of the program was to provide health insurance coverage to all Americans aged 65 years and older. This chapter describes the evolution of Medicare from passage in 1965 to 2011. It is useful for both health-care practitioners and practitioners-in-training to understand the history of Medicare. Medicare has been in constant evolution and will continue to face serious challenges as health-care spending outpaces inflation and as the US elderly population increases.

Passage of Medicare

The Elderly as a Priority

Medicare was passed during an era that was best known for large-scale social programs aimed at combating poverty in the United States. The elderly segment of the population became a target for social intervention when it became apparent that older Americans were significantly poorer than the rest of the population. In the 1960s, the poverty rate for households headed by someone aged 25–54 years was 13 % while the poverty rate for households headed by an elderly head of household was 47 % [1]. This level of impoverishment was thought to be largely due to disproportionate health-care expenditures by the elderly. The elderly faced disproportionately

K.J. Bozic, M.D., M.B.A. (✉)
Department of Orthopedic Surgery, University
of California, San Francisco, CA 94143-0728, USA
e-mail: kevin.bozic@ucsf.edu

B.U. Nwachukwu, B.A.
Harvard Medical School, Oliver Wendell Holmes
Society, Boston, MA 02115, USA
e-mail: Benedict_Nwachukwu@hms.harvard.edu

M.K. Sethi and W.H. Frist (eds.), *An Introduction to Health Policy: A Primer for Physicians and Medical Students*, 15
DOI 10.1007/978-1-4614-7735-8_2, © Springer Science+Business Media New York 2013

higher health-care expenditures in the 1950s and 1960s because health-care insurance at that time was predominantly employer-based. Therefore, as most Americans retired, they could no longer afford coverage and were forced to personally cover medical expenditures.

Support of health-care assistance for the elderly began to gain momentum among politicians in the 1950s. An important first step toward Medicare came in 1960 with the passage of the Kerr-Mills bill which provided federal matching funds to states for health-care provider payments in the treatment of the indigent aged. The program defined indigence as financial hardship causing a person's inability to pay for health-care services [2]. Thus, through federal assistance, the poor elderly could for the first time afford health-care coverage.

Medicare Passes

Despite passage of the Kerr-Mill bill, there was growing support for universal coverage for Americans 65 years and older. In 1962, what would be a precursor bill to the eventual Medicare bill was narrowly defeated (12–11) in committee. The defeated bill, the King-Anderson Bill, proposed coverage of *some* hospital and nursing home costs for patients 65 years and older. The election of Lyndon B. Johnson in 1964, however, proved to be pivotal in the eventual passage of Medicare. With Johnson's election, the Democrats controlled both the Presidency and the Congress with a 2:1 ratio in the House and 32 more seats than Republicans in the Senate. The King-Anderson Bill was revisited and rewritten as Medicare to provide coverage to individuals over the age of 65 for limited hospitalization and nursing home insurance benefits. Johnson proclaimed the new bill as an integral piece to his Great Society program. The new bill was not without opposition, however. Groups previously opposing the original King-Anderson Bill proposed their own versions of Medicare such that three forms of the bill emerged. One of the two opposing bills was outright rejected, and the

Medicare bill that was eventually sent to Congress in March 1965 included several provisions from the other remaining bill.

The final Medicare bill went through more than 500 amendments but was eventually passed on July 28, 1965, as an amendment to the Social Security Act of 1935. The bill, which was known as Title XVIII, included a Part A that provided for hospital insurance for the aged and a Part B that provided supplementary medical insurance.

Of note (and discussed in Chap. 3), Title XIX, also passed at the same time, was known as Medicaid and provided federal matching funds to states in order to assist Americans at or near the poverty line with health-care coverage.

Not Just the Elderly

Over the past five decades, the eligibility of Medicare has been expanded to include specific subsets of Americans younger than 65 years of age. In 1972, Congress expanded the eligibility to include younger Americans who (1) have permanent disabilities or blindness and are eligible for Social Security Disability Insurance (SSDI) or (2) have end-stage renal disease (ESRD). In 2001, coverage was again extended by Congress to include Americans with amyotrophic lateral sclerosis (ALS).

Overview of Medicare

One year after its passage, Medicare was an active program for the 65-and-older population, and by that point, the program already had an enrollment of 19.5 million [3]. By 2008, Medicare had an enrollment of 45 million and was projected to reach 78 million by 2030 [4].

In this section, we provide an overview of the fundamentals and benefit structures within Medicare. In proceeding sections, we chronologically describe the evolution of the program and how the fundamentals have been changed and/or supplemented.

Funding

Medicare benefits are financed primarily by two trust funds. The Part A trust fund is funded through mandatory payroll deductions. 1.45 % of taxable earnings paid by employees and 1.45 % paid by their employers (totaling 2.9 %) accrue to the Part A trust fund. Self-employed individuals pay 2.9 % to the fund [5]. Under this system, these taxes paid each year are used to fund the expenses of current beneficiaries, and those not needed are invested in US Treasury securities. This funding approach thus relies on the current work force to pay for the health-care costs of the elderly, most of who are no longer active members of the work force. This payment structure is noteworthy because Medicare's financial stability thus becomes dependent on preventing health-care expenses incurred by the elderly from exceeding the revenues provided through taxes on the current work force.

Part B (and also Part D which is discussed later in this chapter) is funded through premiums paid by program enrollees and contributions from the general revenue of the US Treasury. The latter revenue source is a significant proportion (approximately 75 %) of the Part B budget.

Eligibility

Age over 65, disability, and end-stage illness are generally the eligibility criteria for Medicare. However, within these major eligibility groups, there are nuanced eligibility requirements.

Age Over 65
Persons over the age of 65 may qualify for Medicare if they are US citizens or have been permanent legal US residents for 5 years *continuously, and* either they or their spouse has paid Medicare taxes for at least 10 years.

Disability
To become eligible to enroll in Medicare, disabled Americans must have received either SSDI benefits or Railroad Retirement Board disability benefits for at least 24 months.

End-Stage Disease/ALS
Patients with ESRD must be getting continuing dialysis for their ESRD or require a kidney transplant. Patients with ALS are eligible for Medicare if they are declared disabled by the Social Security Administration (SSA) and are eligible for SSDI benefits.

Benefits

Part A: Hospital Insurance
Under Medicare Part A, participating institutions (e.g., hospitals, skilled nursing facilities, home health-care services, and hospice services) are reimbursed for a variety of services to the elderly. We briefly review these services.

Inpatient hospital stays are covered under Medicare Part A. Service coverage includes the cost of a semiprivate room, meals, regular nursing services, operating and recovery room, intensive care, and other medically necessary services.

Skilled nursing facility care is also covered under Medicare Part A; however, certain criteria must be met: (1) preceding hospital stay of at least 3 days, (2) admission to nursing home facility for a condition diagnosed during main hospital stay or condition that was cause for hospital stay, and (3) need for skilled nursing care (i.e., custodial and long-term care activities are not covered). Medicare also limits the nursing facility stay to 100 days per benefit period (i.e., per ailment). Medicare covers the first 20 days in full, while the remaining 80 days requires a co-payment.

Medicare Part A also provides coverage for home health agency (HHA) care and hospice care. HHAs may provide health aides for a homebound beneficiary if some form of skilled nursing is required. Similarly to the skilled nursing facility criteria, Medicare covers the first 100 visits after a 3-day hospital stay (or a skilled nursing facility stay); however, there must be a plan of treatment reviewed by a physician. Part A also provides hospice care to terminally ill persons with life expectancy less than 6 months.

Part B: Supplementary Medical Insurance

Part B (supplementary medical insurance) is often viewed as a means to pay for services not covered under Part A. Traditional Part B services include outpatient physician and nursing services, diagnostic imaging and testing, outpatient hospital procedures, vaccinations, and a variety of services provided by physicians on an outpatient basis. However, to be covered under Part B, services have to be deemed medically necessary. Some services, such as physical and occupational therapy, while covered by Part B, typically require higher cost sharing on the part of the beneficiary.

Coverage under Part B is optional and must be secured by paying monthly premiums. Most people deemed eligible for Medicare Part A simultaneously elect for enrollment in Part B. The large proportion of simultaneous enrollees in Part B is partially due to a lifetime penalty (10 % annual premium per year) imposed for not enrolling. Those eligible for Part A who are still working *and* have health coverage through their employer may defer enrollment in Part B without penalty.

Of note, Part B has a deductible feature. As part of this feature, patients pay up to a certain amount for the cost of their care (hence deductible). After this amount has been reached, Medicare then pays for 80 % of the cost for approved services, while the beneficiary is responsible for the remaining 20 %. The Part B deductible was $140 in 2012 [6].

Evolution of Medicare

Changes to Program Administration

Upon passage of the Medicare law, implementation of the program was originally headed by the Department of Health and Human Services (HHS). However, in 1976, administration of Medicare passed to a newly created special purpose Federal Program—the Health Care Financing Administration (HCFA). This organization was in charge of administering both Medicare and Medicaid. HCFA would eventually become in 2001 the Centers for Medicare and Medicaid Services (CMS). Primary responsibilities of the CMS in overseeing Medicare include program policy and guidelines, contracts with intermediaries and carriers, monitoring of utilization, and general financing of Medicare.

The board is also mandated to report annually to the US Congress on the financial operations and actuarial status of the Medicare Program. The information reported to Congress is included in an annual report entitled "Medicare Trustees Report" [7].

In the 2012 report, the Trustees concluded that in 2011 Medicare costs were 3.7 % of GDP, and these costs exceeded Medicare's Trust Fund revenues by more than $27 billion for that year. The Trustees projected that Medicare expenditures would grow to 5.7 % of GDP by 2035 and would increase gradually thereafter to about 6.7 % of GDP by 2086. The reports warned that Medicare fiscal stability would be reliant on policy changes to increase revenues, decrease expenditures, or both.

Introduction of Managed Care

Soon after Medicare was passed, the government looked to Health Maintenance Organizations (HMOs) as a means to reduce escalating Medicare costs. The goal was to reduce the downstream costs of care by promoting preventative (upstream) care. In 1971, the Nixon administration announced a new health strategy that would establish planning grants and loan guarantees for HMOs. Following this announcement, in December 1973 President Richard Nixon signed the Health Maintenance Organization and Resources Development Act. This Act authorized $375 million in federal funds to aid in developing HMOs and also mandated that employers with businesses of more than 25 employees offer HMOs as a health-care option.

Prior to signing the 1973 Act, a 1972 amendment to the Social Security Act introduced HMO enrollment and contracting as an option *within* Medicare [8]. HMOs had to meet Medicare-mandated standards and also had to provide the full range of Medicare services.

Diagnosis Related Group

Diagnosis Related Groups (DRGs) were originally introduced in 1983 as a payment system that classified hospital services into one of 467 groups. It was assumed that patient care episodes falling into each group would be clinically similar, would utilize hospital resources to the same extent, and thus could be reimbursed the same amount. Prior to the introduction of DRGs, Medicare institutional reimbursements were based on a fee for service model in which institutions were reimbursed based on their stated daily costs. As part of the overall compensation, hospitals were also permitted to factor in their overall operating costs into each patient bill. Thus, there was an incentive toward overbilling and overutilization of medical resources. DRGs were introduced to curb this trend in overutilization by paying a preset average cost to treat a patient with a particular diagnosis.

Since its introduction in 1983, DRGs have evolved, and today there are several systems of patient classification that were developed to refine disease classification and include risk adjustment for important cost drivers such as disease severity. Medical Severity (MS)-DRGs have since been widely adopted as the standard beyond the Medicare system and today are the focal point of many health-care industry reimbursement models.

Medicare Advantage

Throughout the 1990s, escalating costs continued to be a source of major concern for Medicare. To address escalating costs in health care, in 1997, the US Congress passed the Balanced Budget Act of 1997—a legislative package designed to balance the federal budget by 2002. As part of the package, the Congressional Budget Office promised $112 billion in Medicare spending reduction [9]. As part of the Act's efforts to control costs and reduce spending, Medicare worked with private insurers to provide beneficiaries with an alternate avenue to access medical services. Medicare hoped to incent more beneficiaries to participate under privately run and lower cost-

managed care contracts rather than in the original fee for service plan created through Parts A and B.

Following passage of the Balanced Budget Act, the Medicare + Choice (M+C) Program (now known as Medicare "Part C") was introduced in 1997. Under M+C, new plans were introduced which were approved by Medicare but run by private insurance entities. Initially M+C was only available to Medicare eligible beneficiaries already enrolled in Parts A and B. M+C plans were required by Medicare to offer benefit packages with similar or better coverage than the original Medicare program. M+C plans did this and a little more. The newly created programs offered choice through diversification in how benefits were covered. For example, under one plan, a beneficiary could pay less for nursing facility stay but might then pay more for a regular doctor's visit. Under another plan, this relationship might be reversed. In general, in absolute terms, M+C plans offered more benefits (such as added dental and vision coverage) than the original Medicare program, and they also offered more attractive financing terms.

For those choosing to enroll in M+C, Medicare would pay the selected M+C plan's private insurance company a set amount every month for each member (payment amount was determined by Medicare based on beneficiary comorbidity and likely health-care use per month). The Medicare member enrolling in M+C would then still have to pay the Medicare Part B premium directly to Medicare—the rationale being that beneficiaries should still retain their original primary care physician who would oversee and coordinate the various benefits of the M+C plan.

By 1998, 17 % of Medicare enrollees (6.9 million) were enrolled in one of 346 M+C plans available nationwide [10]. However, between 1999 and 2001 nearly half of the plans participating in M+C program cancelled their contracts with Medicare. Medicare payment levels and poor profitability (as a result of rising input costs) were thought to be the major impetus for cancelled contracts. During the same time period, there were virtually no new M+C plan entrants. The withdrawals affected 1.6 million beneficiaries and M+C enrollment dropped to 5.5 million [11].

Medicare Prescription Drug, Improvement, and Modernization Act 2003 (Part D)

To stimulate more robust health-care insurance industry participation in Medicare and also to provide even greater coverage and more options to beneficiaries, the Medicare Prescription Drug, Improvement, and Modernization Act (MMA) was enacted in 2003. MMA added a prescription drug benefit (Medicare Part D) and introduced several changes to M+C (M+C was renamed Medicare Advantage [MA] with the new changes). At that time, the changes introduced as part of MMA were the most significant changes introduced into Medicare since its inception.

Upon introduction of MMA, there was explosive growth in the number of participating Medicare Advantage organizations providing benefits. Several key Medicare changes spurred the growth in participating programs. Firstly, payment levels were increased on a per county basis to each county's traditional Medicare costs (some counties realized payment increases up to 20 % from pre-MMA levels). Further, risk-adjusted payments were incorporated into the payment model such that Medicare would pay a premium to the private plan providers for enrollees with greater comorbidities. MMA also introduced a regional preferred provider organization (PPO) option. Benefit providers could offer PPO-style benefits in which a beneficiary signing up for a program could have their care limited to a network of physicians. Finally, MMA also allowed Medicare Advantage programs to target dual eligible (those qualifying for Medicare and Medicaid) beneficiaries via the Special Needs Plan (SNP) option. Medicare Advantage organizations could offer benefit plans targeted to special needs populations—i.e., those with chronic diseases qualifying for Medicaid coverage (see Chap. 3).

MMA also introduced prescription drug coverage. In light of increasingly unaffordable prescription drug costs for the elderly, the most significant change (and thus the genesis of the Act's name) that stemmed from the introduction of MMA was Medicare Part D—a prescription drug benefit program that subsidized the costs of prescription drugs for Medicare beneficiaries. This program went into effect on January 1, 2006.

Beneficiaries were eligible for prescription drug coverage under Part D if they were entitled to benefits under Part A and/or enrolled in Part B. Plans under Part D came in two varieties. The first was a Prescription Drug Plan (PDP), which provided drug coverage *only*. Under PDPs, not all drugs are covered at the same level; thus beneficiaries have the option of picking a PDP that best suits their prescribing patterns. The second option was a Medicare Advantage Prescription Drug plan (MA-PD). MA-PDs were plans that provided medical coverage under Medicare Advantage while *also* providing prescription drug coverage.

The MMA established a standard benefit package for Part D plans. Packages were standardized based on beneficiary contributions as opposed to drug coverage. In 2010, the standard benefit consisted of a $310 initial deductible with a coverage limit of $2,830. Once beneficiaries reach their coverage limit, he/she then pays the full cost for their drugs out of pocket (OOP) up until they have spent a total of $4,550. Once OOP expenses exceed $4,550, beneficiaries become eligible for catastrophic coverage that involves minimal cost sharing—beneficiary pays the greater of 5 % coinsurance or $2.50 for generic drugs and $6.30 for brand-named drugs. The coverage gap (OOP expenses) existing between initial and catastrophic coverage is referred to as the "donut hole" in Part D (Fig. 2.1).

Although the benefit package as described is considered the standard, programs vary widely in the formularies used. For example, some plans may remove the deductible and instead offer stratified co-payments in which cheaper drugs have lower co-pays, whereas costlier medications have a higher co-pay.

Medicare Improvements for Patients and Providers Act 2008

In the wake of Medicare reforms under MMA, the costs associated with payments to MA

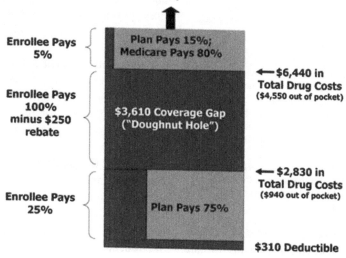

Fig. 2.1 Medicare donut hole (Note: Amounts rounded to nearest whole dollar) (Accessed at http://facts.kff.org/chart.aspx?cb=58&sctn=164&ch=1748; The Henry J. Kaiser Family Foundation illustration of Medicare Part D Standard Prescription Drug Benefit, 2010, Fast Facts. This information was reprinted with permission from the Henry J. Kaiser Family Foundation. The Kaiser Family Foundation, a leader in health policy analysis, health journalism, and communication, is dedicated to filling the need for trusted, independent information on the major health issues facing our nation and its people. The Foundation is a nonprofit private operating foundation, based in Menlo Park, California)

plans began to escalate. The Medicare Improvement for Patients and Providers Act (MIPPA) took preliminary steps to curb increases in payment to MA plans. MIPPA measures aimed at cutting MA plan costs included controlling the proliferation of skilled nursing facilities (SNPs) and private fee for service plans, as well as cutting MA payments for indirect medical education. MIPPA also sought to protect patients from aggressive brokers and agents by codifying consumer protections. Restrictions on program marketing efforts included no door-to-door sales, unsolicited calls, and a restricted marketing locale.

Legislating in favor of providers, MIPPA blocked a 10.6 % cut in Medicare payments to physicians in 2008 and instead increased the physician fee schedule by 1.1 % in 2009. Through the Act, providers were also given pecuniary incentive toward quality reporting and e-prescribing.

Patient Protection and Affordable Care Act 2010 and Medicare

For a detailed discussion on the Patient Protection and Affordable Care Act (PPACA), please see Chap. 19. The following discussion focuses on the law as it pertains to Medicare. With continually escalating health-care costs and beneficiary cost sharing throughout the first decade of the twenty-first century, the government looked to enact health-care reforms that would again drastically restructure Medicare. In 2010, President Barack Obama passed the Patient Protection and Affordable Care Act (PPACA). The legislature is best known by the public for introducing an individual mandate for health insurance and expanding access to insurance for Americans. The program however has profound implications for the Medicare Program. The goal of Medicare provisions under PPACA was both to prolong the time frame of Medicare financial solvency and to reduce beneficiary expenses.

In describing the relationship between PPACA and Medicare, President Obama said:

> This new law recognizes that Medicare isn't just something that you're entitled to when you reach 65; it's something that you've earned. It's something that you've worked a lifetime for, having the security of knowing that Medicare will be there when you need it. It's a sacred and inviolable trust between you and your country. And those of us in elected office have a commitment to uphold that trust—and as long as I'm President, I will. And that's why this new law gives seniors and their families greater savings, better benefits and higher-quality health care. That's why it ensures accountability throughout the system so that seniors have greater control over the care that they receive. And that's why it keeps Medicare strong and solvent—today and tomorrow. [12]

Programs introduced under PPACA aimed to reduce costs via improving the quality of care, reforming the system of care delivery, appropriately pricing/financing health-care systems, and reducing waste within the system. We briefly elaborate on these measures next.

Improving the Quality of Care in Medicare

The PPACA introduced a number of measures seeking to improve quality of care through value-based purchasing (VBP) programs within the Medicare program. VBP programs were introduced as a means to change how health-care providers are paid. The goal is to align payments with performance measures in order to improve the quality of care. For example, the Hospital VBP program is an example of new VBP measures under PPACA. As part of the Hospital VBP, starting fiscal year 2013, incentive payments are made to hospitals that meet (or exceed) Medicare performance standards. Target performance standards focus on efficiently managing high-volume medical conditions (e.g., acute myocardial infarction and heart failure) and limiting hospital-associated complications (e.g., health-care-associated infections).

Further, in an attempt to create even greater accountability, transparency, and incentive toward quality, the PPACA created multiple tools for the public dissemination of health-care provider performance. On the website www. healthcare.gov/compare, the public is readily able to compare a variety of quality measures for health care and service providers. Specifically, quality information on hospitals, medical practices, physicians, nursing homes, home health agencies, and dialysis facilities are available through the website.

PPACA also enacted a "hospital readmissions reduction program," which rewards hospitals for reducing avoidable readmissions and is projected by the CMS Office of the Actuary to reduce Medicare costs by $8.2 billion through 2019 [13].

Reforming the System of Care Delivery and Medicare

PPACA introduced the concept of Accountable Care Organizations (ACOs). ACOs are health care delivery systems in which preassigned teams of physicians, hospitals, or other health-care providers collaborate to manage and coordinate the care of Medicare beneficiaries. Under the Medicare shared savings program, if providers meet certain quality/efficiency benchmarks, they receive a share of any savings resultant from reducing duplicative work. Although budget neutral in principle, the program has been projected to cumulatively reduce Medicare expenditures by $5 billion within 10 years [12].

To provide further oversight of Medicare fiscal health, the PPACA established the Independent Payment Advisory Board (IPAB)—the board's primary goal being to monitor Medicare fiscal health and recommend policy revisions to Congress on how to keep pace with cost growth. Cost projections suggest that IPAB could reduce Medicare costs by almost $24 billion by 2019 [12]. However, IPAB has been highly criticized by many stakeholders for its lack of accountability to publicly elected officials and the fact that practicing physicians are prohibited from serving on IPAB.

Improving Pricing/Financing of Medicare

Cost estimates of payments to new MA plans suggested that Medicare grossly overpaid these plans. It was estimated by the Medicare Payment Advisory Commission (MedPAC) that Medicare paid MA plans 14 % (~$1,000 per person more on average) more for health services than they did under traditional Medicare. The additional payments could not be explained by health differences among service recipients [12]. Although there is no clear explanation for the MA plan overpayments, it can be speculated that MA plans are a more costly way to deliver care given that they require higher marketing/administrative costs than traditional fee for service plans. Further, it has also been suggested that the Medicare disease severity coding formula inappropriately allows MA plans to claim a patient as "sicker" than would be possible under a fee for service plan. PPACA introduced cost-cutting measures aimed at equalizing costs between MA plans and traditional Medicare benefits.

PPACA also introduced the concept of market-based adjustments to provider payments, the goal of these adjustments being to take health-care provider location into consideration and to appropriately adjust provider annual payment based upon region.

Two other smaller-scale financing measures also introduced as part of PPACA include competitive bidding for durable medical equipment (DME) and modified equipment utilization factor for advanced imaging. Under competitive bidding, suppliers submit bids to become Medicare contract suppliers. In competitive bidding areas, the bidding process de facto drives down the price at which the suppliers provide DME. Competitive bidding was already under consideration prior to PPACA; however, the Act accelerated its enactment. The program is projected to reduce Medicare spending by more than $17 billion [12]. Under the modified equipment utilization factor for advanced imaging provisions, the PPACA applied a discount to physician fee schedules for performing advanced imaging services. In essence, the PPACA altered the physician payment schedule such that physicians would be paid less for using advanced imaging modalities. This provision represents a projected $2 billion over 10 years cost savings [12].

Reducing Medicare Fraud and Abuse

PPACA also introduced measures aimed at preventing fraud and abuse within the Medicare system. Screening processes were implemented to verify and validate providers making Medicare claims. More resources were allocated to anti-fraud activities such as prepayment reviews and "boots on the ground" to conduct site visits. The PPACA specifically looked to reduce fraudulent billing in two areas in which Medicare had been historically vulnerable: home health and DME. PPACA imposed tighter restrictions on providers' ability to refer for home health or DME.

The PPACA also expanded the Recovery Auditor Contractor (RAC) program, which had been created in 2003 under the MMA. RACs were independent collection agencies that worked in collaboration with Medicare to implement "claw-backs" through retrospective reviews of claims, thereby reclaiming improper payments. Since the passage of the PPACA, there have been several attempts to implement RAC related demonstrations so that recovery auditors could review hospital claims before they are paid, thereby prospectively identifying improper payments. In 2011, the CMS announced a list of 15 procedures that would be subject to prepayment review. All 15 procedures related to cardiovascular and orthopedic services.

Medicare Beneficiary Provisions Under PPACA

PPACA attempts to enhance Medicare prescription coverage. The Act phased down coinsurance rates in the Medicare Part D donut hole from 100 % to 25 % by 2020. This was accomplished via federal subsidies and Medicare-mandated pharmaceutical manufacturer discounts. These reduced cost-sharing initiatives are projected to save beneficiaries about $43 billion within 10 years [14]. PPACA also removed beneficiary cost sharing for Medicare-covered preventative services such as colorectal screenings.

PPACA measures did not, however, result in across-the-board positive impacts for beneficiaries. PPACA introduced income-related Medicare Part B premiums such that higher-income beneficiaries began to pay higher premiums. Beneficiaries enrolled in MA plans also saw their number of benefits reduced. With a scaling down of government subsidies to MA programs, the programs responded by reducing the array of additional benefits offered to plan enrollees.

Evolution Beyond 2011?

The biggest challenge facing Medicare remains controlling costs in order to ensure the financial health and long-term sustainability of the program. With increased life expectancy and the aging of the baby boom generation, the 65 and older population in the USA is expected to double by 2030 [4]. This phenomenon, in addition to increased health-care utilization, rise in prices, and adoption of new technologies, is expected to place an unbearable strain on the Medicare budget.

Many of the programs and measures described in this chapter have taken aim at improving Medicare's long-term fiscal viability. More steps must be taken, however. Much of the future debate will center upon which shareholder group should bear the fiscal burden of the Medicare program. Some policymakers suggest that seniors should begin to play a greater role in the cost sharing and that they should be made financially responsible for the benefits that they receive. Others argue, however, that limiting payments to providers would effectively decrease costs and could encourage more judicious use of resources.

The medical profession has an obligation to remain abreast of the constantly evolving Medicare landscape and to provide leadership and input into strategies to ensure the viability of the Medicare program. As such, we may better understand the impact of Medicare policy changes on our profession and the health-care accessibility options for those under our care.

Conclusion

In this chapter, we presented an overview of the Medicare program. Medicare is a social security program passed in 1965 that since passage has provided health insurance coverage to Americans aged 65 years and older. We described the evolution of Medicare from its original format - Part A and B - to the addition of Medicare Advantage plans and prescription drug benefits. Given how closely Medicare history is tied to legislative acts of Congress, we outlined and presented the key

pieces of legislature that have shaped Medicare since 1965. Most recently, such acts have included the Balanced Budget Act of 1997; the Medicare Prescription Drug, Improvement, and Modernization Act of 2003; and the Patient Protection and Affordable Care Act of 2010. Medicare has evolved to provide US seniors with choice and access to care unparalleled in American history. Going forward, the program will inevitably continue to evolve as necessitated by the financial strains of an aging population and escalating medical costs.

References

1. Moon M. Medicare now and in the future. Washington, DC: The Urban Institute Press; 1996.
2. Kulesher RR. Medicare—the development of publicly financed health insurance: medicare's impact on the nation's health care system. Health Care Manag. 2005;24:320–9.
3. Stevens RA. History and health policy in the United States: the making of a healthcare industry, 1948–2008. Soc Hist Med. 2008;21:461–83.
4. The 2009 Annual Report of the boards of trustees of the federal hospital insurance and federal supplementary medical insurance trust funds. 2009. http://www.cms.hhs.gov/Research-Statistics-Data-and-Systems/Statistics-Trends-and-Reports/ReportsTrustFunds/downloads//tr2009.pdf. Accessed 30 May 2012.
5. Hoffman E, Klees B, Curtis C. Overview of the medicare and medicaid programs. Health Care Financ Rev—Medicare and Medicaid statistical supplement. 2003:1–22.
6. Medicare Part B (Medical Insurance). 2012. http://www.medicare.gov/navigation/medicare-basics/medicare-benefits/part-b.aspx?AspxAutoDetectCookieSupport=1. Accessed 30 May 2012.
7. Trustees report and trust funds. 2012. http://www.cms.gov/Research-Statistics-Data-and-Systems/Statistics-Trends-and-Reports/ReportsTrustFunds/index.html?redirect=/ReportsTrustFunds/. Accessed 15 May 2012.
8. Zarabozo C. Milestones in Medicare managed care. Health Care Financ Rev. 2000;22:61–7.
9. Putting Medicare in context: how does the Balanced Budget Act affect hospitals? 2000. http://www.urban.org/UploadedPDF/medicare-context.pdf. Accessed 30 May 2012.
10. Overview of the Medicare advantage program. 2010. http://www.hapnetwork.org/medicare-advantage/ship-resource-guide/overview.pdf. Accessed 30 May 2012.
11. Medicare+Choice withdrawals: understanding key factors. 2002. http://www.kff.org/medicare/loader.

cfm?url=/commonspot/security/getfile. cfm&PageID=14173. Accessed 30 May 2012.

12. Affordable Care Act update: implementing Medicare cost savings. 2010. http://www.mmapinc.org/pdfs/ ACA-Update-Implementing-Medicare-Costs-Savings.pdf. Accessed 30 May 2012.

13. Estimated financial effects of the "Patient Protection and Affordable Care Act" as amended. 2010. https:// http://www.cms.gov/Research-Statistics-Data-and-Systems/Research/ActuarialStudies/downloads/ PPACA_2010-04-22.pdf. Accessed 30 May 2012.

14. How will the Patient Protection and Affordable Care Act affect seniors? – timely analysis of immediate health policy issues. 2010. http://www.rwjf. org/files/research/65648seniors.pdf. Accessed 30 May 2012.

Medicaid and the State Children's Health Insurance Program

Vasanth Sathiyakumar, Jordan C. Apfeld, and Manish K. Sethi

Learning Objectives

After completing this chapter, the reader should be able to answer the following questions:
- What is Medicaid and who qualifies for it?
- What are the origins of the Medicaid program?
- What were the original structure and benefits when Medicaid was first enacted?
- How has Medicaid changed to its present form today?
- What were the proposed changes to Medicaid under the Affordable Care Act?
- What are the current and future challenges that Medicaid needs to address?

Introduction

Congress enacted the original Medicaid program in 1965 under Title XIX of the Social Security Act [1]. Medicaid was established as a voluntary, collaborative effort between the federal and state governments to jointly fund medical services and treatments required by low-income Americans. Although the federal government sets broad guidelines for the overall structure of the Medicaid program, individual states have the authority to specify who is eligible and what services are provided under Medicaid [2].

Originally passed to improve health care access for low-income citizens who were already receiving governmental support through cash assistance or "welfare," Medicaid has since expanded to cover more uninsured citizens – such

V. Sathiyakumar, B.A.
Department of Orthopedic Trauma, Vanderbilt University Medical Center, Nashville, TN 37232, USA
e-mail: vasanth.sathiyakumar@vanderbilt.edu

J.C. Apfeld, B.A.
Vanderbilt Orthopedic Institute Center for Health Policy, Vanderbilt University Medical School, Nashville, TN 37232, USA
e-mail: jordan.c.apfeld@vanderbilt.edu

M.K. Sethi, M.D. (✉)
Director of the Vanderbilt Orthopaedic Institute Center for Health Policy, Assistant Professor of Orthopaedic Trauma Surgery, Department of Orthopaedic Surgery and Rehabilitation, Vanderbilt University School of Medicine, Nashville, TN 37232, USA
e-mail: manish.sethi@vanderbilt.edu

M.K. Sethi and W.H. Frist (eds.), *An Introduction to Health Policy: A Primer for Physicians and Medical Students*, DOI 10.1007/978-1-4614-7735-8_3, © Springer Science+Business Media New York 2013

as children of low-income-bracket families, disabled Americans, and seniors – as it has evolved to its current structure today. Currently, Medicaid is the largest payer of health-care services and medical treatments for low-income citizens regardless of welfare status. Nearly one-half of all current program participants are children, and nearly one-fifth of all beneficiaries are disabled Americans [3]. Medicaid also serves as a safety net during economic recessions and covers more people than any other insurance program in the country, including Medicare and private insurance programs.

This chapter specifically provides an overview of the Medicaid program, including its origins, overall structure, eligible participants, benefits provided, funding for services, and governmental oversight on both the federal and state levels. The specific changes proposed to Medicaid under the 2006 Massachusetts Reform and the Affordable Care Act will also be described, as Medicaid is a common component in most health-care reforms. Finally, the chapter will conclude by addressing the current and future challenges of the program as well as where the program is headed in terms of potential changes after the 2012 Supreme Court's ruling that expanding Medicaid under the Affordable Care Act is unconstitutional.

Passage of Medicaid

Before Medicaid

Prior to the establishment of Medicaid, governments on the state and federal levels in the 1920s attempted to provide low-income citizens with public assistance for required health-care services. However, these attempts were limited in scope. Certain provisions in the Social Security Act of 1935 allowed for some state-sponsored health-care assistance for low-income mothers and children requiring mandatory health-related treatments [4]. Nevertheless, Americans who carried health insurance at the time were largely covered through private insurance plans that gained a large foothold in the insurance market during World War II. As discussed in Chap. 1, a variety of payroll-tax-sponsored public health insurance plans were introduced to Congress in the 1940s as a way to finance health care for low-income Americans, but none of these bills ever came to fruition [4]. For the first time, in 1950, the federal government directly helped state governments fund health-care expenses for citizens who were on public assistance. But these efforts were also limited in that only citizens who were already receiving some sort of public assistance would be compensated [5].

Medicaid Passes

National debates in the late 1950s and early 1960s under Harry Truman's presidency centered on whether health insurance for low-income Americans should be publicly or privately funded [6]. Although passage of a public health insurance plan for low-income Americans failed under President Truman's Fair Deal program, Congress in 1965 passed Title XIX of the Social Security Act as an amendment to establish an entitlement insurance program for Americans who were already receiving cash payments or "welfare." President Lyndon Johnson signed the amendment to the Social Security Act as part of his Great Society movement that expanded the federal government's role and placed a larger emphasis on public-sponsored health needs [6]. The federal government for the first time provided assistance to state governments that covered health-care costs for low-income Americans by matching state-allocated funds. Although the American Medical Association initially opposed the passage of the plan, the organization soon backed the plan along with the American Nurses Association and the National Association of Social Workers. In its original form, Medicaid was a voluntary program, meaning that each state could make an independent decision as to whether or not to enroll in the program. However, since Arizona became the final state to enact its version of Medicaid in 1982, all states now have some form of Medicaid.

Overview of Medicaid

Role of Medicaid and Coverage

Since its original enactment, Medicaid has expanded to cover more uninsured Americans than any other insurance program. After 1996, Medicaid enrollees no longer were required to receive welfare support in order to be a Medicaid beneficiary. Medicaid essentially serves as a broad net that covers those Americans living close to the federal poverty level who are not covered by private insurance plans or Medicare. However, some beneficiaries do jointly have both Medicare and Medicaid. These beneficiaries are known as "dual eligible" [7]. Medicaid provides extra assistance for long-term services excluded under Medicare and further helps these citizens cover Medicare premium costs. Nearly 20 % of all Medicare recipients are dual-enrolled in Medicaid [7]. Medicaid also covers seniors and nursing home residents, low-income children with working or unemployed parents, a wide range of disabled Americans with mental and physical health conditions, and Americans requiring long-term care. Medicaid is currently the nation's largest source of long-term care funding.

In 2010, nearly 66 % of the nation's poor or near poor were enrolled in Medicaid, including 1 out of every 5 adults in the country [8]. In terms of children, nearly one-third of all children are enrolled in Medicaid, and over one-half of children born to low-income families are Medicaid recipients. For Americans with severe disabilities, almost 20 % are Medicaid recipients, and the vast majority (nearly 70 %) of nursing home residents currently have Medicaid. Medicaid currently covers approximately 42 million low-income individuals in the United States and covers nearly nine million people with disabilities [9].

Furthermore, Medicaid serves an expanded role during economic recessions. As more Americans lose jobs and occupation-related health insurance during recessions, they subsequently become eligible for enrollment within Medicaid. The program has no enrollment caps or waiting lists and can therefore absorb more Americans at any given time. According to a report formulated for the Kaiser Foundation, nearly one million more Americans are eligible for Medicaid for every 1 % increase in the nation's unemployment rate [10]. This cyclical nature of Medicaid enrollment consequently places a strain on public hospital systems. As a result, Medicaid is currently accountable for nearly 33 % of public hospital revenues and nearly 40 % of public health center operating revenues at any given time [10].

Structure

Medicaid is a joint program between the federal government and the state governments. The federal government, through its Centers for Medicare and Medicaid Services (CMS) agency under the US Department of Health and Human Services, authorizes each state-sponsored Medicaid program. States in turn have the responsibility of implementing and administrating Medicaid. CMS specifically sets guidelines and regulations, recommends policy changes, and implements amendments to state-level plans. However, the states have the ultimate responsibly of drafting a Medicaid plan that details eligibility categories and requirements, benefits that will be covered for Medicaid recipients, and how the Medicaid program will be administered in each state, as long as these guidelines fall within the minimum guidelines established by the CMS [11]. States are also responsible for maintaining transparency by providing readily accessible information about the rules, policies, eligibility requirements, and benefits received for potential Medicaid beneficiaries. Furthermore, each state is required to run a "medical care advisory committee" which oversees the development of new policies and any changes in Medicaid administration on the state level [5].

Due to the freedom that states have in operating individual Medicaid programs, eligibility requirements and benefits may often widely vary from state to state. For example, seven states including Nevada, Utah, and Colorado have less than 7 % of residents enrolled in Medicaid, whereas 12 states including New York, California, and Massachusetts have over 15 % of their residents enrolled in Medicaid [12]. Furthermore, states have the options to either contract with private health insurance companies to provide approved "Medicaid" plans that cover mandatory benefits or pay health-care providers such as doctors and physicians directly without contracting to private insurance companies.

Funding

Federal funding for Medicaid is termed "federal financial participation (FFP)" and is unique to each state based on that state's needs. Federal funding can either finance administrative costs associated with the Medicaid program or reimburse treatment or coverage costs. States receive funding based on comparing each state's per capita income to the national average. The minimum federal assistance for any state is 50 % of the FFP but may increase up to 76 % for poorer states [13]. There is no cap on federal funding, ensuring that both the federal government and state governments share the costs for Medicaid beneficiaries. Overall federal contributions for all state Medicaid programs average to about 60 % of total Medicaid spending, with states covering the remaining 40 % of costs [14].

During times of economic recessions when more Americans are eligible for Medicaid due to loss of occupationally related health insurance, the federal government may temporarily increase the FFP contribution to help those states that need greater assistance [15]. For example, the American Recovery and Reinvestment Act was passed in 2009 to temporarily increase Medicaid spending by approximately $87 billion by increasing FFP rates from 56 % to 85 % [16].

Medicaid is also the largest source of revenue for states and comprises 44 % of all federal grants. These grants help create Medicaid-related jobs and help stimulate state-level economies through the flow of federal dollars into state economies. On the other hand, states average nearly 16 % of their annual budgets on Medicaid expenses [17]. This makes the program the most expensive public program offered by states second only to education programs.

Waivers

States may apply for a "Section 1115 waiver" that allows them to implement "experimental" or "pilot" demonstrative programs that coincide with the goals and visions of Medicaid but do not necessarily fit within the strict guidelines and regulations set forth by the CMS on how Medicaid should be structured [18]. For example, a Section 1115 waiver in Massachusetts allowed for the development of "MassHealth" (see Chap. 18), which allowed for greater eligibility expansions for Medicaid recipients. Similar waivers are also seen in California ("Medi-Cal"), Maine ("MaineCare"), Oregon ("Oregon Health Plan"), Oklahoma ("Soonercare"), and Tennessee ("TennCare"). States may apply for more than one Section 1115 waiver if they would like to implement different aspects of experimental Medicaid programs. Currently, a total of 95 waivers are on file with the Department of Health and Human Services [19]. Section 1115 waivers essentially allow states to test new delivery models that expand coverage to individuals, provide new types of services, or develop policy changes that increase efficiency while reducing medical costs. However, the Secretary of Health and Human Services as well as the CMS have authority to approve or negate these waivers.

Waivers are typically issued for 5-year periods but may be subsequently renewed for another 3 years [19]. Furthermore, these "pilot" Medicaid programs are instructed to be "budget neutral" with respect to the federal government. This stipulation dictates that federal government assistance for Medicaid should remain unchanged as if the pilot programs were not in place at all in order to curtail costs associated with potentially expensive experimental programs.

Medicaid and CHIP

Some states have elected to combine Medicaid with other programs, such as the Children's Health Insurance Program (CHIP), in order to have one central entity control these programs. CHIP was established in 1997 to provide coverage for uninsured children whose families earn high enough incomes that make them ineligible for Medicaid, but not enough to afford a private health insurance plan. CHIP has also been called "Children's Medicaid," although this terminology may be confusing since CHIP is a separate entity altogether from Medicaid. Typical Medicaid cutoffs for the eligibility of children are family incomes that are within 100 % of the Federal Poverty Line [20]. Children in families that make greater than 100 % of the Federal Poverty Line are not technically eligible for Medicaid, but they are eligible for coverage under CHIP. Overall CHIP provides similar benefits compared to Medicaid.

CHIP specifically provides coverage to an additional seven million children. Combined together, CHIP and Medicaid cover most children (43 million) whose families earn up to 200 % of the Federal Poverty Line [20]. Of the remaining uninsured children, nearly 70 % qualify for either Medicaid or CHIP. In recent years, most states have extended qualifications under CHIP by including children whose families earn up to 250 % of the Federal Poverty Line. From 1996 to 2002, the rate of uninsured children dropped 4 % due to coverage expansions under Medicaid and the enactment of CHIP [18].

Unlike for Medicaid, states have the ability to set caps on the number of children enrolled in CHIP and can charge premium or enrollment fees since CHIP is a separate program from Medicaid. For example, 33 states currently charge premiums or enrollment fees for children joining CHIP as of 2004, and 16 of these states have historically increased these premiums [16]. Studies have suggested that, when an entire family obtains coverage, children are more likely to be enrolled, thereby limiting out-of-pocket costs for these children and treating all medically relevant conditions. However, when states set limits on CHIP enrollments, the number of CHIP-eligible children increases.

In 2009, states were incentivized through the Children's Health Insurance Program Reauthorization Act (CHIPRA) to encourage enrollment of uninsured children in either Medicaid or CHIP [20]. CHIPRA also provided

incentives to enroll more children in Medicaid than original target goals set aside by the CMS. States reaching these goals were provided additional "federal performance bonuses" based on the number of children enrolled. Nearly $73 million in these federal bonuses were allocated to nine states in December 2009 [19]. CHIPRA also established the Medicaid and CHIP Payment and Access Commission, which has the responsibility to review Medicaid and CHIP eligibility requirements and policies and to suggest changes to the Secretary of Health and Human Services, to individual states, and to Congress on how to further enroll uninsured children into either Medicaid or CHIP.

Eligibility

Individuals and families are eligible for Medicaid on the following provisions: if they fall into one of several "eligibility categories," if they meet income and resource eligibility requirements, and if they are American citizens, as proven through documentation. Examples of these categories defined by the CMS include [21]:

- Pregnant women and children under the age of 6 if family income is within 133 % of the Federal Poverty Line
- Children between the ages of 6 and 18 years whose family incomes are within 100 % of the Federal Poverty Line
- Individuals who receive Supplemental Security Income (SSI) due to disabilities or elderly individuals over the age of 65 years who receive SSI
- Children who are in foster care and certain children in adoption assistance programs
- Young adults between the ages of 18 and 21 years who were formerly in foster care through the Foster Care Independence Act of 1999
- Medicare recipients who have low annual incomes
- Designated "medically needy" individuals who have annual incomes that are higher than normal eligibility for Medicaid but have incurred so many medically related costs that they are now eligible for Medicaid

Within these broad categories, there are numerous sub-criteria that individuals can meet that may make them eligible for Medicaid coverage. For example, if an individual can demonstrate that he or she needs long-term nursing home care and if that person earns an income that is within 300 % of the Federal Poverty Level, then that individual may be eligible for Medicaid-sponsored nursing home services [21].

The CMS has decided that states can establish their own methods for checking income levels of potential recipients of Medicaid, although most states have turned to an "asset test" in order to appraise the value of all assets that an individual has [1]. Although children are not subjected to asset tests, most states still require these tests for disabled and elderly participants, and nearly half of all states have asset tests for parents. Furthermore, those who are not American citizens but are immigrants must wait 5 years before being eligible to enroll in Medicaid due to the 1996 Personal Responsibility and Work Opportunity Reconciliation Act [8]. The federal government has since given states the freedom to choose whether they want to impose a 5-year wait period for immigrant pregnant women and immigrant children.

In addition to the "categories" for coverage listed previously that states must meet, states have the option to expand coverage for additional groups such as elderly and disabled Americans with incomes within 100 % of the Federal Poverty Line. Furthermore, pregnant women, children, or adults with incomes that are over the Federal Poverty Line-based thresholds may also be eligible for Medicaid [8].

Although most children in low-income families fall into one of the outlined "categories," their parents unfortunately are often not eligible for coverage. Parents may face much stricter income thresholds for Medicaid eligibility, such as income levels within 50 % of the Federal Poverty Level. Furthermore, only five states provide coverage for adults without children [8].

Those who are denied entry into Medicaid have the right to a fair hearing and may be represented by an attorney.

Benefits Covered

Similar to how the CMS defines categories of eligible Americans, the CMS also defines a set of 14 "mandatory" service categories that must be covered through Medicaid insurance plans [11]. States may also choose from 34 optional categories in order to extend coverage for Medicaid beneficiaries (Table 3.1). Some of these coverage benefits are typically found in most private insurance plans, although Medicaid also provides coverage for a

Table 3.1 Comparison of mandatory and optional categorical coverage

Mandatory coverage	Optional coverage
Inpatient hospital care	Case management services
Nursing facility services	Chiropractic services
Home health-care services	Clinic services
Early and periodic screening, diagnosis, and treatment	Dental services
	Dentures
Labs and x-rays	Diagnostic services
Vaccines for children	Emergency hospital services
Prenatal care	Home and community services
Outpatient hospital care	For the disabled
Family planning services	Hospice care [11]
Physician services	Psychiatric services
Health center services	Intermediate care facility services
Transportation services	Nursing facility services under 21
Rural health clinic services	Occupational therapy
	Optometrists' services
	All-inclusive care for elderly
	Personal care services
	Physical therapy
	Podiatrists' services
	Prescribed drugs
	Preventive services
	Private duty nurses
	Prosthetic devices
	Rehabilitative services
	Respiratory care services
	Screening services
	Speech, hearing, and language therapy

number of services not found in private insurance plans such as transportation coverage, dental care, and long-term care services. Nearly one-third of all Medicaid expenditures are attributable to these optional categories [11]. However, these optional categories are prone to being cut during recession periods.

States are prohibited from limiting coverage of benefits to any specific geographic area within the state. Furthermore, all Medicaid beneficiaries under a specific eligibility category should receive similar benefits without any forms of discrimination or limitations [11]. However, through the Deficit Reduction Act, Congress has given states the ability to limit coverage of certain "benchmark" benefits to some groups of people based on their health behaviors. Nevertheless, most Medicaid-eligible groups (such as pregnant women and children) are exempt from this Act. States do, however, have the freedom to limit drug coverage, including fertility drugs and non-prescription drugs. Furthermore, while the CMS requires states to provide coverage for all medically required services and requires that states have reasonable standards in place to determine which benefits are eligible for coverage, states can define what constitutes "medically necessary" [11]. However, this definition is often tied to standard treatment of care practices.

In order to cover services not authorized by the CMS, such as home modifications and nonmedical transportations, states may request a waiver under Section 1915 of the Social Security Act to cover some home- and community-based services [22].

In terms of children, states are mandated to provide early and periodic screening, diagnosis, and treatment (termed "EPSDT") services to children under the age of 21 years [23]. These services include all mandatory and optional services listed earlier. States must specifically follow set schedules to check children's medical conditions, including vision, hearing, and dental conditions, in order to prevent any potential problems from progressing into future complications. EPSDT also provides coverage for all medically required treatments resulting from the successful detection and diagnosis of early disease states. In order to be more effective, EPSDT instructs

states to reach out to families and their children and inform them of the importance of early screening and diagnosis. While states may limit services offered to its Medicaid adults, they are prohibited under EPSDT from cutting these services to children.

Overall, with the exception of EPSDT, states show considerable variation in the benefits offered to recipients due to the number of optional services provided by each state.

Evolution of Medicaid

Relationship with the Private Market

Medicaid is a joint venture between the federal government and the state governments. However, the private insurance market nevertheless plays a large role in this relationship. Most medical services for Medicaid recipients are obtained through private market plans that provide minimum Medicaid-approved benefits. Medicaid costs are subsequently reimbursed by state and federal funds that are set aside for Medicaid. Furthermore, more than half of Medicaid beneficiaries are enrolled in managed care plans in comparison to fee-for-service plans, in which Medicaid directly pays health providers based on the services that they provide [24]. To entice care providers to accept Medicaid patients, Medicaid chooses high reimbursement rates for care providers. Also, states must pay hospitals that serve an increased number of Medicaid inpatients additional funds through "disproportionate share hospital" adjustments.

Recent trends show that nearly 70 % of enrollees are in managed care plans contracted with private insurance companies in comparison to fee-for-service plans [24]. Managed care plans are insurance plans that are contracted between the insurance company and a network of cooperating physicians to provide care. Variations of managed care plans include health maintenance organizations (HMOs), in which enrollees choose a primary care physician who serves as a gateway for all other specialist services and enrollees must choose among physicians in the network;

preferred provider organizations (PPOs), in which the plan will cover physicians outside of the primary network for the enrollee to a limited extent; and point-of-service (POS) plans, in which enrollees choose between an HMO or a PPO plan at the time they need service. These managed care plans have been established to increase access to quality care for enrollees through cost-effective measures. Furthermore, states may apply for Section 1915(b) waivers under the Social Security Act [13]. These waivers allow states to create new reimbursement schemes that would further contain costs, such as contracting directly with private insurance companies to reduce costs with innovative techniques.

Patient Protection and Affordable Care Act of 2010 and Medicaid

Due to the individual mandate in the 2010 Patient Protection and Affordable Care Act (PPACA), Medicaid was set to absorb most of the newly insured low-income Americans who were now mandated to obtain health insurance. This expansion in Medicaid included approximately 16 million more Americans at a cost of $434 billion in health-care expenditures [25]. One major mechanism of expansion of Medicaid that was proposed within PPACA included loosening eligibility requirements. Under PPACA, historical "eligibility categories" that were once used to determine whether an individual would be allowed to enroll in Medicaid would be eliminated. Instead, Medicaid eligibility would be solely based upon income levels. This stipulation would allow more low-income uninsured adults to enroll, such as those without children. States furthermore were instructed to use a uniform, across-the-board system on calculating income levels without using the "asset" test. As a result of this expansion, Medicaid was set to absorb nearly every uninsured person below the age of 65 years who had an income level within 133 % of the Federal Poverty Level [25]. The federal government would increase the amount of revenue provided to states to help cover these costs, although states would have to contribute a portion of the new costs as well.

Furthermore, PPACA called for increased use of technology and other services that make it easier for potential enrollees to join Medicaid. Beneficiaries would also face an improved access to care, such as increased reimbursements to primary care physicians, enticing these physicians to accept Medicaid patients, and providing financial incentives to states that cover preventive services as well as at-home and community-based long-term care services.

In essence, under PPACA Medicaid was poised to serve as a vector to absorb most uninsured Americans. However, if states did not comply with PPACA's new eligibility requirements, they faced the risk of losing not only new funds allocated towards covering uninsured Americans but all of the existing Medicaid funds provided by the federal government. The Supreme Court, on June 28, 2012, ruled that it was unconstitutional for the federal government to cut *all* Medicaid funding to states if they did not comply with new eligibility requirements [26]. The Court deemed it is constitutional for the federal government to curtail new Medicaid funds provided to states, but the Court deemed it unconstitutional for the federal government to cut all Medicaid revenue if states do not comply with this expansion. As a result, PPACA's vision of expanding insurance coverage is now limited because states are not mandated to comply with this expansion and would not face threats of cuts to existing federal Medicaid funds [26].

Current and Future Challenge: Costs, Fraud, and Quality

One major challenge with Medicaid is the cost of the program. In 2009, total Medicaid expenditures were $384.3 billion, with a projected increase to $627.5 billion by 2015 [13]. As the percentage of disabled and aged Americans increases at a rate faster than the percentage of younger Americans, Medicaid will incur increased costs since Medicaid is the largest source of disability benefits and long-term nursing care. Nearly 75 % of Medicaid costs are used to cover costs for a quarter of Medicaid enrollees, who include disabled and elderly

Americans [27]. Furthermore, new legislation over the years that has increased benefits for enrollees-benefits such as increased prescription drug options and expanded services-has also contributed to increasing Medicaid costs. Nearly 50 % of all Medicaid services are spent for 5 % of Medicaid enrollees due to increased coverage benefits and costs [28]. State expenditures on Medicaid currently amount to approximately 10 % of each state's budget. To deal with increasing Medicaid costs, the federal government has historically increased its share of revenues to states for cost-sharing purposes. For example, in 2009 the American Recovery and Reinvestment Act increased Medicaid matching by nearly 14 % to states between 2009 and 2011 [29]. Furthermore, states that combine CHIP with Medicaid are provided with higher average federal revenue rates. These increased federal dollars persisted into the latter months of 2011 under the Education, Jobs, and Medicaid Assistance Act of 2010.

In addition, dual enrollees who are members of Medicare and Medicaid plans account for nearly 45 % of all Medicaid costs [7]. Medicare covers additional services not provided through Medicare such as hearing aids, visual aids, and extended nursing-care services. Coverage of care by these two programs is largely uncoordinated and inconsistent. Therefore, Medicaid has often disproportionately covered services for patients that should have been covered under Medicare. The establishment of the Coordinated Health Care Office under PPACA may help to facilitate this relationship with Medicare in order to ensure that the correct program is paying for a particular service [30]. Furthermore, certain groups of Americans who have Medicare have their Medicare premiums, coinsurance, and deductibles covered through Medicaid dollars. As more Americans will be covered under Medicare and eligible for dual-Medicaid enrollment, costs in Medicaid will subsequently increase as well. The Coordinated Health Care Office in theory should help reduce the expansion of these costs.

In order to address fraud under Medicaid – such as hospitals temporarily admitting a high proportion of Medicaid patients to receive "disproportionate share hospital" adjustment funds – Congress formed the Medicaid Integrity Program (MIP) in 2006 [11]. MIP specifically identifies fraudulent use of the Medicaid program on the federal level. Furthermore, the Payment Error Rate Measurement (PERM) program was formed in 2008 to randomly check claims and eligibility requirements each year in a selected sample of states to ensure that states are not abusing federal funds [28]. PERM has the additional goal of increasing state accountability for its allocation of Medicaid funds.

In order to improve health quality measures, Medicaid encourages states to use electronic medical records to improve coordination of care among providers and to reduce overhead costs. Furthermore, Medicaid data – both from managed care organizations and fee-for-service arrangements in the form of resource utilization data and patient surveys – are often used to form evidence-based guidelines that will provide the best care for the most patients. Monetary incentives are provided to hospitals and physicians that provide high-quality care for enrollees at low costs. Further federal funding is available for care providers who implement technological reforms that improve patient care.

Conclusion

Medicaid is the current safety net for low-income uninsured adults and also serves as the primary source of coverage for a variety of other Americans. From its original form to its current structure today, Medicaid covers more Americans than any other insurance program in the country and also provides more benefits than any private insurance program. Although the Supreme Court ruled it is unconstitutional for the federal government to limit Medicaid revenue to states that do not broaden eligibility requirements as called for under PPACA, the costs of the Medicaid program as well as improvements in technology and quality must be addressed in order to create a solvent future for the program.

References

1. Title XIX – grants to states for medical assistance programs. Social Security. Accessed 5 Oct 2012.
2. Medicaid: a primer. Kaiser Family Foundation. www.kff.org/medicaid/7334.cfm. Accessed 5 Oct 2012.
3. Medicaid: overview and policy issues. American Academy of Family Physicians. Accessed 5 Oct 2012.
4. Brief summaries of medicare & medicaid. Centers for Medicare and Medicaid Services. November 1, 2010. Accessed 5 Oct 2012.
5. State medicaid program administration: a brief overview. CRS Report for Congress. May 14, 2008. Accessed 5 Oct 2012.
6. Tracing the history of CMS programs: from president Theodore Roosevelt to president George W. Bush. Centers for Medicare and Medicaid Services. Accessed 5 Oct 2012.
7. Medicaid coverage of medicare beneficiaries (dual eligibles) at a glance. Centers for Medicare and Medicaid Services. 2012 Jan. Accessed 5 Oct 2012.
8. Chapter I: medicaid eligibility. Kaiser Commission on Medicaid and the Uninsured. Accessed 5 Oct 2012.
9. Medicaid coverage and spending in health reform. Kaiser Commission. May 2012. Accessed 5 Oct 2012.
10. Medicaid: overview of a complex program. Urban Institute Research of Records. Accessed 5 Oct 2012.
11. Chapter II: medicaid benefits. Kaiser Commission on Medicaid and the Uninsured. Accessed 5 Oct 2012.
12. Medicaid enrollment by state. Medicaid.gov. Accessed 5 Oct 2012.
13. Financing & reimbursement. Medicaid.gov. Accessed 5 Oct 2012.
14. Federal Medicaid Funding Reform. National Center for Policy Analysis. July 31, 2006. Accessed 5 Oct 2012.
15. Moving ahead amid fiscal challenges: a look at medicaid spending, coverage and policy trends. Kaiser Family Foundation. October 2011. Accessed on 5 Oct 2012.
16. The high cost of capping federal medicaid funding. AARP Public Policy Institute. Accessed 5 Oct 2012.
17. Medicaid today; preparing for tomorrow: a look at state program spending, enrollment and policy trends. Kaiser Family foundation. Accessed 5 Oct 2012.
18. The role of Section 1115 Waivers in Medicaid and CHIP: looking back and looking forward. Kaiser Family Foundation. Accessed 5 Oct 2012.
19. Medicaid Section 1115 Waivers. Kaiser Family Foundation. 2005 Jan. Accessed 5 Oct 2012.
20. Children's Health Insurance Program (CHIP). Medicaid. www.medicaid.gov/Medicaid-CHIP-Program-Information. Accessed 5 Oct 2012.
21. Eligibility. Medicaid.gov. Accessed 5 Oct 2012.
22. Understanding Medicaid Home and Community Services. U.S. Department of Health and Human Services. 2000 Oct. Accessed 5 Oct 2012.
23. About medicaid for children and families. Georgetown University Health Policy Institute. Accessed 5 Oct 2012.
24. Medicaid and managed care. Department of Health Information New York. Accessed 5 Oct 2012.
25. Medicaid expansion. US Government Accountability Office. 2012 Aug. Accessed 5 Oct 2012.
26. How the supreme court PPACE decision upholding medicaid expansion costs states. State Budget Solutions. 2012 June 22. Accessed 5 Oct 2012.
27. Medicare, medicaid – The 2012 statistical abstract. US Department of Commerce. Accessed 5 Oct 2012.
28. Medicaid benefits: online database. Kaiser Family Foundation. 2008. Accessed 5 Oct 2012.
29. National health care reform: the new medicaid. BlueCross of Michigan. Accessed 5 Oct 2012.
30. Medicaid: overview and impact of new regulations. Kaiser Family Foundation. January 2008. Accessed 5 Oct 2012.

Breaking Down Health Care Insurance from HMO to PPO and Beyond

4

David Polakoff and Audrey Smolkin

Learning Objectives

After completing this chapter, the reader should be able to answer the following questions:
- Understand the history of the health care insurance industry in the United States.
- Understand how the development of health maintenance organizations (HMOs) and the managed care industry affected the US health care system.
- Understand what caused the decline of HMOs and the affect this had on the health care landscape.
- Understand the effect on the future of the health care industry of the introduction of Accountable Care Organizations (ACOs) and payment reform initiatives.

Historical Underpinning of Insurance

The health care insurance industry in the United States is arguably the most maddeningly complex and confusing system in the world. Other chapters will examine some of the quality, equity, access, and consistency challenges of America's hydra-headed approach to health insurance; this chapter attempts to reduce the complexity by tracing the historical origins and examining the structure and processes of our health insurance system.

We begin by providing a basic glossary of terms (Table 4.1) that will help you understand this system. Like many complex systems, the health insurance industry has its own language and jargon, and this table will serve as a basic English to "health insurance language" dictionary. Next, we provide background on the history of health insurance in this country from its origins in the late 1920s to its expansion and sophistication today. While the focus of this chapter is on private commercial insurance, we also refer to Chapters 2 and 3 and the interconnection of the private insurance system with publically funded insurance programs. We will then segue into the rise of health maintenance organizations and managed care in the 1980s, which morphed into a variety of coverage options in the 1990s, including Preferred Provider Organizations (PPOs), Administrative Services Only (ASOs), and some degree of return

D. Polakoff, M.D., M.Sc. (✉) • A. Smolkin, MPP
University of Massachusetts Medical School,
Shrewsbury, MA 01545, USA
e-mail: david.polakoff@umassmed.edu;
audrey.smolkin@umassmed.edu

M.K. Sethi and W.H. Frist (eds.), *An Introduction to Health Policy: A Primer for Physicians and Medical Students*,
DOI 10.1007/978-1-4614-7735-8_4, © Springer Science+Business Media New York 2013

Table 4.1 Glossary of health insurance terms

Term	Definition	Citation
Accountable care organization (ACO)	A group of providers and suppliers of services (e.g., hospitals, physicians, and others involved in patient care) that will work together to coordinate care for the Medicare fee-for-service patients they serve	Center for Medicare & Medicaid Services. (2012). Accountable care organizations. Accessed April 24, 2012 https://www.cms.gov/Medicare/Medicare-Fee-for-Service-Payment/ACO/index.html
Administrative Services Only (ASO)	An arrangement in which an employer hires a third party to deliver administrative services such as claims processing and billing; the employer bears the risk for claims. This is common in self-insured health care plans	U.S. Department of Labor. (2011). Glossary of Employee Benefit Terms. Washington, DC: U.S. Bureau of Labor Statistics
Adverse selection	People with a higher than average risk of needing health care are more likely than healthier people to seek health insurance. Health coverage providers strive to maintain risk pools of people whose health, on average, is the same as that of the general population. Adverse selection results when the less healthy people disproportionately enroll in a risk pool	Kaiser Family Foundation. (2009). Glossary of health reform terms. Menlo Park, CA: The Henry J. Kaiser Family Foundation
Capitation	Method of paying for health care where the provider of services receives a set amount of money per person for all care the person receives during a set time period (usually a year). Payment is "capped" and therefore creates an incentive for providers to provide the best care at the lowest cost	Barr, D. (2007). Introduction to US Health Policy: The Organization, Financing, and Delivery of Health Care in America. Baltimore, MD: Johns Hopkins University Press
Coinsurance	A form of medical cost sharing in a health insurance plan that requires an insured person to pay a stated percentage of medical expenses after the deductible amount, if any, was paid. Rates may differ: • If services received from an approved provider or if received by providers not on the approved list • For different types of services	U.S. Department of Labor. (2011). Glossary of Employee Benefit Terms. Washington, DC: U.S. Bureau of Labor Statistics
Copayment	A form of medical cost sharing in a health insurance plan that requires an insured person to pay a fixed dollar amount when a medical service is received. The insurer is responsible for the rest of the reimbursement. Two things to remembers: • There can be separate copayments for different services • Some plans require that a deductible first be met for some specific services before a copayment applies	U.S. Department of Labor. (2011). Glossary of Employee Benefit Terms. Washington, DC: U.S. Bureau of Labor Statistics
Deductible	A fixed dollar amount that an insured person pays before the insurer starts to make payments for covered medical services	U.S. Department of Labor. (2011). Glossary of Employee Benefit Terms. Washington, DC: U.S. Bureau of Labor Statistics

Term	Definition	Reference
Employee Retirement Income Security Act (ERISA)	The Employee Retirement Income Security Act of 1974 (ERISA) is a federal law that sets minimum standards for most voluntarily established pension and health plans in private industry to provide protection for individuals in these plans. Important amendments made to ERISA: • Consolidated Omnibus Budget Reconciliation Act (COBRA) provides some workers and their families the right to continue their health coverage for a limited time after certain events, such as the loss of a job • Health Insurance Portability and Accountability Act (HIPAA) provides important new protections for working Americans and their families who have preexisting medical conditions or might otherwise suffer discrimination in health coverage based on factors that relate to an individual's health • Newborns' and Mothers' Health Protection Act • Mental Health Parity Act • Women's Health and Cancer Rights Act	U.S. Department of Labor (2011). Health Plan & Benefits – Employee Retirement Income Security Act (ERISA). Accessed from http://www.dol.gov/dol/topic/health-plans/erisa.htm
Fee-for-service (FFS) plan	Health coverage in which doctors and other providers receive a fee for each service (office visit, test, procedure, or other health care service). There are no restrictions on physician, hospital, or ancillary services. The amount the plan plays dependent upon established fee schedule. Usually considered the most expensive type of health insurance	U.S. Office of Personnel Management. (2012). Health and insurance glossary. Washington, DC: U.S. Office of Personnel Management
First dollar coverage	Coverage for an insured individual who is not required to make an initial payment for care before insurance benefits is available. Limited to eligible charges or duration of coverage for specific procedure or expense	Scofea LA. (1994). The development and growth of employer-provided health insurance. Monthly Labor Review 117(3), 3–10
Flexible spending account (FSA)	Savings account offered and administered by employers for employees to set aside funds, on a pretax basis, for employee's share of insurance premiums or medical expenses not covered by employer's health plan. Funds must be used within a benefit year or employee loses funds	U.S. Department of Labor. (2011). Glossary of Employee Benefit Terms. Washington, DC: U.S. Bureau of Labor Statistics
Health maintenance organization (HMO) plan	A health care system that assumes both the financial risks associated with providing comprehensive medical services (insurance and service risk) and the responsibility for health care delivery in a particular geographic area to HMO members, usually in return for a fixed, prepaid fee. Financial risk may be shared with the providers participating in the HMO	U.S. Department of Labor. (2011). Glossary of Employee Benefit Terms. Washington, DC: U.S. Bureau of Labor Statistics
	Restrictions on physician, hospital, and ancillary services. A primary care physician must provide referrals for specialty care. Preapprovals are necessary for procedures and tests in order to be covered by HMO	Torpy JM, Burke AE, Glass RM. (2007). Health care insurance: The basics. The Journal of the American Medical Association 297(10), 1154

(continued)

Table 4.1 (continued)

Term	Definition	Citation
Health savings account (HSA)	Tax-exempt accounts that can be used to pay for current or future qualified medical expenses. Employers may make HSAs available to their employees, and if the employer contributes to the HSA, the contributions are excluded from employee gross income. In order to open an HSA, an individual must have health coverage under an HSA-qualified high deductible health plan (HDHP), which can be provided by the employer or purchased from any company that sells health insurance in a state	Claxton G. (2008). How Private Health Coverage Works: A Primer, 2008 Update. Menlo Park, CA: The Henry J. Kaiser Family Foundation
Indemnity insurance	Coverage of some health expenses and allows individual to select a physician or a hospital without restrictions. Patients are responsible for paying the portion of a medical bill not covered by insurance	Torpy JM, Burke AE, Glass RM. (2007). Health care insurance: The basics. The Journal of the American Medical Association 297(10), 1154
Independent practice organization (IPO)	Organized entity that contracts with individual physicians from an array of specialties. IPOs do not conduct marketing, financing, or pricing. IPOs are not licensed as an HMO; therefore, they cannot sell directly to employers and usually cover a specified (and limited) geographic area. Therefore, IPOs usually contract with an HMO	Taylor RJ, Taylor SB. (1994). The AUPHA manual of health services management. Gaithersburg, MD: Apsen Publishers, Inc
Integrated care organization (ICO)	A group of providers and suppliers of service that has as its hub either a primary care center or a small group practice and also includes APRNs, specialists, hospitals, pharmacists, behavioral health practitioners, and providers of long-term care that will work together to coordinate care for individuals who are dually eligible for Medicare and Medicaid	
Managed care plans	Managed care plans generally provide comprehensive health services to their members and offer financial incentives for patients to use the providers who belong to the plan. Examples of managed care plans include: • Health maintenance organizations (HMOs) • Preferred provider organizations (PPOs) • Exclusive provider organizations (EPOs) • Point-of-service plans (POSs)	U.S. Department of Labor. (2011). Glossary of Employee Benefit Terms. Washington, DC: U.S. Bureau of Labor Statistics

Term	Definition	Reference
Maximum dollar limit	The maximum amount payable by the insurer for covered expenses for the insured and each covered dependent while covered under the health plan	U.S. Department of Labor. (2011). Glossary of Employee Benefit Terms. Washington, DC: U.S. Bureau of Labor Statistics
Medical savings account (MSA)	Savings account designated for out-of-pocket medical expenses. Employers and individuals are allowed to contribute on pretax basis and carry over unused funds at end of year	U.S. Department of Labor. (2011). Glossary of Employee Benefit Terms. Washington, DC: U.S. Bureau of Labor Statistics
Moral hazard	Additional health care that is purchased when a person becomes insured	Nyman JA. (2004). Is 'Moral Hazard' Inefficient? The Policy Implications Of A New Theory. Health Affairs 23(5), 194–199
Point-of-service (POS) plan	HMO/PPO hybrid. POS plans resemble HMOs for in-network services. Out-of-network services are usually reimbursed like an indemnity plan	U.S. Department of Labor. (2011). Glossary of Employee Benefit Terms. Washington, DC: U.S. Bureau of Labor Statistics
Primary care physician (PCP)	A physician who serves as the primary contact within the health plan for a group member. The PCP provides general medical care and coordinates and authorizes referrals for specialized services	U.S. Department of Labor. (2011). Glossary of Employee Benefit Terms. Washington, DC: U.S. Bureau of Labor Statistics
Preferred provider organization (PPO) plan	A network of selected health care providers (such as hospitals and physicians) working for specific health insurance company. The enrollees may go outside the network but would incur larger costs in the form of higher deductibles, higher coinsurance rates, or non-discounted charges from the providers	Torpy JM, Burke AE, Glass RM. (2007). Health care insurance: The basics. The Journal of the American Medical Association 297(10), 1154
Risk pooling	Large groups of individual entities (individuals or employers) whose medical costs are combined in order to calculate premiums	American Academy of Actuaries. (2009). Critical issues in health reform: Risk pooling. Washington, DC: American Academy of Actuaries
Usual, customary, and reasonable (UCR) charges	The charge is the provider's usual fee for a service that does not exceed the customary fee in a specific geographic area and is reasonable based on the circumstances. Indemnity plans operate on UCR charges	U.S. Department of Labor. (2011). Glossary of Employee Benefit Terms. Washington, DC: U.S. Bureau of Labor Statistics

to Fee-For-Service (FFS)/indemnity plans. Finally, we will examine the degree to which we may have moved "back to the future" with the current discussions and movement toward accountable/integrated care organizations.

Health insurance in the United States, and elsewhere, is a relatively recent concept. Several factors contributed to the lack of health insurance offerings before the twentieth century including a lack of expensive (and effective) health interventions and the lack of interest by insurance companies. For example, it was only in 1895 that X-rays were invented and they were not in routine use until 1917 during World War I in aid stations and hospitals [1]. X-ray services were not covered by Blue Cross Blue Shield or other insurance providers until the 1930s [1]. The first vaccine for polio came in 1955. Most women had children at home; for example, only half of the US births were in hospitals in 1938; by 1955, 99 % of women were giving birth in hospitals as a result of the expansion of private health insurance [2]. Well into the twentieth century, surgery was a relatively rare intervention. It would be many years before the explosive advances in medical and pharmaceutical technology would lead to interventions that people would want and need. For much of the period through World War I, families needing medical assistance paid for it out of pocket and, if anything, purchased "disability" insurance that would provide income supplementation or replacement in the event of crippling illness or accident [3].

Even for families interested in paying for this concept of "health insurance," most commercial insurance companies were uninterested in offering such a product. The prevalent line of thought was that health was not an insurable commodity as a result of two concerns that continue to complicate health insurance discussions even today: moral hazard and adverse selection. Moral hazard is the notion that individuals would engage in more dangerous (or hazardous) activities because they believed they were covered by a safety net (in this case, the safety net being that insurance would cover any medical costs arising as a result of risky behavior). Insurance companies wanted to avoid covering people who would then be free

to treat their health as risk that someone else covers the cost of treating. Today, one will often hear it said that "the consumer/patient must have skin in the game." Adverse selection is the concept that the most unhealthy, and thus costly, individuals would disproportionately purchase insurance, making it difficult to correctly calculate risks and determine appropriate pricing considering the variation in baseline health and needs of the intended population.

While moral hazard and adverse selection could have been addressed, at least in part, by making health insurance compulsory or publically funded (as many European nations did by the 1920s), physicians and pharmacists strongly resisted this option as they believed it would significantly reduce their power and profits. The disinterest of the commercial insurance industry, the lack of demand from consumers, and the resistance of the medical professionals combined to delay the formation of an active US health insurance market. But slowly, things began to change.

Workers' Compensation and Health Insurance:

Workers in the late 1800s and early 1900s often faced difficult, unsafe, and life-threatening conditions [4]. This was challenging both for the workers themselves and for their employers. In order to address this situation, the first workmen's compensation law was passed, entitled the Federal Employer's Liability Act in 1908 to protect railroad workers. Slowly, individual states began to adopt workers' compensation laws, and today all American workers have some type of compensation benefits including provision of some medical costs and partial wages for work-related injuries. In this way, workers' compensation was one of the earliest forms of health care insurance in the United States.

Several demographic, scientific, and economic advances accrued to make medical care more expensive, and the possibility of commercial

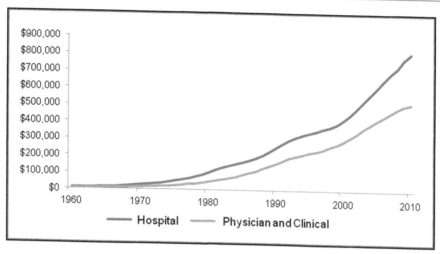

Fig. 4.1 US National Health Expenditures, 1960–2010 (Data from Centers for Medicare and Medicaid. National Health Expenditure Data. Washington, DC: Centers for Medicare and Medicaid; 2010)

insurance began to seem more profitable and necessary. This section briefly outlines some of those factors:

1. More faith in medicine: By the 1920s and 1930s, breakthroughs in medicine and science [5] made medical care more innovative, more trusted, and more expensive. With the rise of standardization in medical education, medical schools became more costly, and these higher costs were passed through in the pricing of medical services. At the same time, hospital costs were also rising dramatically. In addition, many women began to choose hospitals to deliver their babies, at a significant and uncovered cost for many families.

   See Fig. 4.1 for an overview of US National Health Insurance Expenditures (1960–2010).

2. Rising incomes: Increasing incomes and a sense of general prosperity in the years before the Great Depression stimulated more demand for health care services [6].

The Baylor Plan and Blue Cross

While these factors were brewing, a group of teachers in Dallas, Texas came together to make health insurance history. In 1929, Dr. Justin Kimball became an administrator at Baylor Hospital and, as a result of his prior experience as school superintendent, noted that many Dallas school teachers were unable to pay their bills. He created the "Baylor Plan" which allowed participants to pay $.50 a month into a fund for care at Baylor Hospital. The plan was guaranteed to provide 21 days of hospital care for $6 a year.

The plan was limited and small and was considered an experiment. Today, it is considered to be the origin of modern health insurance and quickly spread to other cities and towns under the name Blue Cross. This bold experiment was considered a great success and was quickly spread and modified in important ways including an expansion to multiple hospitals (the first multi-hospital plan began in New Jersey in 1931). Within a decade, it further expanded to provide payment for medical services under the name Blue Shield. Before we turn to the development of Blue Shield and the later merging of hospital (Blue Cross) and medical care (Blue Shield) insurance programs, it should be noted that Dr. Kimball's decision to link payment to a specific hospital put hospital care at the center of health insurance, a placement that significantly continues to shape health insurance, health care delivery, and health care costs today.

> *"A godsend to thousands."*
> —Brian Twitty, Assistant to Dr. Justin Kimball regarding the Baylor Plan.
>
> More than 1,300 teachers initially signed up for the Baylor plan, and within 5 years, more than 408 employee groups with more than 23,000 members were covered by this new type of plan [7].

Blue Shield

Almost exactly a decade after Dr. Kimball began his grand experiment, the Blue Shield concept was developed by employers in the lumber and mining camps of the Pacific Northwest. While paying for services instead of hospital stays was different, the basic concept was the same. A monthly payment was made to "medical service bureaus" that included groups of physicians who would provide all needed care. A key feature, and one that continues to shape the most basic structure of American health insurance to this day, was that fees were paid by the employers, not the employees. This key new worker benefit made certain employers more appealing and also had the potential to reduce missed days of work for illness or disability. This first official Blue Shield Plan began in 1939, and in 1948, the symbol was informally adopted by nine plans and called the Associated Medical Care Plan, which was later renamed the National Association of Blue Shield Plans. It was not until several decades later, in 1982, that Blue Shield merged with the Blue Cross Association and formed the Blue Cross and Blue Shield Association.

World War II and the Rise of Nationally Subsidized Employer-Based Insurance

While Blue Shield and similar plans were beginning to spring up across the country, before World War II, few people were covered. However, during the war, the federal government placed a freeze on wages [8], making the ability to offer fringe benefits appealing. Employers began offering health insurance as a key benefit. The fact that this benefit was not subjected to taxation for either the employee or the employer made it highly appealing. Today, the majority of Americans receive their health insurance as a nontaxable fringe benefit of employment.

The seeds of the managed care revolution were planted about 10 years after Baylor was beginning its grand experiment, by another inventive doctor named Sidney Garfield. This experiment took place in the late 1930s in middle of the Mojave Desert.

Dr. Garfield built the Contractors General Hospital in an effort to treat sick and injured workers associated with the construction of the Los Angeles Aqueduct. Though some workers had health insurance, most did not. Dr. Garfield did not turn away any worker needing care. The result was a rise in hospital expenses. Harold Hatch, an insurance agent, advised insurance companies to pay Dr. Garfield a fixed amount per day, per covered worker in advance, introducing the concept of prepayment. Thousands of workers enrolled for five cents per day and received the treatment needed, making the Contractors General Hospital a success. Another massive construction project, the Grand Coulee Dam, signaled a need for a new hospital and the recruitment of physicians in a "prepaid group practice" to provide care to 6,500 workers and their families. This first "replication" was again well received, and, hearing of Dr. Garfield's success, Henry J. Kaiser created the ultimate test, providing health care for 30,000 shipyard workers. The association formed between Dr. Garfield's innovative health system and Kaiser's extensive industries created Kaiser Permanente, the organization which still exists today [9]. See Fig. 4.2 for a diagram depicting the development of employer-based health care plans.

HMO Era

The development and history of health maintenance organizations (HMOs) and other related managed care organizations in the United States

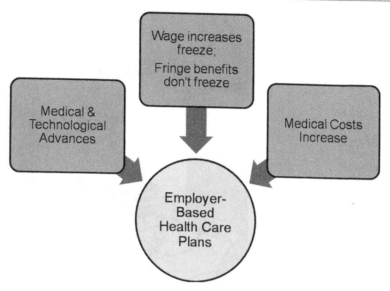

Fig. 4.2 Development of employer-based health care plans

span decades. The concept began to develop as early as 1929 with Blue Cross and 1937 with the Kaiser Foundation Health Plans and Group Health Association (GHA). It continued to evolve and expand in the 1960s and 1970s, and its influence in the delivery of health care peaked in the 1980s and 1990s. But by the late 1990s, that influence on health policy began to decline as a direct reflection of its failure to restrain growing health care costs. The cartoon in Fig. 4.3 depicts this.

The 1970s

Since 1965 when President Lyndon B. Johnson signed amendments to the Social Security Act creating Medicare and Medicaid, the US economy continued to grow. Congress became frustrated with the combination of inflation, uncontrolled health care costs, and utilization of the Medicare program. In 1971, President Nixon enforced control on wages and price freezes to curb further inflation [10]. In an effort to limit further growth in the Medicare budget, the Nixon Administration requested the assistance of Dr. Paul Ellwood to present his ideas for reducing

health care spending [11]. Dr. Ellwood was a close colleague of Dr. Philip Lee, Assistant Secretary of Health during the Johnson Administration, and knew too well the health care situation that was unfolding. Dr. Ellwood proposed the concept of the health maintenance organization as a strategy to improve the existing health care system, using government funding to support the growth of prepaid health plans [12]. The underlying concept was essentially the same as that introduced decades earlier by Drs. Kimball and Garfield. A group of providers are "prepaid" a fixed sum for all of the care required by an individual. This creates an incentive for the doctors and other providers to keep that person healthy, limiting the amount needing to be spent on "sick care." In insurance parlance, it also shifts the utilization risk to the providers.

By 1973, health care costs increased from 4 % of the federal budget in 1965 to 11 % [10]. The discussions with Dr. Ellwood laid the groundwork for the Health Maintenance Organization (HMO) Act of 1973. Signed by President Nixon in December 1973, the HMO Act provided start-up funding in the form of grants and loans for new HMOs and access to employer-based insurance markets [11]. The Act provided $325 million

Fig. 4.3 HMO cartoon (Used with permission. Copyright © John McPherson J. Distributed by Universal Uclick via CartoonStock.com. That's how much time your HMO allots for bypass surgery [image on the Internet]. 2005 Dec 25 [cited 2012 Apr 17]. Available from: http://www.cartoonstock.com/cartoon-view.asp?catref=jmp060725)

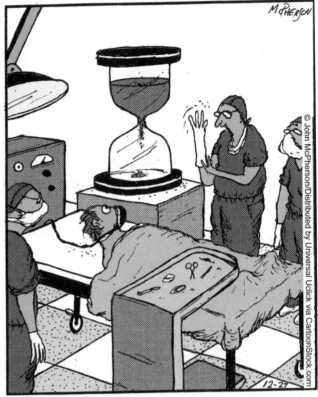

"That's how much time your HMO allots for bypass surgery."

in appropriations, spread over 5 years, a fraction of the $3.9 billion proposed during initial discussions. It also assisted new HMOs with marketing, initial operating costs, and facility design [13].

However, the establishment of the HMO Act of 1973 and further amendments in 1976 did not accomplish the initial vision of Dr. Ellwood and President Nixon's HMO strategy. Health care spending did not decline. The Act caused HMOs, particularly federally funded HMOs, to be heavily regulated by federal and state regulations and legislation [13]. The HMOs that were established through federal funding were limited. Rather than continue to support additional spending, Congress passed a bill in 1981 to phase out and end both the grant and loan programs created by the HMO Act of 1973. Though federally funded HMOs were limited in number and enrollment, both government and nongovernment interests

continued to search for a more effective and less expensive health care system. This led to continued and widespread development of HMOs without federal assistance in the later part of the 1970s and early 1980s and generated new models of insurance, collectively referred to as "managed care" [13].

The Development of HMOs

The economic recession in the early 1980s reinforced the need to control costs and expenditures. HMOs were developed to reduce health care utilization and expenses and were widely adopted during the 1980s and 1990s. Beyond their original focus on prevention (health maintenance), HMOs supported the imperative to reduce health care spending by controlling hospital utilization, the specialist referral process, and selecting providers. Provider competition grew as HMOs implemented "selective contracting" with providers as an effective cost-containment strategy, limiting their subscribers to specific providers and hospitals and negotiating lower fees with those limited groups [14]. Many of the HMOs (formerly called prepaid group practices) that were developed during this era reflected the models of the Kaiser Permanente and Group Health plans. Initially, this model led to reduced utilization, created some efficiencies, and limited payments to physicians [15].

As the pressures for cost containment continued, the managed care movement shifted from the management of care by a primary care physician (PCP) to the management of physicians by HMO administrators "intent on reducing costs, limiting services and increasing margin" [16]. This signaled a shift of authority and control from physicians to the HMOs as the managers of care and services. Many consumers perceived a transformation in health care into a "corporate industry" with HMOs working with employers to provide cost-effective health care to their employees through managed care plans. The employee benefit created in the 1930s to attract and retain employees, in lieu of increased pay, had become an enormous and uncontrollable financial liability for employers. Employer selection of the HMO model grew from 5 % in 1984 to 50 % in 1993 as companies sought to control these costs [17].

The Rise of PPOs and POS Plans

With the rise in HMO adoption came a significant backlash against the core features and management techniques of this type of plan, as well as what many saw as excesses in their application. By 1985, managed care organizations began to restructure and evolve. The Preferred Provider Organizations (PPOs) and point-of-service (POS) plans that were created became competitors to HMOs in the provision of health care coverage. PPOs consist of a network of selected health care providers (such as hospitals and physicians) working for a specific health insurance company.

Patients are given strong financial incentives to stay within this set network of providers. Care outside the network costs more, often significantly more, in the form of higher deductibles, higher coinsurance rates, or non-discounted charges from the providers. From the provider perspective, PPOs may be appealing because patients not in the PPO network can still be seen, and providers may charge more than PPO network providers for services. Providers agree to discounted rates for in-network services in exchange for increased volume of referrals. Though PPOs do not require referrals from the primary care physician for specialty care, this could promote uncoordinated care as patients may receive care from specialists without the knowledge of the primary care physician.

Another variant that developed at about the same time as the PPO was the point-of-service (POS) plan. A POS plan is a type of managed care that is a hybrid of the HMO and the PPO. Members of a POS plan do not have to decide which system (in network or out of network) to use until the point in time when the service is being used. However, as a managed care plan, the individual is required to choose a primary care physician (PCP) to be the main "point of service" and care coordinator. There are cost and convenience incentives for the member to choose providers within the network, but either choice is permitted. See Table 4.2 for a listing of types of health insurance plans and their descriptions.

As HMOs began to offer PPO and POS products, PPOs obtained HMO licenses, and HMOs contracted with employers on a self-funded rather than capitated or fully insured basis, shifting more risk back to employers [11]. The differences between the various types of managed care plans began to blur.

With this restructuring and rapid HMO growth, enrollment grew from 3 million in the 1970s to 13 million in the early 1980s and to over 80 million in 1995 [12]. While enrollment continued to increase, the number of licensed HMOs peaked in 1986 and has since declined [15]. The rapid growth in HMOs had outpaced their ability to manage costs. By the 1990s, the influence of HMOs began to diminish rapidly.

Table 4.2 Types of health insurance plans

Type of plan	Key characteristics	What it means for providers
HMO	• Members must choose primary care physician (PCP) from provider network	• Shared financial risk
	• Referrals are required to utilize specialty services	• Medical group paid on negotiated rate
	• Members pay fixed monthly fee	• Primary care physician provides referral for specialty services
	• Low out of pocket expenses	• May provide services to HMO and non-HMO members
	• Various models: group, staff, network, individual practice association (IPA)	
PPO	• Member not required to select primary care physician	• Payment incentives for providers (through a variety of mechanisms)
	• Receive care from any physician in PPO network or out of network	• Prompt payment features for favorable payment rates
	• No referrals from PCP necessary	• Utilization management services to control utilization and cost of health services provided
	• Member may use non-PPO providers, at additional (usually higher) cost	
	• Members pay for services as they are rendered	
POS	• Hybrid of PPO and HMO plans	• Reimbursement through capitated payments/fee schedule
	• Member must choose a PCP	• Primary care physician "gatekeeper" of referral and medical services
	• PCP provides referrals	• Physician payments paid upon achieving utilization and cost targets
	• Resembles HMOs for in-network services	
	• Out-of-network services are reimbursed on fee schedule	
ACO	• Group of providers responsible for group of patients	• Shared responsibility for treatment of a group of patients
	• Provider payments based on the care the ACO as a whole provides to patients	• Providers must coordinate care with other physicians
		• Providers share any cost savings received

The Fall of HMOs

There were a number of factors that contributed to the decline of HMOs in the late 1980s and 1990s. Many providers objected to risk contracting terms, which pressured them to take on more risk. Patient and provider backlash against managed care business practices became widespread. New regulations to limit unfavorable HMO practices provided patients with more legal rights to sue HMOs. A number of class litigation actions were brought by consumers, physicians, and other providers against managed care business practices that included injury or death resulting from alleged decisions to withhold or limit

medical care. As a result, physician relationships with HMOs and managed care organizations, a descriptor that had become prevalent by the mid-1990s, soured sharply.

Responding to pressures from purchasers (the employers who purchase most commercial health insurance on behalf of their employees) to control rising premiums, managed care organizations adopted a variety of techniques to limit utilization of health care services or shift their costs to consumers. Under the heading of utilization management, health plans implemented prior authorization, specific benefit restrictions, quantity limits, referral requirements, and retrospective review and denials. Among the cost-shifting techniques that were developed or expanded during this era were annual and specific-service deductibles, copayments and coinsurance. While all were part of a rational effort to control the national rise in health care costs, the cumulative effect was perceived by consumers as intrusive and burdensome and by providers as an abrogation of the prerogatives reserved by law and tradition for the medical profession. Ultimately, this prompted a substantial backlash by a consumer movement and organized medicine.

This backlash prompted changes in the business approaches of HMOs, which in turn significantly transformed the business model of the health insurance industry. Anything that was perceived as a limitation on access to or choice of providers was softened or eliminated. On the other hand, use of all forms of cost shifting intensified and accelerated. These moves could be portrayed as "consumers have access to any provider or service they wish, as long as they are willing to pay for it." Insurance product design also evolved further. More and more HMOs began to offer products that were similar to PPOs and POS plans [18]. The choice of providers was not limited to a finite network. Cost shifting to the consumer took the place of utilization controls.

Despite these changes in the business model, health plans did not succeed in restraining rising health care costs for very long. The annual percent change in per capita health care spending increased from 2 % in 1996 to 10 % in 2001 [17]. The retreat from traditional cost controls by HMOs resulted in a resumption of the previous growth curve in medical spending and a search for new ways to restrain it.

What's Next for HMOs and Managed Care

In recent years, the persistent and inexorable rise in health care costs has become one of the United States' most persistent and vexing economic issues. While previously much of the pressure to restrain rising costs had come from purchasers, cost shifting to consumers has activated them and

increased the national level of frustration around health care. The nexus of these pressures from consumers, employers, providers, and government regulators falls on health plans. A careful examination of the history outlined here revealed that among the cost control methods that have been successful in the US in previous decades were government price controls, capitation, and what was previously termed "managed care." The former is unacceptable in contemporary politics. The second failed because providers were in many instances unprepared to accept and manage risk. And the latter, while successful in controlling costs, ultimately sank under the weight of a mixture of corporate excesses in failed implementation. The next generation of cost control initiatives is drawing from the best of these, while learning from recent experiences.

> "If all we're doing is adding more people to a broken system then costs will continue to skyrocket, and eventually somebody is going to be bankrupt, whether it's the federal government, state governments, businesses or individual families."
> –President Barack Obama, White House Health Care Summit, 2/2010 [19]

Back to the Future: Accountable Care Organizations (ACOs) and Integrated Care Organizations (ICOs)

Among a wide number of sweeping changes, the Patient Protection and Affordable Care Act signed into law on March 23, 2010, contains a provision to develop accountable care organizations (ACOs) as one of the first new payment reform initiatives. Though initially established as a new way of paying for health care provided to Medicare beneficiaries, there is significant opportunity for pilot programs to test this payment model by private payers and Medicaid agencies [20]. ACOs are organizations comprised of physicians, hospitals, and other health care providers who accept prepayment and risk to manage a group of patients. They are responsible (accountable) for all, or a contractually defined range, of health care services. As part of this management, they assume many of the functions previously performed by managed care organizations or health plans, including utilization management, care and case management, and cost control. The reimbursement system often includes rewards for attainment of quality of care and outcome benchmarks, as well as cost control [21].

The implementation of the ACO model will need to overcome several challenges to be successful. The ACO will need to build trusting relationships among physicians, payers, and other partners. This trust may prove difficult to reconcile as the turbulent relations between physicians, patients, and insurers during the late 1990s created an unfavorable climate. Individual physicians may be reluctant to accept responsibility for the care of an unselected panel of patients within an organization. Hospitals and health care organizations may experience difficulty in aligning their medical staff to promote accountability [22]. And hospitals, the financially dominant partners within an ACO, will be driven by conflicting incentives: reducing utilization to achieve savings and keeping their beds filled. But a full collaboration among the provider, health-care organization, patient, and payer is critical to the success of the ACO. Data management and data sharing present further challenges. Organizations will be required to develop data-sharing agreements and exchange performance and financial data between providers and payers [21]. These data will also be critical for providers to understand their patient populations and health care patterns and to establish performance measures.

The implementation of health information technology (HIT) is vital for ACOs. HIT, including electronic health records and care management systems, will be the basis for data sharing across providers, organizations, and payers [23]. Without such technology, the coordination of care, establishment of performance measures and metrics, and management of care spending will remain difficult. Health information exchanges, currently under development in many states, will support these efforts. But they are currently in their infancy. It will be critical to ensure that solutions to these challenges are available if ACOs will be successful.

At this time, the ACO as a payment model is relatively new; the benefits to improving the health care system and reducing health care costs are still undetermined. Pilot programs are being implemented between providers, health care organizations, and payers, both government and commercial, to determine the viability and cost effectiveness of ACOs as a payment and care model.

Conclusion

Since its earliest roots in the 1920s, health insurance in the United States has evolved into the costliest and one of the most complex in the world. This chapter traces the history and evolution of the employer-based system of health insurance and documents shifts both into and away from a managed care and health maintenance systems (Fig. 4.4). The massive growth in number of plans and complexity of payment systems has contributed to higher costs and to some modest improvements in quality and access. The most recent shift, brought about by the passage and imminent implementation of the federal health care reform law (Patient Protection and Affordable Care Act) will significantly shift the health insurance landscape toward a model based on some form of "accountable care organizations." If past is prologue, the ultimate impact of the dramatic changes envisioned in the new law will surprise us and will not be fully understood for many years.

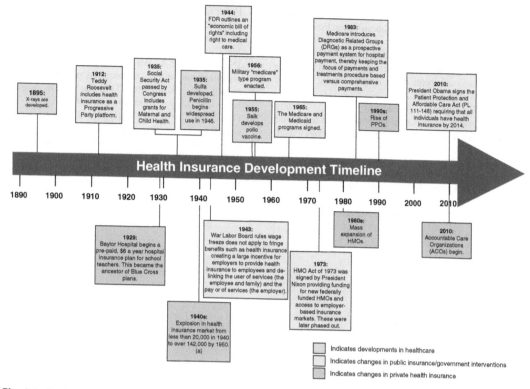

Fig. 4.4 Health insurance development timeline (a: Data from Health Insurance Institute. Book of Health Insurance Data, 1965. New York: Health Insurance Institute; 1966)

References

1. Linton O. Medical applications of X-rays. Beam Line. 1995;25(2):25–34.
2. Cassidy T. Birth: the surprising history of how we are born. New York: Atlantic Monthly Press; 2006.
3. Field MJ, Shapiro HT. Employment and health benefits: a connection at risk [internet]. Washington, DC: Institute of Medicine. 1993. Chapter 2, Origins and evolution of employment-based health benefits. [cited 2012 May 25]. http://www.nap.edu/openbook.php?record_id=2044&page=49.
4. Befort SF, Budd JW. Invisible hand, invisible objectives: bring workplace law and public policy into focus. Palo Alto: Stanford University Press; 2009. p. 83.
5. Rosenberg C. The care of strangers: the rise of America's hospital system. New York: Basic Books; 1987.
6. Barr D. Introduction to U.S. health policy: the organization, financing, and delivery of health care America. Baltimore: The Johns Hopkins University Press; 2007.
7. Pollard C. Blue cross and blue shield: a historical compilation. Consumer Union-Policy & Action from Consumer Reports. Retrieved from consumersunion.org/research/blue-cross-and-blue-shield-a-historical-compilation/, 2007.
8. Hall R, Jones C. The value of life and the rise in health spending. Q J Econ. 2007;122(1):39–72.
9. Kaiser Permanente [Internet]. Oakland (CA): Kaiser Pernamente; c2012. History of Kaiser Permanente; 2012 Jan 1 [cited 2012 Apr 23]; [about 2 screens]. http://xnet.kp.org/newscenter/aboutkp/historyofkp.html.
10. Hoffman C. Focus on health reform: national health insurance – a brief history of reform efforts in the U.S. Menlo Park, CA: Kaiser Family Foundation; 2009. 8 p. Publication no. 7871.
11. Fox PD. An overview of managed care. In: Kongstvedt PR, editor. The managed health care handbook. Gaithersburg: Aspen Publishers; 1996. p. 3–15.
12. Shapiro S. An historical perspective on the roots of managed care. Curr Opin Pediatr. 1996;8(2):159–63.
13. Coombs JG. The rise and fall of HMOs: an American health care revolution. Madison: The University of Wisconsin Press; 2006.
14. Drake DF. Managed care: a product of market dynamics. JAMA. 1997;277(7):560–3.

15. Barton PL. The health services delivery system: managed care. In: Health Administration Press, editor. Managed care essentials: a book of readings. Chicago: Health Administration Press; 2000. p. 25–53.

16. Porter ME, Teisberg EO. Redefining health care: creating value-based competition on results. Boston: Harvard Business School Press; 2006.

17. Lagoe R, Aspling D, Westert G. Current and future developments in managed care in the United States and implications for Europe. Health Res Policy Syst. 2005;3(1):4.

18. Jensen GA, Morrisey MA, Gaffney S, Liston DK. The new dominance of managed care: insurance trends in the, 1990. Health Aff (Millwood). 1997;16(1):125–36.

19. White House Health Care Summit. Bipartisan Meeting on Health Reform. 2010 Feb 25.

20. Fisher ES, Shortell SM. Accountable care organizations: accountable for what, to whom, and how. JAMA. 2010;304(15):1715–16.

21. Van Citters AD, Larson BK, Carluzzo KL, Gbemudu JN, Kreindler SA, Wu FM et al. Four health care organizations' efforts to improve patient care and reduce costs. Washington, DC: The Commonwealth Fund; 2012. 14p. Publication no. 1571 Vol. 1.

22. Fisher ES, Staiger DO, Bynum JP, Gottlieb DJ. Creating accountable care organizations: the extended hospital medical staff. Health Aff (Millwood). 2007; 26(1):w44–57.

23. Shortell SM, Casalino LP. Implementing qualifications criteria and technical assistance for accountable care organizations. JAMA. 2010;303(17): 1747–8.

Understanding Quality and Cost from a Health Policy Perspective

5

Jason D. Keune and Bruce Lee Hall

Learning Objectives

After completing this chapter, the reader should be able to answer the following questions:

- Understanding the cost and quality of health-care proposals is fundamental to the central problem of health policy: the need to make decisions about health-care resource use, given the constraint on health-care resources.
- It is impossible to make a reasoned health policy decision without either knowing both the cost and the quality of a health-care proposal explicitly or else by making implicit judgments about one or both of those quantities.
- Most health policy decisions in the United States heretofore have been based on implicit judgments about cost and quality.
- The most complete economic evaluation of health-care proposals for use in health policy is the cost-benefit analysis, which monetarizes outcomes, allowing both relative and absolute benefit to be characterized. The cost and effort of this type of analysis, however, is not always justified.
- Quality reporting is becoming more prominent in the present era: appropriate use of quality data is essential to appropriate decision making regarding health-care resource use.

J.D. Keune, M.D., M.B.A.
Department of Surgery, Barnes-Jewish Hospital,
St. Louis, MO 63110, USA
e-mail: keunej@wudosis.wustl.edu

B.L. Hall, M.D., Ph.D., M.B.A. (✉)
Washington University in St. Louis—Barnes Jewish
Hospital and BJC Healthcare, St. Louis, MO 63130, USA
e-mail: hallb@wustl.edu

As part of the health care reform law that I signed last year, all insurance plans are required to cover preventive care at no cost. That means free check-ups, free mammograms, immunizations and other basic services. We fought for this because it saves lives and it saves money – for families, for businesses, for government, for everybody. That's because it's a lot cheaper to prevent an illness than to treat one. President Barack-Obama [1]

M.K. Sethi and W.H. Frist (eds.), *An Introduction to Health Policy: A Primer for Physicians and Medical Students*,
DOI 10.1007/978-1-4614-7735-8_5, © Springer Science+Business Media New York 2013

Introduction

Health-care policy makers in the United States face a myriad of challenges in the contemporary era. The recent Patient Protection and Affordable Care Act (PPACA) sought to address three fundamental goals underlying the deficits of the American health-care system: lowering cost, improving quality, and increasing access. Of these, the first two can be thought to represent the central problem of health-care policy today: cost versus quality. How should health-care resources best be used given the constraints on these resources ("cost") to achieve the highest overall utility for the populace ("quality")? The question is one of opportunity cost: the cost and return of one activity measured against what could be achieved with the next best alternative foregone. Understanding the cost and quality of health-care proposals is a necessary step in applying the principle of opportunity cost. Every proposal ever considered would, ideally, be compared to the next best option. In this chapter, we discuss health-care decision making in the setting of limited resources, differences between implicit and explicit knowledge of cost and quality, and the notoriously difficult problem of determining and appropriately using health-care quality data.

In 2008, in the context of presidential candidates' statements on the issue at the time, Cohen and colleagues examined whether or not preventative care saves money [2]. They analyzed 599 cost-effectiveness studies published between 2000 and 2005 that properly discounted future costs and benefits. Of these studies, 279 cost-effectiveness ratios were identified that related to interventions to avert disease or injury ("preventative care"). Cost-effectiveness ratios were reported in terms of dollars per quality-adjusted life-year (QALY). A QALY is a measure of disease burden that takes into account both the quantity and the quality of the life being measured. A QALY of less than 1.0 reflects a year of life that has been either shortened or had its quality lessened by a disease or ailment. A change in QALY is a standardized way of reporting the effect of a health-care proposal. From the ratios in the Cohen article,

only 20 % of proposals were found to be both cost saving and to improve health. The majority of proposals (>75 %) were successful at improving health (increasing QALYs) but were found to actually cost money rather than save money. The remainder of proposals (approximately 3.5 %) were found to both worsen health and increase cost (Fig. 5.1). The assumption that all preventive care improves health while simultaneously saving money is clearly challenged!

Recognizing which proposals save money and which cost money might at first seem a very basic task with regard to health-care policy. Proposals that truly save money (while achieving the same or better health outcome) are obvious choices: they should always be implemented. Likewise, proposals that increase cost and worsen health are also obvious: they should never be implemented. The rub is in deciding among those health-care proposals that, despite costing some resources, still might be acceptable. It is in this middle area that the concept of opportunity cost becomes the fundamental guiding principle, and challenge, underlying a health-care policy decision.

If resources were unlimited, policy makers would choose to implement all proposals that augmented QALYs at any cost. However, most governments face a limit on just how much money can be spent on health care. In the United States, the budget is limited by the realities of the taxation and deficit spending mechanisms. Within the overall federal budget, health-care spending faces competition for resources from other areas, such as defense and education. Therefore, by necessity, policy makers must work within some limit of "cost acceptability." Somehow, this level of acceptability must be derived or established by the society that the policy makers represent. This limit has at least two important aspects: (1) Is the spending level on this one proposal or intervention acceptable to society? (2) Are there any available resources in the total budget? The analogy to any other consumer good should be clear: (1) Is the price of this car acceptable to us? (2) Is there enough money in the budget for this car? In theory, for health care, these two aspects should be tightly linked by a societal willingness to raise taxes to

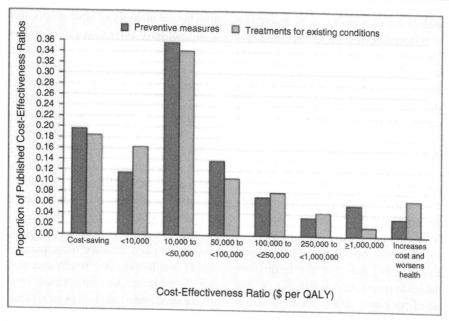

Fig. 5.1 Distribution of cost-effectiveness ratios for preventive measures and treatments for existing conditions. QALY denotes quality-adjusted life-year (Data are from the Tufts-New England Medical Center Cost-Effectiveness Registry. Reprinted with permission of Massachusetts Medical Society from Cohen JT, Neumann PJ, Weinstein MC. Does preventive care save money? Health economics and the presidential candidates. N Engl J Med 2008; 358(7):661–3)

pay for all "acceptable" interventions; in other words, what is "acceptable" is framed partly in terms of willingness to pay taxes at that level. In practice, this link is not always understood, and, in any case, in the setting of loose deficit spending, the emphasis often rests on the price acceptability of the individual item rather than on its fit into the overall budget.

Given, then, some ultimate limitation on resources, the challenge for policy makers is to take those proposals that cost money but improve life and rank them in order of the most valuable as compared to the next best alternative. Once this is done, they can be examined in order to determine which proposals have an "acceptable" cost to society and at what point the cost becomes unacceptable. Finally, among those that are acceptable, starting with the highest-value proposal, they should be implemented until the budget is consumed (leaving some acceptable proposals not implemented) or until all acceptable proposals have been implemented (leaving some residual in the budget). In Cohen's study, the proposals are distributed on a scale of dollars spent per QALY achieved (Fig. 5.1). If one accepts that the QALY does indeed represent a reasonable measure of health and that it can be adequately standardized across studies (one QALY is just as good as any other QALY), then policy makers who are interested in implementing preventive care programs should select first those proposals that are obviously cost saving (far left in Fig. 5.1); then (moving rightward) those in the <$10,000/QALY range; then, when those are exhausted, the ones in the $10,000 to <$50,000/QALY range; and so on. This should continue until one of two things happens: either a threshold is reached where the $/QALY is no longer deemed acceptable based on societal standards or the entire available budget accorded to prevention has been spent. To get a sense for what the $/QALY limit on any particular intervention might be, one might reference the cost that Great Britain's National Institute for Health and Clinical Excellence (NICE) considers acceptable for one QALY: roughly £30,000 (~$39,261 at a rate of $1.31/1£). Alternately, one could consider what the Centers for Medicare and Medicaid Services (CMS) in the USA pays for the lifesaving treatment of dialysis: roughly $130,000 per patient per year (see additional discussion to come in this chapter). This maximum price which policy makers are willing to pay for another increment of health is known as the shadow price, and obviously it can vary!

Though this seems complete, there are several layers of complexity to this decision process. What pressure makes it so necessary for policy makers to be tuned in to the cost and quality of health-care proposals? The answer to this question is one of chilling sobriety. According to an analysis performed by Peter Orszag and colleagues at the beginning of the health-care debates that led to recent ACA legislation [3], the growth rate of per capita cost of medical care is the single most important factor driving the future financial health of the United States. At the time that the study was performed, federal spending on Medicare and Medicaid was approximately 4.6 % of gross domestic product (GDP). The Congressional Budget Office estimated that, if the laws were not changed, the trajectory of spending would increase the proportion of spending on Medicare and Medicaid to 20 % of GDP by 2050, approximately the same absolute amount as the entire federal budget at the time the article was published. The study also asserted that this growth would not be due to the aging of the population nor to any growing disease burden in the population but rather due to the expansion of expenditures on new medical technologies and therapies. Policy makers, then, should be interested in knowing the cost and quality of health-care proposals, not only because of the dominance of health care in the federal budget but also because discerning among choices regarding therapies could address the core issue of rising expenditures. Whether or not the ACA will be successful in "bending the cost curve" remains to be seen.

Cohen and coworkers' summary of the cost-effectiveness of preventive care is unusual. It aggregates the results of hundreds of studies about prevention that use the same basis for measuring cost (dollars) and the same variable for measuring quality (QALYs). Policy makers

studying the majority of other proposals probably would not have such a wealth of published and relevant data available to them. Therefore, at this point, a distinction must be drawn with regard to the modes that data can be incorporated into policy decisions: data can be incorporated either "explicitly" or "implicitly." Explicit data are those which are determined through empirical research. They consist of specific and concrete values representative of measurable aspects of health-care cost and quality. Explicit data are objective values which are published or stated prior to being applied to any particular decision process. Cohen's article reviews explicit data. In contrast, implicit data are those pieces of information which underlie a health-care policy decision when explicit data are not used. Implicit data are assumed under, implied in, or revealed by any particular decision when explicit data are not stated "a priori."

Explicit knowledge of cost and quality data is valuable in the sense that it allows direct comparisons between health-care proposals. Clear statements of explicit criteria lend transparency to a decision process and allow criteria underlying decisions to be individually examined or modified. They also serve to communicate shared values and priorities. Keeping in mind that the fundamental problem of health-care policy making is to assess opportunity costs, there is no better way to make comparisons between one proposal and the next best alternative than to examine explicit cost and quality data. Policy decisions commonly proceed, however, without explicit data. When decisions are made regarding health-care expenditures in the absence of explicit data about cost and quality, then the cost and quality of the proposal are being assumed implicitly. *No reasoned decision is possible without at least implicit assumptions about costs and results.*

Why Are Cost Data Critically and Unavoidably Important in Health Policy?

Imagine a health-care proposal for which policy makers must decide between funding two competing drugs. Assume that the drugs are designed to lower blood pressure. The literature regarding these two drugs is reviewed, and drug A is found to lower blood pressure by 18 mm of mercury while drug B is found to lower blood pressure by 22 mm of mercury. Without review of any cost data, it would seem that drug B is the better one and therefore should be adopted. However, without either explicit knowledge about the costs of the drugs or implicit assumptions about those costs, such a decision would be empty and unfounded. Cost data must be included in the decision: *it is impossible to make any decision that does not involve costs.* The policy maker who states that he/she will not consider cost at all and thus chooses drug B has in reality assumed implicitly that the drug costs are equal!

Suppose now that each drug costs $1 million per month. This information probably obviates consideration of either drug, since neither drug cost would be independently "societally acceptable" (in all likelihood). It would also obviate the need for *serious study* of either drug, the quality of which have already been determined (we know that each drug lowers blood pressure and by what degree). The study of these drugs in itself is costly, and therefore the decision about what studies should be undertaken should itself be scrutinized. Under this cost scenario, we would know that drug B was more effective per dollar (just like when we assumed the costs were equal), but now we know that in reality neither drug is acceptable.

Now suppose that the cost of drug A (the one with worse performance) was only one-fifth the cost of drug B and that the costs of the drugs were generally in the range of other blood pressure lowering drugs on the market. This distribution of costs would put both drugs in need of a reasoned health-care policy decision. Whether the extra expenditure going from drug A to drug B was worthwhile could only be judged if it were known how reductions in blood pressure translated into measures of overall health and how valuable that change in health might be. Now the policy maker is in need of a standardized measure of health outcome or quality, such as the QALY, to make good use of the cost data they do have!

Explicit Values and Implicit Assumptions About Cost and Quality

It should now be clear that a fallacy occurs when policy makers claim that either cost or quality data are not needed for a health-care policy decision. It is impossible to make a reasoned health policy decision without either knowing the cost and the quality of a health-care proposal explicitly or else assuming one or both implicitly. For any health-care decision that does not acknowledge contributing factors in an intentional and explicit fashion, the underlying assumptions about cost and quality can always be inferred. Often, these underlying hidden or implicit values are referred to as the "revealed preferences."

One way of calling attention to explicit (and thus implicit) data is to examine what society considers a human life to be worth—an important reference point when deciding health-care policy. The value of one anonymous, or "statistical," life can be deciphered in different ways. One common approach is to ask how much value individuals place on the ability to change their risk of death. For instance, the Environmental Protection Agency (EPA) uses such a determination in its calculations when deciding what environmental efforts to promote. The EPA readily discloses the value it uses, often to a great deal of commotion in the media if the value should be decreased [4]. The value stated in July 2008 was $6.9 million per life. Keep in mind this is for an entire life, not a single year of life as stated for QALYs. Fundamentally, though, the value could be raised or lowered for either economic or political reasons.

In health care, possibly due to fears of misinterpretation, but also because analyses are not always carried out to determine explicit cost levels, such values are not as commonly publicly reported as they are by the EPA and other agencies. As noted earlier, however, they can always be inferred. In 1972, legislation was passed in the United States to allow patients with stage V chronic kidney disease (CKD) to enroll in Medicare regardless of age, a program that had previously been open only to those 65 years old or older. The primary need of patients

Fig. 5.2 Tail distribution of incremental cost-effectiveness ratios published in this work asymptotically approaches zero probability (Reprinted with permission of Elsevier from Lee CP, Chertow GM, Zenios SA. An empiric estimate of the value of life: updating the renal dialysis cost-effectiveness standard. Value Health 2009, 12(1):80–7)

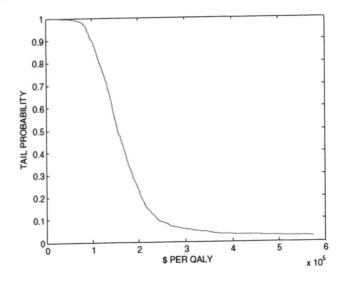

with stage V CKD is routine dialysis, a costly procedure that is lifesaving. Without dialysis, patients with such advanced kidney disease would die. Since the time of its inclusion into federal law, the program has been very stable with no lapses in coverage for patients with advanced renal disease.

Lee and colleagues have interpreted the statistical value of a human life when it comes to health care by examining what the United States government (Medicare) pays for dialysis [5]. These researchers created a model comparing cost, life expectancy, and quality-adjusted life expectancy for those on dialysis to patients undergoing less costly alternatives, including no dialysis. The populations studied were Medicare patients and patients enrolled under the healthcare provider Kaiser Permanente, Northern California. Though the federal government has not opted to publish the statistical value of a human life, there is such a value that is discernable through such methods. In this case, Lee and coworkers determined that the incremental cost-effectiveness ratio of a statistical year of life implied by dialysis practice currently averages $129,090 per QALY (published in 2009). In publishing this data, Lee and colleagues demonstrate that even though no explicit data are available

regarding the acceptable cost of a QALY, such data can certainly be revealed. Cost is part of a health-care policy decision whether explicitly or not.

Interestingly, Lee also attributes significance to the distribution of values that was determined. Figure 5.2 shows that the tail distribution of incremental cost-effectiveness ratios published in this work asymptotically approaches zero probability. This is consistent with a wide range of possible cost-effectiveness values. Lee interprets this in a Rawlsian context, stating that such a distribution is consistent with an interpretation that there is not one single value that can be used as a threshold but rather a continuum of values that reflects resources being allocated to benefit everyone, "including the most vulnerable individuals." In other words, the implication is that we (society) purposefully use a wide distribution of acceptable costs under different circumstances. Such behavior is actually somewhat difficult to rationalize! An alternative interpretation might be that the wide range of values reflects a lack of explicit data usage or intentional reliance on implicit approaches. If true, this would be quite a criticism of contemporary health-care policy, for it would reflect a substantial and undesirable lack of consistency.

Making Decisions Based on Explicit Data

Making decisions based on explicit data has several advantages that, when recognized, can lead to powerful consequences. Some of these have already been raised. *Consistency* across multiple programs can be achieved with explicit data. For example, for proposals involving the evaluation of different vaccination campaigns, an explicit data set with consistent entries regarding cost and quality for each will allow careful comparisons of different campaign strategies. Not only can individual vaccines for the same virus be compared, but comparisons can be made at a certain time point between vaccination plans for different pathogens and longitudinally over time for newly developed vaccines or new pathogens. The consistency that can be achieved is valuable for its efficiency. Components contributing to a decision are clearly identified, consistently valued across evaluations, and can be modified with ease. Since established methods can be used, evaluation of new proposals can be made part of a system rather than inventing a whole new system every time a new proposal arises for consideration.

Efficiency is realized in ways other than through consistency of data. An important benefit of the use of explicit data is that relevant alternatives can be systematically identified and elucidated, often by calling attention to the components contributing to a decision [6]. The use of implicit data in health-care decision making can be haphazard, and the chance that an important alternative is inadvertently excluded from consideration is increased under an implicit approach. The explicit data approach adds an analytic perspective that is difficult to obtain any other way. A decision about health care is richer and more well founded when more component factors are delineated and discussed transparently.

Furthermore, when decisions are made with explicit data and approaches, it enhances the ability to communicate values, improve understanding, and share priorities across society. The difference might be shown in a policy proposition of providing students free school lunches over the summer months. If decisions are made implicitly, policy makers might simply state something like "I think that school lunches served to students over the summer months would be good for them." With explicit data, policy makers could pronounce: "Based on the data analyses we have discussed, if school lunches are made available to students over the summer months, we expect that students will come to school in the fall with significantly higher ability to focus, which will lead to significant measurable increases in reading skill by early November, at a cost of X dollars per student…." The richness afforded to a health-care decision with the addition of explicit considerations is valuable in the sense that it is communicative: policy makers are able to more clearly explain why a particular policy is valuable and what costs and benefits are involved.

Finally, decisions that are made with explicit data might be less prone to error. Duncan Neuhauser and Ann Lewicki's now classic article "National Health Insurance and the Sixth Stool Guaiac" demonstrated just how much more a 6th stool guaiac test would cost, compared to the first in a colon cancer screening program [7]. The American Cancer Society had just come out with an endorsement of the six sequential stool guaiac tests as a reasonable way to screen for cancer. Though the concept of marginal cost per case detected was understood, Neuhauser and Lewicki's explicit conclusions came as a surprise to the health policy community. Sequential tests for screening were generally accepted to have higher marginal cost per case detected as the prevalence of disease went down, and the prevalence of colon cancer in patients who already had five negative stool guaiacs was quite low. Since the rate of detecting colon cancer on the 6th guaiac was 0.0003 cases out of 10,000 persons tested, the researchers claimed that the marginal cost of this 6th stool guaiac was $47 million per case detected; an unacceptable level of cost! Without this explicit data analysis, the magnitude of this cost and the subsequent insight into the problem might not have been appreciated by health-care policy makers. However, a cost analysis such as this always involves figures and calculations that require careful consideration and could themselves be incorrect. A subsequent analysis by Brown and Burrows claimed that the aforementioned analysis had two fundamental errors and that, once corrected, the marginal cost of the sixth test was defensible and acceptable [8]! Thus, while no single analysis is ever immune to error, at least an explicit analysis benefits from transparency; it can be carefully considered, challenged, modified, and tested.

Economic Evaluations of Healthcare Interventions: The Concept of Efficiency

Given that knowing cost and quality in an explicit fashion and in a way that allows comparisons from one treatment modality to another is important, what, then, is the best way to perform such evaluations? There is a wide range of economic evaluations that are available to policy makers. Review of some basics of different strategies for evaluations and discussion of ramifications ensures that options and nomenclature are consistently understood. This section is based largely on the excellent text by Drummond and colleagues [6].

At the very beginning of the spectrum, the most elemental health-care evaluation is probably the toxicity study. In this study, the simple question is whether an intervention can be conducted or administered without causing harm or at what intervention level harmful effects arise. A good example of the toxicity study is testing for side effects of a new drug entity.

The next type of study is the efficacy study, which asks whether an intervention can have the desired results under ideal circumstances. Ideal circumstances means this is often a study conducted under controlled laboratory circumstances, with full compliance (perfect cooperation) on the part of the subjects. If an intervention can have the desired results in the ideal circumstance, it has "efficacy" or is "efficacious."

The next study is the effectiveness study, which builds in real-world limitations such as imperfect compliance with instructions by subjects or other reasons for the circumstances of the study to be less than perfect. Thus, this study often reflects the "real-world" results that should be expected for the intervention, and these results are called the "effectiveness" of the intervention. It should be obvious that an intervention might have "efficacy" but in the real world lack "effectiveness." Effectiveness studies, with real-world imperfections of treatment built in, are usually viewed as a better basis for decision making than efficacy studies, unless it is believed that a result closer to full efficacy could somehow be achieved in the future.

Neither toxicity nor efficacy nor effectiveness studies alone address the critical question of "efficiency." Efficiency is achieved when a particular result is accomplished at the lowest possible cost or, in terms of a health-care policy decision, the highest level of utility (QALYs) is achieved per unit expenditure. Sometimes people refer to the concept of "utility per unit expenditure" as "value." Of course, it is possible that the highest level of utility achievable with any one intervention is still not acceptable in terms of societal thresholds for cost, but then that intervention should not be implemented. For an efficiency analysis to be most useful, there should be a comparison of a new proposal to some existing standard intervention (or "next best alternative"), and there should be descriptions of both the costs and the outcomes of the interventions. When studies meet these criteria, they can be considered "full" economic evaluations.

When an efficiency study compares one proposal to an alternative, describes costs, and describes the resulting outcomes in terms of "natural units" (i.e., millimeters of mercury reduction of blood pressure achieved), the study is called a "cost-effectiveness analysis" or CEA. With a CEA, it can be simple to decide which intervention achieves the more improvement per cost unit, but the results are in terms of "natural units" that are sometimes difficult to make sense of. Furthermore, comparisons across studies are limited. Few studies discuss outcomes that are fortuitously framed in the same natural units, and comparisons, when possible, are typically limited to outcomes only from the single perspective of those natural units. For example, a CEA of two drugs reducing blood pressure can only be compared to another CEA also examining reduced blood pressure. A CEA of two blood pressure interventions cannot be compared to a CEA of two baldness remedies, for the outcomes studied will be in different natural units (millimeters of mercury vs. hair follicles)! A CEA also has difficulty assessing more than one outcome for a subject, since those outcomes are also typically in different units. For instance, a CEA might have difficulty handling one blood pressure drug that reduces pressure but causes headaches versus another drug that reduces pressure but causes impotence!

To circumvent some of the limitations of the CEA, outcomes under study are often translated into a more standardized measure of "utility" to the subject, resulting in a "cost utility analysis" or CUA. The term "utility" in the traditional economic sense means any kind of value. The common measure of utility we have already discussed is the QALY. Using a standardized QALY, interventions with different effects can now be compared, as long as the assignments of utility or QALYs is carefully done. Now a drug that reduces blood pressure can be translated into an improvement of QALYs and a drug that reduces baldness can also be translated into an improvement of QALYs, and now the two can be compared on this standardized outcome. In addition, now even undesired side effects on multiple different axes can be taken into account in the assignment of QALYs, so multiple types of outcomes or effects can be incorporated at once. There are many different methods for assigning utility to a particular outcome or "state." The methods are beyond the scope of this chapter but include approaches such as evaluating willingness to pay, time trade-offs, standard gambles, and risk premiums. The assignment of utility values within a CUA, however, is a critical feature of this evaluation method and must be carefully done or the end results will be questioned.

While a properly performed CUA can tell you which of two interventions results in more utility per unit spending, it still does not tell you if you are spending too much. For this, the end result of the CUA needs to be monetarized in some fashion, meaning it needs to be translated into a currency value that can be further examined. The typical approach to this challenge is to determine the societally acceptable level of spending for the utility gained. When dealing with QALYs, this means determining how much society agrees is worthwhile to spend on achieving one QALY. As mentioned previously, this could be ~$40,000 (according to NICE) or it could be ~$140,000 (according to CMS dialysis spending). The challenge is to derive or generate a value which the stakeholder audience will agree with so that the end result of the analysis will be accepted. The resulting analysis, with a monetarized outcome, is referred to as a "cost-benefit analysis" or CBA. Sometimes a CBA will be put forward using multiple different conversion numbers as a sensitivity analysis, or the results can be put forward as a range of cost that would be spent on the intervention, and the audience can decide for themselves whether the result is acceptable. For instance, an analysis might state: "Reducing the amount of sulfur dioxide in the water will result in improved population health at a cost of $1,100,000 per QALY." The audience is left to make the final judgment of acceptability or not. The beauty of the CBA is that it is ultimately comparable to all other studies or interventions that are translated into the same monetary outcome (i.e., dollars per QALY). Importantly, the CBA can actually help determine that the intervention simply "costs too much" by societal standards (however those are determined). All of the other economic efficiency analyses are limited to telling you which of two outcomes is more efficient, but do not tell you whether the cost per outcome unit achieved meets acceptability standards like the CBA does. In this sense, the CBA can prevent you from making a "bad investment," according to societal standards. The weakness of the CBA is that it ultimately relies on some level of agreement about what constitutes acceptable cost standards, which might be lacking in society or, at a minimum, might be controversial.

Adding back the concept of explicit versus implicit approaches to decision making, it is now possible to state that the most complete economic evaluation of health-care proposals would be the explicit cost-benefit analysis (CBA), which monetizes outcomes, allowing both relative and absolute benefit to be characterized. The explicit approach lends transparency and the ability to revise assumptions and values as indicated. However, all of the approaches described have limitations and cost resources to carry out. Thus, in every decision circumstance, it is important to consider what type of analysis is warranted and how many resources should be expended generating data and insight to support the decision at hand. Explicit cost-benefit analysis is itself costly and therefore need not be used in every instance.

The Use of Explicit Cost and Quality Data in Health-care Policy

The overall quality of health care delivered to Americans, or at least a substantial portion of them, is arguably worse than it should be or could be. And this care likely comes at costs that are too high. Of course, "too high" means different things to different people. To some, it means the USA expends more resources in terms of %GDP than most or all other developed countries without clear resulting benefits. To others, "too high" is not conceived in terms of GDP but rather simply that for some expenditures, there were better, perhaps more efficient, opportunities that were bypassed.

As one examines recent policy decisions regarding health care, it becomes evident that cost and quality data are rarely known explicitly and that health-care decisions are commonly based on implicit assumptions. Whatever failures there are in the US health-care system could be interpreted in part as failures of those implicit assumptions and thus failures to drive more robust decisions with explicit data. There is a variety of reasons why this might be the case. In this section, we will review reasons why health-care decision makers in the United States might not use explicit data regarding cost and quality.

Health care in the United States prior to the health maintenance organization (HMO) era was marked by expansion in a setting where resources were perceived as virtually unconstrained. For additional detail on the history of American health care, the reader is directed to Chap. 1. However, a brief summary of some important points is useful here. After World War II, a period of worldwide growth and optimism saw the establishment of national state-sponsored health-care plans in a number of countries. The predominant payment model in the United States was via an insurance mechanism, and the dominant insurance model was "fee-for-service" (FFS). With FFS, every time a service was rendered, a new fee could be generated, which created inflationary pressure to deliver more and more care (services). In addition, the typical charge structure at the time could be described as "cost plus." Under this paradigm, hospitals and providers would charge insurance companies for the full cost of care delivered for an insured patient, plus some margin. This meant there was virtually no risk in expending resources on a patient, since all claims would be reimbursed at the "cost plus" a margin. This was also inflationary, driving delivery of more and more services. Since reimbursements were at cost plus a margin, hospital balance books remained flush, and expansion was an obvious strategy. Hospitals had incentive to buy new equipment and expand infrastructure. As a result, the expanded hospitals' care would become increasingly expensive but would continue to be reimbursed with a margin, and health-care costs rose in an ascending spiral. Furthermore, since World War II, in the USA, health insurance provided through an employer had favorable, tax-exempt treatment (codified into tax law in 1954). This drove purchases of generous insurance plans and also drove the practice of community rating. These phenomena accelerated penetration of health insurance, feeding back into the inflationary spiral.

This upward pressure on the costs of health care in the United States coincided with another macroeconomic phenomenon. The 1970s saw a period of inflation at the same time as a slow economic growth rate and high levels of unemployment, a situation known as stagflation. Not only did prices rise in response to the inflationary pressures of the FFS and cost-plus structures of the widespread insurance mechanism, but the buying power of money was also decreasing. Since unemployment was high and the growth rate low, more health-care expense fell to the government. Paying for this, however, was not trivial, and as government health-care expenditures began to consume a larger share of the GDP, the pressure was on politicians to raise taxes. Of course, politicians are loathe to raise taxes since this can threaten their electoral support. Thus, there was rise of the concept of cost control but mainly in the form of government pressures on health-care plans to keep costs low. This top-down approach initially had little to do with relationships between cost and quality, and therefore the relationships between cost and quality were not emphasized as relevant to policy makers. At this point, an alternative payment and delivery structure for health care came to prominence: "managed care," as embodied by the health maintenance organization or HMO.

In 1973, the United States Congress passed the HMO Act. The Act provided funding in the form of grants and loans to insurance companies that wanted to expand into the HMO domain, allowed for federal certification of HMOs which freed them of state-level restrictions, and required employers with 25 or more employees to offer a federally certified HMO along with more classic indemnity or service benefit plans. The concept of "managed care" was attractive because it promoted carefully considered and delivered health care as a way to control costs *but also* provide better care. The fundamental concept of "managed care" is to move resources up to the front of the care process and to use these resources to keep people healthy from the start (health maintenance and preventive care) rather than wait passively for a disease to develop and then use resources to react. There was belief that this would not only keep people healthier but also that the approach would save money in the long run. The HMO proposition was for patients who enrolled to be covered for the entirety of their medical care subject to restrictions and guidelines established by the organization and typically with care delivered by a restricted, specified

group of physicians. The patients would choose such a plan to obtain comprehensive care, including preventive care, at reasonable cost. The physicians would agree to such a plan because it could guarantee them a steady and constant stream of patients and could mitigate their business risks. It also enabled providers to advocate the noble aim of promoting health and wellness, as opposed to merely reacting to disease.

Though the system took root and supplanted much FFS insurance in the United States in the 1980s, it was problematic in that it often focused on cost control and at times did not encourage a sufficient focus on quality of care (health maintenance and prevention of disease). In the name of management, HMOs limited patients' access to certain expensive therapies, which was very unpopular in the public eye. The effect was that public trust of HMOs diminished over time. Famously, the treatment of metastatic breast cancer with bone-marrow transplantation, when initially thought to be efficacious, was often denied by HMOs. This served as the font of a myriad of critiques of the managed care business model. Many other similar examples came to public attention.

Despite the original hope that managed care would help heal a broken system, the health-care cost bubble continued to grow. The limitations on care that so characterized the HMO model of the time eventually were regarded by physicians, and in turn by the general public, to be draconian. In response to public pressure, such regulations and guidelines were made less restrictive. For example, in backlash against cost controls, establishing a "Patients' Bills of Rights" became commonplace. The result was that the reigning in of the FFS structure, which was still a dominant mode of payment to physicians under managed care, was not accomplished.

The dominant FFS system deemphasized any need to focus on health-care quality. Under the FFS model, contracted physicians receive payments based on the quantity of services provided, without regard to quality. And, as already noted, the system was also inflationary, since neither the physicians nor patients bear much responsibility for costs: physicians have incentives to provide and patients have incentives to consume health-care services without much regard to quality or effectiveness. In addition, FFS does not encourage coordination of care, as physicians are driven only to provide the care for which they are specialized and are not encouraged to synchronize what they do with other physicians.

There were several efforts to control upwardly spiraling costs from within the framework of managed care involving payment mechanisms such as fee-bundling, global payment structures, capitation, and fixed physician salaries. Under fee-bundling and global payment structures, HMOs contract with physicians to provide a set payment for a specified episode of care. The arrangement is meant to cover all care provided to the patient for that diagnosis or at least for a certain time horizon and thus should create incentives to control costs via efficient care. Similarly, under capitation, HMOs provide a set payment to a provider to cover all of a patient's medical needs for a specified period of time, whether the patient actually requires care or not. Under the fixed salary (or "staff") model, physicians are given a salary for an agreed-upon work commitment, with minimal or no relation to the amount of services that a physician provides within that work commitment.

Though it may be possible that such payment methods would introduce the matter of quality into the thought processes of individual physicians (a physician would now have incentive to treat the patient in the most cost-efficient fashion possible), they have not been overwhelmingly successful. Fee bundles, global payments, and capitation are subject to actuarial limitations and risks that can make providers wary. For example, if a payer rates a patient at a certain level of health and pays the physician for the care of that patient under that assumption, then the physician must assume that the rating is correct or that the company has underestimated the patient's level of health, lest the physician end up providing more care than predicted. Furthermore, under these structures, conflicts of interest become evident because physicians can have incentives to minimize the number of diagnostic tests and treatments rendered, which can be viewed by the public as unacceptable. Physicians who attempt quality control under these conditions are met

with another problem: a lack of comparative data that can be used for medical decision making. As Marcia Angell has pointed out, the Food and Drug Administration approval process does not test drugs "head to head" and approves drugs with only studies that show efficacy with respect to placebo, so comparative effectiveness trials are left to larger society to complete [9].

For these reasons, attempts to place quality control in the hands of individual physicians have been generally unsuccessful. Calls for explicit cost and quality data to support provider decision making have met with inadequate responses. In the current era, it has become recognized that the FFS model does not emphasize quality, which might be detrimental to American health care. The question for US policy makers is just how a move *towards* quality care should be achieved. The recently released 2012 American College of Physicians Ethics Manual states:

> Physicians have a responsibility to practice effective and efficient health care and to use health care resources responsibly. Parsimonious care that utilizes the most efficient means to effectively diagnose a condition and treat a patient respects the need to use resources wisely and to help ensure that resources are equitably available. [10]

The statement continues that it is unreasonable to put decisions about parsimonious care in the hands of individual physicians; rather, such decisions should be made at the policy level by institutions.

Why Are Explicit Data Not Used More Often in the Contemporary Era?

Why would any society accept an implicit and not transparent approach to policy decision making if explicit modes are more satisfying? Most often, the reason that health-care decisions are based on implicit assumptions is that explicit data about cost and quality do not exist. The fundamental reason for this, in turn, is that making data explicit is itself a costly endeavor. Britain's NICE evaluates treatments to determine cost efficiency and approval status within their system. However, NICE does not randomly select treatments to be studied, nor does it study all available treatments, but instead relies on direction from the National Health Service (NHS) as to the most important decisions warranting study. The NHS determines what will be comparatively studied based on the burden of disease, the impact on resources, and the degree of practice variation across Great Britain [11].This is done at an annual budget of £32 million ($55 million) [12]. Endeavors to research comparative effectiveness and cost-effectiveness in the United States are distributed across public and private institutions, and therefore costs are more difficult to assess. However, every institution performing such research has some limited budget, which must be respected. Here, the concept of opportunity cost manifests itself well in the problem of selecting which health-care proposals should be studied explicitly. Decisions are ultimately required to study an intervention, pay for the intervention without study, or deny the intervention without further study. Both of the latter two would be based on implicit underlying assumptions. In this way, the system of cost-effectiveness analyses is itself subject to cost-effectiveness analysis. Yet, the need for study of the costs of such analyses is relatively underemphasized and underappreciated.

Explicit data cannot be produced for every treatment; therefore, a system must be in place to evaluate and choose which analyses should be performed. As Drummond and colleagues point out in their text on the economic evaluation of health-care proposals, resources for performing evaluations, being scarce, should be used efficiently [6]. The authors offer a systematic way of deciding which proposals ought to be studied with the objective of minimizing the need for evaluators to become involved with inappropriate or ineffective evaluations or spending longer than is appropriate on any one evaluation. Central criteria pertinent to the selection of health-care proposals to study should include the criticality of the decision at hand, the total disease and cost burdens involved, and the potential implications of making a decision error on the topic. There is always a need to avoid of errors of omission in which certain proposals that are being studied might be supported in ignorance of other proposals that have not been explicitly compared.

At times, explicit data might not be used in policy decisions because it can be politically risky to do so. The recent Affordable Care Act created a Patient-Centered Outcomes Research Institute (PCORI), the primary charge of which is to examine the "relative health outcomes, clinical effectiveness, and appropriateness" of competing therapies by examining present published data and also performing new studies. The legislation stipulates, however, that results of PCORI's findings cannot be used to develop explicit "dollars per quality-adjusted life-year" assessments in the same way that Britain's NICE does. It also does not have the power to endorse coverage rules, as might be adopted by Medicare or state payers. The reason for this legislated disconnect between data and practice stems from a political argument about rationing that was attributed to the advocates for health-care reform. Opponents of the reform movement were successful at publicizing the concept of "death panels" to criticize the stipulated requirement for doctors to speak to patients about end-of-life care, which was represented as a way to lower costs [13].

Another manifestation of politics discouraging the use of explicit data in health-care decision making is demonstrated in the following example. When President George Bush signed Medicare Part D into law in 2003 as part of the Medicare Modernization Act, around 80 % of Medicare seniors already had some form of prescription coverage. Medicare Part D represented a huge new expenditure (projected to be $400 billion over the 10-year period from 2004 to 2013) that would have to be covered with tax dollars. There was not a clear cost-quality-related justification for the legislation; the new bill encouraged private payers to make prescription plans available to seniors. The number of senior citizens with prescription coverage was similar after the law was enacted, but now senior citizens were not paying for much of their prescription coverage. Rather, the costs had been transferred into the Medicare program. One theory is that the politicians who enacted the law wanted to shift resources towards a block of active voters who would keep them soundly in office: senior citizens. This explanation is consistent with the political economy model of policy making: the idea that political forces affect the choice of economic policies just as often, or more often, than a focus on maximizing the well-being of the entire population. Optimizing the well-being of the entire population is referred to as the "public interest" model, and this concept would be more consistent with the use of explicit data in health-care decision making.

A third reason why explicit data may not be used more commonly in policy is that available data are not always established or appropriately up to date. Medical therapy is constantly changing, with thousands of research articles published per year. The Medline database, maintained by the National Library of Medicine, attempts to catalogue all new publications in the life sciences and biomedical literature. In 2009, Medline added 778,683 new articles to its database [14]! In a very real sense, what is considered to be "quality" or "state of the art" in health care is a moving target.

Furthermore, according to the Donabedian model of health-care quality assessment, quality can be evaluated along the axes of structure, process, or outcome [15]. Thus, quality and its assessment can be viewed quite differently by different parties. For example, the Surgical Care Improvement Project (SCIP) is a quality data collection project led by a national partnership of organizations that focuses on process measures in surgery. At its start in 2006, the project, focusing on surgical site infections and thromboembolic and cardiac events, had a stated goal of reducing these complications by at least 25 %. Different process measures proved easier to meet than others, but most centers reached extremely high compliance for some measures within a relatively short period of time. In one study of Veterans Affairs hospitals and a group of private US hospitals, it was found that compliance was greater than 90 % for most measures [16]. Some measures reached even higher compliance levels; for example, one recommended process measure, hair removal from the surgical site at the time of operation, reached 99 % compliance in one study [17]. As compliance levels rose over time, achievement targets were raised. And yet, while standards for compliance have been escalating, it has not been clear that corresponding improvements in patient outcomes have been realized. Thus, in this constantly shifting environment, notions of quality can be hard to pin down.

Quality Reporting and a Vision for Future Health-care Policy

Health care in the United States has reached a new era with respect to quality reporting. The Institute of Medicine (IOM) published a consensus report in 2001 entitled "Crossing the Quality Chasm: A New Health System for the 21st Century" [18]. The report stated: "The development of a more effective infrastructure to synthesize and organize evidence around priority conditions would also offer new opportunities to enhance quality measurement and reporting." In the current era, data storage and processing abilities have reached a level high enough to support the emergence of reporting initiatives that can synthesize and organize evidence such as the IOM recommends. Questions that those who would report on health-care quality face, though, include just how such large amounts of data should be aggregated, by whom, at what costs, and who should bear those costs?

Peter Pronovost and Richard Lilford [19] have made five recommendations to advance quality measurement. First, validity and transparency should be ensured. The authors suggest three levels on which this should be done. Face validity requires that the thing being measured have relevance and recognition to those being measured. Criterion validity requires that the things being measured have a concrete correlation to things that manifest in the "real world." Convergent validity requires that a measure being used has similar predictive capabilities as other measures that are more highly established. Second, the authors suggest that surveillance be highly standardized. As Susan Dentzer recently pointed out, as we get better at measuring health-care quality, that quality often appears to be worse [20]. Standardization would require quality reporting systems to look no harder at one hospital than at another, to limit biases that could result from differences in intensity of scrutiny. Third, performance data should not be measured at a single time point, but rather change should be demonstrated over time. This is primarily in response to a problem of statistics. It is difficult to make strong, statistically significant statements based on the small sample sizes often available for quality measurement. An emphasis on trends over time can mitigate this problem, though it is not guaranteed to do so. Furthermore, sophisticated statistical methods should be used for such demonstrations of change, and many hospitals lack the technical expertise to perform such analyses themselves. Pronovost and Lilford advocate for systems that involve biostatisticians, academic centers, government agencies, and private vendors to overcome these challenges. Fourth, tools should be built to prioritize measures. As already discussed, determining what should be measured is not a trivial issue and should be subject to a rigorous and formal process. Finally, an independent agency should be created to advance this entire process. This agency should be independent of individual hospitals and should promote development of measures by the private sector, transparency, private sector analyses, reporting that is accessible to the public, auditing, and feedback.

The National Surgical Quality Improvement Program of the American College of Surgeons (ACS-NSQIP) is a reporting system that analyzes outcomes for surgery patients for member hospitals and in many ways satisfies Pronovost and Lilford's recommendations. The system works by collecting a variety of perioperative data and 30 days of postoperative data on a systematic sample of surgical patients from participating hospitals. The ACS-NSQIP aggregates the data, risk adjusts evaluations, and provides reports that compare each hospital to all other member hospitals. The data are risk-adjusted, meaning that the expected risk for each patient is generated from a set of coefficients resulting from multivariate regression analyses of the entire set of patients across all participating hospitals. The reports are updated regularly and are distributed to each hospital demonstrating both how the observed outcomes relate to the expected outcomes for that hospital and how this "O:E ratio" compares to all other participating hospitals. The NSQIP program has been demonstrated to improve surgical quality for participating hospitals. In one study, participating hospitals were evaluated over a 3-year period (2005–2007), and it was concluded that 66 % of hospitals reduced risk-adjusted mortality and 82 % improved risk-adjusted complication rates during this time [21].

One key component of an infrastructure that will support quality reporting is the adoption of improved health information technologies (HIT). The same IOM report that called for an effective measurement and reporting infrastructure pointed out the need for HIT in the form of computerized order entry and electronic health records, especially in order to reduce patient errors. The American Recovery and Reinvestment Act of 2009 included a provision to establish financial incentives for health-care groups who implement HIT in a way that meets "meaningful use" standards as defined by the Secretary of Health and Human Services [22, 23]. The incentive payments made available totaled $27 billion, with $44,000 (via Medicare) or $63,750 (via Medicaid) per provider to accelerate the rate at which HIT is adopted in the USA [24]. The first installment of a three-part set of meaningful use criteria was announced by Kathleen Sebelius in 2010, after a lengthy process in which more than 2000 comments by professionals and the public at large were taken into consideration. The release of the second group of meaningful use criteria is to occur in the summer of 2012.

One group from the University of Minnesota recently reported that the use of computerized physician order entry and electronic health records by physicians was associated with higher quality across a spectrum of quality measures, with significant results found for two pneumonia-related measures. The differences were larger at academic medical centers than they were at non-academic hospitals [25]. The mechanisms by which HIT can improve quality are multiple. Prominent are the ability for medical systems that are digitally integrated to detect potential adverse drug events and interventions to reduce such events, automation of quality data aggregation, provision of decision support logic, and the ability to detect epidemiological issues like infectious disease outbreaks in a timely fashion.

Conclusion

The future of health care in the United States depends largely on the ability of policy makers to control upwardly spiraling costs while simultaneously improving quality. Advances in health-care technology and large-scale quality data aggregation and analysis will allow unprecedented levels of understanding of cost and quality information. The existence of such data alone, however, will not be enough to bend the cost curve. There will always be a need to make value judgments in decision making and policy setting. It is literally impossible to make any decision which does not in some way place values on the costs and consequences of an intervention, whether explicitly or implicitly. Therefore, for important decisions, the link between data and policy making must be made concrete: explicit data should be used in ways that are transparent, publicly acknowledged, and meaningful. Ideally, every proposal or intervention considered should be compared to the next best options to determine the relevant opportunity costs. Only in this way can the maximum benefit for society be achieved with efficiency.

References

1. Remarks by the President on Preventive Care. The White House. Office of the Press Secretary. 10 Feb 2012. http://www.whitehouse.gov/the-press-office/2012/02/10/remarks-president-preventive-care. Accessed 15 Apr 2012.
2. Cohen JT, Neumann PJ, Weinstein MC. Does preventive care save money? Health economics and the presidential candidates. N Engl J Med. 2008;358(7):661–3.
3. Orszag PR, Ellis P. The challenge of rising health care costs–a view from the Congressional Budget Office. N Engl J Med. 2007;357(18):1793–5.
4. "Value On Life 11 Percent Lower Than 5 Years Ago." All Things Considered. Melissa Block (host). National Public Radio; 2008 July 11. http://www.npr.org/templates/story/story.php?storyId=92470116. Accessed 30 June 2012.
5. Lee CP, Chertow GM, Zenios SA. An empiric estimate of the value of life: updating the renal dialysis cost-effectiveness standard. Value Health. 2009;12(1):80–7.
6. Drummond MF, Sculpher MJ, Torrance GW. Methods for the economic evaluation of health care programmes. Oxford: Oxford University Press; 2005.
7. Neuhauser D, Lewicki AM. National health insurance and the sixth stool guaiac. Policy Anal. 1976;2(2):175–96.
8. Brown K, Burrows C. The sixth stool guaiac test: $47 million that never was. J Health Econ. 1990;9(4):429–45.
9. Angell M. The truth about the drug companies: how they deceive us and what to do about it. New York: Random House; 2004.
10. Snyder L, American College of Physicians Ethics, Professionalism, and Human Rights Committee.

American College of Physicians Ethics Manual: sixth edition. Ann Intern Med. 2012;156(1 Pt 2):73–104.
11. "How we work." NHS. National Institute of Clinical and Health Excellence. 2012. http://www.nice.org.uk/aboutnice/howwework/how_we_work.jsp. Accessed 15 May 2012.
12. Steinbrook R. Saying no isn't NICE – the travails of Britain's National Institute for Health and Clinical Excellence. N Engl J Med. 2008; 359(19):1977–81.
13. Daniels N. Review of "just caring: healthcare rationing and democratic deliberation" by Leonard Fleck. Notre Dame Philosophical Reviews; 2010 July 7.
14. Medline Citation Counts by Year of Publication. U.S. National Library of Medicine. National Institutes of Health; 2012. http://www.nlm.nih.gov/bsd/medline_cit_counts_yr_pub.html. Accessed 8 May 2012
15. Donabedian A. The definition of quality and approaches to its assessment, Explorations in quality assessment and monitoring, vol. I. Ann Arbor: Health Administration Press; 1980.
16. Stulberg JJ, Delaney CP, Neuhauser DV, et al. Adherence to surgical care improvement project measures and the association with postoperative infections. JAMA. 2010;303(24):2479–85.
17. Hawn MT, Vick CC, Richman J, et al. Surgical site infection prevention: time to move beyond the surgical care improvement program. Ann Surg. 2011; 254(3):494–9. discussion 499–501.
18. Crossing the Quality Chasm: A New Health System for the 21st Century, the Committee on Quality of Health Care in America and Institute of Medicine. National Academies Press; 2001. ISBN-10: 0309072808, ISBN-13: 978–0309072809.
19. Pronovost PJ, Lilford R. Analysis and commentary: a road map for improving the performance of performance measures. Health Aff (Millwood). 2011;30(4):569–73.
20. Dentzer S. Still crossing the quality chasm–or suspended over it? Health Aff (Millwood). 2011;30(4):554–5.
21. Hall BL, Hamilton BH, Richards K, et al. Does surgical quality improve in the American College of Surgeons National Surgical Quality Improvement Program: an evaluation of all participating hospitals. Ann Surg. 2009;250(3):363–76.
22. Health Information Technology for Economic and Clinical Health (HITECH) Act, Title XIII of Division A and Title IV of Division B of the American Recovery and Reinvestment Act of 2009 (ARRA), Pub. L. No. 111–5, (Feb. 17, 2009).
23. American Recovery and Reinvestment Act of 2009 (ARRA), Pub. L. No. 111–5, (Feb. 17, 2009).
24. Blumenthal D, Tavenner M. The "meaningful use" regulation for electronic health records. N Engl J Med. 2010;363(6):501–4.
25. McCullough JS, Casey M, Moscovice I, Prasad S. The effect of health information technology on quality in U.S. hospitals. Health Aff (Millwood). 2010;29(4):647–54.

Part II

Understanding the Basics II

Prevention and US Health Care

6

Heather A. Smith

Learning Objectives

After completing this chapter, the reader should be able to answer the following questions:
- Be familiar with the concepts of health promotion and disease prevention.
- Understand the parallel but separate evolution of prevention and clinical medicine and its impact on the current state of public health.
- Understand how population health and health policy impact clinical practice.
- Be familiar with the different federal agencies and initiatives aimed to improve both individual and community health.
- Understand concepts behind societal and financial costs and cost-effectiveness of preventive efforts.

Introduction

In the United States, the public health system – a joint effort among federal, state, and private sectors – attempts to accomplish a holistic view of health through incorporation of three components [1, 2]:

- *Community-based essential public health services*: monitoring health indicators, educating the public about health risks and promoting healthy behaviors, and reducing health risks from air, water, food, consumer products, work place, and recreational hazards
- *Clinical preventive services*: immunizations, screening tests, and counseling by physicians and other health professionals
- *Social, economic, and regulatory policies*: promoting healthy behaviors, reducing hazardous exposures, and promoting healthy standards of living including access to medical care

The earliest prevention programs in this country arose in the nineteenth century in the eastern coast port cities with the rapid influx of immigrants and the recognition of potential introduction of epidemic diseases, such as yellow fever and cholera [3, 4]. In the setting of continued endemic conditions of typhoid, typhus, measles, diphtheria, influenza, tuberculosis, and malaria, this initial focus on the use of quarantines

H.A. Smith, M.D., M.P.H (✉)
Department of Obstetrics and Gynecology,
Yale University, New Haven, CT 06520, USA
e-mail: heather.a.smith@yale.edu

M.K. Sethi and W.H. Frist (eds.), *An Introduction to Health Policy: A Primer for Physicians and Medical Students*,
DOI 10.1007/978-1-4614-7735-8_6, © Springer Science+Business Media New York 2013

transitioned to an emphasis on environmental sanitation and disease prevention [3]. The late nineteenth century was then met with significant expansion of social reform movements in both the public and private sectors. Public health departments were created in Massachusetts [5], the U.S. Public Health Service was established [6], and organizations such as the American Public Health Association, the American Red Cross, and the American Tuberculosis Association emerged [7].

The past century has seen public health and prevention measures evolve from a distinct field into being incorporated into routine health and considerations of well-being. Initially, prevention – both community-based and individual preventive services – was considered the sole responsibility of governmental public health agencies [7, 8]. This concept was reinforced by the design of the health system based on identification and treatment of disease. The separation of public health services from clinical medical practice was accentuated during the mid-twentieth century with the introduction of private health insurance, which as the major financier of personal health care did not initially offer preventive services as covered benefits in their plans. The impact of this lack of insurance coverage was then further compounded by the traditional focus of the medical school curriculum on diagnosis and treatment rather than prevention, with minimal incorporation of public health education [9].

Health care today is now moving in the direction of strengthening the public health system and incorporating prevention theory into the general medical care. The practice of prevention has been greatly advanced by the development of academic centers that train both clinical practitioners and scientific researchers in prevention, developing a scientific base for public health practice [7]. Also, both private and public health plans now provide coverage for some preventive services for individuals and have implemented policies to encourage the utilization of such services by both physicians and patients [10, 11]. And, finally, we have seen the greater cooperation among governmental public health agencies and the other public and private organizations in providing population-based and community health services [8, 12, 13].

Preventable Deaths in the USA

Health promotion and disease prevention services are essential for maintaining and improving health on both individual and population levels. An important focus for such preventive measures is on risk factors which have been found to be responsible for premature or preventable deaths. These risk factors fall into three main groups – lifestyle risk factors, dietary risk factors, and metabolic risk factors – and have been shown to be able to be modified through a range of public health and health system interventions [14]. This has further led to the concept of "amenable mortality," referring to deaths from certain causes that should not occur in the presence of timely and effective health care [15].

Previous research has indicated that modifiable risk factors are responsible for a large number of premature deaths in the United States [14, 16]. In 2010, there were an estimated 502 preventable deaths per week [15]. Smoking, high blood pressure, and being overweight are the leading preventable risk factors for premature mortality [17]. Being overweight or obese shortens life expectancy, and half of all long-term tobacco users will die prematurely from a smoking-related condition; in fact, tobacco, smoking, and hypertension alone account for about 1 in 5 deaths in US adults. Other behaviors, such as alcohol use, have mixed benefits and risk [15, 17]. While alcohol use prevented 26,000 deaths from ischemic heart disease, ischemic stroke, and diabetes, researchers estimate that it caused 90,000 deaths from other types of cardiovascular diseases, other medical conditions, and road traffic accidents and violence [17].

Public health and health system interventions have been introduced to address these issues, and the rate of preventable deaths – including cancer, heart disease, and diabetes – has begun to decline [15]. Yet, despite these efforts and the significantly higher per capita amount that the US spends on health care, these rates are declining slower than compared to other industrialized nations [15]. Futhermore, disparities in preventable death rates are exacerbated among racial and ethnic minority populations. Many minorities are more likely to be diagnosed with late-stage breast and colorectal cancers, are disproportionately affected by diabetes and heart disease, and are more likely to die from HIV [18].

Clinical Recommendations

With the goal of reducing and even eliminating such amenable morbidity and mortality, preventive care measures have been introduced into medical management and even daily routines. Examples of such efforts can range from daily healthy activities to medical examinations to screening tests and include hand washing, breastfeeding, cholesterol screening, and immunizations. Preventive recommendations, many of which are aimed towards particular populations, are based on scientific review of empirical evidence showing benefit of such services that outweigh risks [19]. To best discuss the guidance process for screening and preventive actions, one must better understand the different levels of the preventive intervention classification system: universal, selective, and indicated prevention [20, 21]:

- *Universal* – involves whole populations (or) entire populations (nation, local community, school, district) and aims to prevent or delay the onset of undesired outcomes, such as cavities, drug abuse, or tobacco use. This is accomplished through the provision of information and skills to all individuals regardless of exposure or risk factors.
- *Selective* – involves groups whose risk of being negatively impacted or developing a disease is above average, such as having a family history of cardiac disease or multiple sexual partners. Individual members who possess specific risk factors or exposures are then screened for disease presence.
- *Indicated prevention* – involves a screening process and aims to identify individuals who exhibit early signs of disease or behavior

problems, such as substance abuse or need for increasing doses of medication. Individuals with worsening status or behavioral problems are targeted.

In the United States, recommendations for such medical screening and preventive measures are created by multiple public and private agencies. Both medical specialty organizations, such as the American Cancer Society or American Congress of Obstetricians and Gynecologists, and federal agencies provide guidance on appropriate selective and indicated prevention services. The U.S. Preventive Services Task Force (USPSTF), created in 1984, is an independent group of national experts in prevention and evidence-based medicine [22]. The USPSTF develops recommendations utilizing a "grading" system that was introduced in 2007 that accounts for the strength and impact of evidence and provides both a "suggestion for practice" and a level of certainty regarding net benefit [19, 23] (Table 6.1).

As of 2012, the USPSTF has provided guidance on a large number of services among adults, adolescent, and children, currently offering strong recommendations for more than 40 such preventive and screening measures [19]. Just as there are screening tests, vaccines, and services that are recommended for their health benefits, there are those that are recommended against due to the increased risks. The USPSTF in fact has identified 29 preventive services for which the side effects or physical harm from invasive screening or follow-up processes are considered to outweigh the benefits [24]. There are a number of other services that have not had sufficient evidence showing either definite benefit or risk and therefore specifically have not had official recommendations made by the USPSTF.

Recommendations: Challenges and Controversy

In 2009, the USPSTF made updates to their recommendations for breast cancer screening based on evaluation of multiple studies and research findings. The USPSTF aimed to assess the efficacy of reducing mortality from breast cancer by

Table 6.1 What the grades mean and suggestions for practice

Grade	Definition	Suggestions for practice
A	The USPSTF recommends the service. There is high certainty that the net benefit is substantial	Offer or provide this service
B	The USPSTF recommends the service. There is high certainty that the net benefit is moderate or there is moderate certainty that the net benefit is moderate to substantial	Offer or provide this service
C	Note: The following statement is undergoing revision. Clinicians may provide this service to selected patients depending on individual circumstances. However, for most individuals without signs or symptoms there is likely to be only a small benefit from this service	Offer or provide this service only if other considerations support the offering or providing the service in an individual patient
D	The USPSTF recommends against the service. There is moderate or high certainty that the service has no net benefit or that the harms outweigh the benefits	Discourage the use of this service
Statement	The USPSTF concludes that the current evidence is insufficient to assess the balance of benefits and harms of the service. Evidence is lacking, of poor quality, or conflicting, and the balance of benefits and harms cannot be determined	Read the clinical considerations section of USPSTF Recommendation Statement. If the service is offered, patients should understand the uncertainty about the balance of benefits and harms

Source: US Preventive Services Task Force. The guide to clinical preventive services. Rockville, MD 2009

screening with film mammography, clinical breast examination, breast self-examination, digital mammography, and magnetic resonance imaging. The commissioned group completed a targeted systematic review of the evidence on the benefits and harms of screening as well as a decision analysis that used population modeling techniques to compare the expected health outcomes and resource requirements [25, 26].

Following this new assessment, the USPSTF introduced significant changes, at times contradicting the current practice and the recommendations of other medical organizations, including a recommendation against routine screening mammography for women ages 40–49 years who are not at increased risk for breast cancer. Additionally, the USPSTF also recommended a switch from annual to biennial screening mammography in women ages 50–74 years, as well as recommended against self-breast exams. Based on their concern of negative impact of screening itself, that from overdiagnosis as well as that of false-positives, these changes were made with the intent of reducing by half the potential harms of screening [25–27].

Utilization of Preventive Services

Despite their proven effect to decrease both morbidity and mortality [28], preventive services are not utilized by many people as recommended, even when they may have health insurance. In fact, Americans in general use preventive services at about half the recommended rate [28, 29]. It has been shown that design of health insurance plans can impact the utilization rates of such screening and preventive services [10, 11, 30, 31] with decreased likelihood of use with increasing levels of cost-sharing [32, 33]. People with health insurance are more likely than those without to obtain preventive services in a timely manner [34–36], with insured people being four times more likely to have their blood pressure checked regularly than people who are uninsured [37]. This lack of appropriate and recommended care can have significant health consequences, which is seen when those without insurance are much less likely to be screened for different types of cancer and, as a result, are more likely to have their cancer diagnosed in later stages [38].

Even though there has been a recognized positive impact on health from appropriate screening, neither private insurance nor Medicare benefits reflect the full complement of USPSTF recommendations [24]. With the implementation of the provisions included in the 2010 Patient Protection and Affordable Care Act (PPACA), health plans will be required to provide preventive services as guided by the USPSTF, CDC, and HRSA recommendations, without cost-sharing obligations [39].

Prevention, Spending, and Cost-Effectiveness

Preventive measures in health care have been discussed as a means of avoiding disease or providing early detection for improvement in health with a concurrent minimization of health care expenditures [28]. Inherently, it initially makes sense that, if a disease can be detected early or prevented altogether, the cost of treating it can be reduced or eliminated and overall health care spending should decrease. Yet, this has not been borne out, and debate about potential savings and value of clinical preventive services has become more polarized. Some preventive services can reduce health care costs, but many do not, and others may actually increase health care costs over a lifetime [40–42]. In a review of the cost-effectiveness of selected clinical preventive services, the evidence does not support the idea that global prevention reduces medical spending [43], and the vast majority of other clinical preventive services do not save money [40]. In fact, overall costs to the health care system typically go up when disease-preventing strategies are put into practice [44].

Despite potential overall increased costs, some experts have suggested that clinical preventive services are still worthwhile when they provide good value, defined as substantial health benefit per dollar spent net of any savings [45–47]. Applying this concept, many preventive services are cost-effective, even when they do not reduce lifetime total cost [48, 49]. The National Commission on Prevention Priorities reviewed recommended preventive services known to improve health and found that 16 of them

increased costs while only five services decreased cost [41]. Only a limited number of services have since been shown to decrease costs *and* enhance life-years saved: childhood immunization series, smoking cessation advice and assistance, discussion of daily aspirin use to prevent cardiovascular disease, and breast and colorectal cancer screening [43, 44]. Today, research continues to evaluate not only the value of disease prevention and health promotion efforts but also the most effective manner of dissemination and adoption of recommendations. It has been shown that combining targeted campaigns to increase access to preventive services with more comprehensive community programs may yield even greater cost savings [41].

Federal Agencies and Initiatives

Within the federal government, there are a number of agencies and bodies dedicated to recommending and implementing clinical prevention policies and programs. These range from federal departments and appointed committees to Presidential designees. A number of these agencies and bodies are housed under the umbrella of U.S. Department of Health and Human Services (HHS) comprising the U.S. Public Health Service, the largest public health program in the world. These agencies – including the Centers for Disease Control and Prevention (CDC) and the Agency for Healthcare Research and Quality (AHRQ), as well as the U.S. Preventive Services Task Force (USPSTF) and the Office of Disease Prevention and Health Promotion (ODPHP) – are dedicated to serving public health, disease prevention, and health promotion efforts.

The Centers for Disease Control and Prevention

The Centers for Disease Control and Prevention (CDC), the United States' national public health institute, serves under the auspices of HHS working to protect public health and safety through its research, national programs, and partnerships with state health departments and other organizations [50]. While the focus of the CDC's activities are on developing and applying disease prevention and control – especially to infectious diseases, foodborne pathogens, and microbial infections – other programs include injury prevention, occupational safety and health, environmental health, and health education [51].

The CDC was initially established in 1946 stemming from the wartime agency Malaria Control in War Areas under the moniker the Communicable Disease Center [52, 53]. Since then, the agency has been renamed and has grown and evolved into the nation's health promotion, prevention, and preparedness agency. Today, the CDC is globally recognized for its research, disease surveillance and monitoring, prevention guidelines, and preparedness work [51, 54, 55]. The CDC works closely with states and other partners in these aims and has distinguished itself with its commitment to improving health on a daily basis as well as in times of emergency [50, 51].

The Prevention Research Centers – a network of academic, community, and public health partners – were established by the CDC to further this mission, promoting applied public health research and more broadly disseminating findings and recommendations [56]. Supporting its mission and promoting continued, meaningful research, the CDC houses a number of national, publicly-available databases, including the *CDC Data and Statistics* [57] and the *Behavioral Risk Factor Surveillance System* (BRFS) [58], and publishes well-respected, peer-reviewed reports in their *Emerging Infectious Diseases* [59] and *Morbidity and Mortality Weekly Report* (MMWR) [60].

The U.S. Preventive Services Task Force

The U.S. Preventive Services Task Force (USPSTF) is an independent advisory panel of experts in prevention and primary care in the United States. The agency conducts systematic, evidence-based assessments of the effectiveness of a broad range of clinical preventive services, including screening, counseling, and preventive medications [22]. Today, the USPSTF, while remaining politically independent, is housed at the Agency for Healthcare Research and Quality (AHRQ), through which it is provided administrative, research, technical, and communication support [61].

The USPSTF is an independent group of national experts – a panel of currently 16 volunteer members – who are mostly practicing clinicians in the fields of preventive medicine and primary care [22]. The formation of the USPSTF was authorized by Congress in 1984, with the stated purpose to "develop recommendations for primary care clinicians on the appropriate content of periodic health examinations" [62].

Following a 1990 reconstitution, the USPSTF were charged with their now current mission to evaluating the effectiveness of clinical preventive services that were not previously examined, to reevaluate those for which there is new scientific evidence or new technologies, and to publish their findings [62]. It is important to note that the USPSTF is an independent body, and, while supported by federal agencies and funds, its work does not require AHRQ or HHS approval.

For the past 20 years, these evaluations have been submitted to the USPSTF for consideration by medical organizations, specialty societies, government agencies, and other groups concerned with the delivery of clinical preventive services [22]. Additionally, the USPSTF collaborates with other federal agencies, including the Task Force on Community Preventive Services and the CDC's Advisory Committee on Immunization Practices. The importance of the role of the USPSTF in promoting prevention was acknowledged through the legislated increased financial and administrative support by AHRQ in the 1998 Public Health Service Act and again in 2010 through the Patient Protection and Affordable Care Act [22, 61].

The Office of the Surgeon General and the Public Health Service Commissioned Corps

Initially established in the nineteenth century as the Supervising Surgeon to the Marine Hospital System, the role of the Surgeon General has evolved into the leading spokesperson on issues in public health and serves as America's Doctor [63]. Appointed by the President, the Surgeon General serves 4-year terms and reports to the U.S. Assistant Secretary for Health (ASH) in the Office of the Secretary, U.S. Department of Health and Human Services (HHS). The Surgeon General is charged to protect and advance the health of nation. Among many activities, the Surgeon General accomplishes this through administering the Public Health Service Commissioned Corps, chairing the National Prevention Council, and providing advice to the President and Secretary of HHS on public health and health system issues. An informal albeit more well-known duty of the Surgeon General includes the education of the American public about health issues and advocating for healthy lifestyle choices [64], including the campaign for increased awareness of family history and warnings on tobacco packages [63, 65].

The Office of the Surgeon General, under the direction of the Surgeon General, oversees the operations of the Commissioned Corps of the U.S. Public Health Service (PHSCC) [66]. Established more than 200 years ago [4], the PHSCC is one of the seven uniformed services of the USA and holds the mission to protect, promote, and advance the health of the country [6, 66]. The 6,500 members of the Commissioned Corps are health professionals who are trained in medical fields including disease control, emergency response, and biomedical research. In the event of a public health emergency, either natural or man-made, the Corps members are available 24 hours per day and can be dispatched as needed by the Secretary of HHS or the ASH. Recent examples of such deployment include the anthrax attacks in 2001 [67], Hurricane Katrina in 2005 [68], and the earthquake in Haiti in 2010 [4].

Office of Disease Prevention and Health Promotion

The Office of Disease Prevention and Health Promotion (ODPHP) [69], initially created in 1976, plays a vital role in developing and coordinating a wide range of national disease prevention and health promotion activities. Housed within HSS, the ODPHP manages many of the federal prevention initiatives, providing the at-large American population with recommendations for leading healthier lives and preventing disease.

Specifically, ODPHP provides information on dietary recommendations and physical activity, as well as serves as a depot of resources for more information and contacts. The *Dietary Guidelines for Americans,* jointly published every 5 years with the U.S. Department of Agriculture, provides evidence-based nutrition information and advice for people age two and older and serves as the basis for federal food and nutrition education programs [70]. The ODPHP is also dedicated to improving health care through improving health communication and health literacy [71], facilitating access to appropriate recommendations and correct information [72, 73], and educating providers and researchers [74, 75].

Federal Initiatives

National Prevention Strategy

The National Prevention and Health Promotion Strategy is a comprehensive plan that aims to increase the number of Americans who are healthy at every stage of life [76]. As legislated in the 2010 Patient Protection and Affordable Care Act, this National Prevention Strategy was released by the National Prevention, Health Promotion, and Public Health Council in June 2011 and serves as a roadmap outlining actions that public and private partners can take to improve the nation's health [77]. The four strategic directions include building healthy and safe community environments, expanding quality preventive services in both clinical and community settings, empowering people to make healthy choices, and eliminating health disparities [76].

Healthy People 2020

Healthy People, the well-known federal initiative with the most recent iteration of *Healthy People 2020,* is managed by ODPHP under the umbrella of HHS [78]. For three decades, *Healthy People* has established benchmarks to guide national health promotion and disease prevention efforts. *Healthy People* aims to identify nationwide health improvement priorities and address them through increasing public awareness and understanding of the determinants of health, disease, and disability, as well as identifying opportunities for progress. By providing measurable objectives and goals at the national, state, and local levels, this initiative is geared towards improving the health of all people in the United States. Currently, *Healthy People 2020* contains about 1,200 science-based objectives in 42 topic areas, including access to health services, public health infrastructure, cancer, diabetes, and sexually transmitted infections [79].

State Agencies

While significant actions and funds are dedicated to disease prevention and health promotion at the federal level, much work continues to be performed at the state and local levels [80, 81]. Each state has designed and manages its health agency differently. Some state health departments are top-level administrative agencies, while in other states, they are a division or bureau of another office. Most share the common purpose to promote public health through policy initiatives, research, and service programs. Often, a state's public health administration is combined with the provision of social services.

Health departments are usually responsible for public health issues, including preventive medicine, epidemiology, vaccinations, environmental health (sometimes including health inspections), and the licensing of health care professionals. They can also serve as a warehouse for data, including the collection and archiving of vital records such as birth and death certificates, sometimes marriage and divorce certificates, and health statistics. Furthermore, the state agencies act as stewards for public safety, recording occupational safety and health data, releasing notifications on notifiable diseases, and publishing health warnings [80, 81].

The Field of Preventive Medicine

Officially established in 1954, the field of preventive medicine is a unique medical specialty that focuses on health promotion and disease prevention not only for individual patients but also for communities and defined populations. Its goal is to protect, promote, and maintain health and well-being and to prevent disease, disability, and death. Recognized by the American Board of Medical Specialties, Preventive Medicine encompasses multiple population-based and clinical approaches to health care. Specialists in Preventive Medicine are uniquely trained in both clinical medicine and public health, and they work in a variety of settings. Preventive Medicine has three specialty areas with common core knowledge, skills, and competencies that emphasize different populations, environments, or practice settings: aerospace medicine, occupational medicine, and public health and general preventive medicine [82, 83].

Conclusion

The concept of prevention alongside health promotion in the USA has evolved significantly from the time of the Marine Hospital System, giving rise to the public health infrastructure as we know it today. Different federal and state initiatives are incorporated into collaborative efforts across the private and public sectors. With the inclusion of prevention by the traditional medical care system, there has been a surge in an integrated concept of health and well-being at both the individual and community level. Additionally, we will likely see a continued evolution of the standards for screening and prevention recommendations, with an increased emphasis on value and quality-of-life years gained rather than the sole idea of costs. As we continue to move forward with the aim of a healthier nation in the setting of persistent disparities and a globalized economy, public health – and thus the government and policy makers – will play a significant role in addressing health and illness outside of clinic and hospital walls.

References

1. Omenn GS. Prevention policy: perspectives on the critical interaction between research and policy. Prev Med. 1994;23(5):612–7.
2. Scott HD, Shapiro HB. Universal insurance for American health care. A proposal of the American college of physicians. Ann Intern Med. 1992;117(6):511–9.
3. Fee E. The origins and development of public health in the United States. In: Detels R, Holland W, McEwen J, Omenn GS, editors. Oxford textbook of public health. 3rd ed. New York/Toronto: Oxford University Press; 1991.
4. U.S. Public Health Service Corps. History. http://www.usphs.gov/aboutus/history.aspx
5. Shattuck L. Report of the commission of Massachusetts 1850. Cambridge, MA: Harvard University Press; 1850.
6. Mullen F. Pagues and politics: the story of the U.S. public health service. New York: Basic Books; 1989.
7. Gordon RL, Baker EL, Roper WL, Omenn GS. Preventing and the reforming U.S. health care system: changing roles and responsibilities for public health. Annu Rev Public Health. 1996;17(1):489–509.
8. Health Care Reform and Public Health: A paper on population-based core functions: the core functions project, U.S. Public Health Service, 1993. J Public Health Policy. 1998;19(4):394–419.
9. Fani Marvasti F, Stafford RS. From Sick Care to Health Care — Reengineering Prevention into the U.S. System. New England J Med. 2012;367(10):889–91.
10. Faulkner LA, Schauffler HH. The effect of health insurance coverage on the appropriate use of recommended clinical preventive services. Am J Prev Med. 1997;13(6):453–8.
11. Freeman JD, Kadiyala S, Bell JF, Martin DP. The causal effect of health insurance on utilization and outcomes in adults: a systematic review of US studies. Med care. 2008;46(10):1023–32.
12. Pickett G. The future of health departments: the governmental presence. Annu Rev Public Health. 1980; 1:297–321.
13. Baker EL, Melton RJ, Stange PV, et al. Health reform and the health of the public. Forging community health partnerships. JAMA. 1994;272(16):1276–82.
14. McGinnis JM, Foege WH. Actual causes of death in the United States. JAMA. 1993;270(18):2207–12.
15. Nolte E, McKee CM. Measuring the health of nations: updating an earlier analysis. Health Aff (Millwood). 2008;27(1):58–71.
16. Mokdad AH, Marks JS, Stroup DF, Gerberding JL. Actual causes of death in the United States, 2000. JAMA. 2004;291(10):1238–45.

17. Danaei G, Ding EL, Mozaffarian D, et al. The preventable causes of death in the United States: comparative risk assessment of dietary, lifestyle, and metabolic risk factors. PLoS Med. 2009; 6(4):e1000058.
18. Agency for Healthcare Research and Quality (AHRQ). National healthcare disparities report. Rockville: U.S. Department of Health and Human Services; 2011.
19. U.S. Preventive Services Task Force (USPSTF). The guide to clinical preventive services. Rockville: Agency for Healthcare Research and Quality; 2012.
20. Gordon R. An operational classification of disease prevention. Rockville: U.S. Department of Health and Human Services; 1987.
21. Kumpfer KL, Baxley GB. Drug abuse prevention: what works? Rockville: National Institute on Drug Abuse; 1997.
22. U.S. Preventive Services Task Force (USPSTF). http://www.uspreventiveservicestaskforce.org/. Accessed 20 July 2012.
23. U.S. Preventive Services Task Force (USPSTF). Grade definitions after May 2007. http://www.uspreventiveservicestaskforce.org/uspstf/gradespost.htm. Accessed 21 July 2012.
24. Salinsky E. Clinical preventive services: when is the juice worth the squeeze? Issue Brief George Wash Univ Natl Health Policy Forum 2005 Aug 24; (806):1–30.
25. Screening for breast cancer: U.S. Preventive services task force recommendation statement. Ann Intern Med. 2009 Nov 17;151(10):716–6, W-236.
26. Summaries for patients. Screening for breast cancer: U.S. Preventive services task force recommendations. Ann Intern Med. 2009;151(10):I44.
27. Nelson HD, Tyne K, Naik A, Bougatsos C, Chan BK, Humphrey L. Screening for breast cancer: an update for the U.S. Preventive services task force. Ann Intern Med. 2009;151(10):727–37. W237-742.
28. Jhu E, Nowakowski J. Benchmarking preventive care utilization. Millman healthcare reform briefing paper. 2011.
29. McGlynn EA, Asch SM, Adams J, et al. The quality of health care delivered to adults in the United States. N Engl J Med. 2003;348(26):2635–45.
30. Newhouse JP, Manning WG, Morris CN, et al. Some interim results from a controlled trial of cost sharing in health insurance. N Engl J Med. 1981;305(25):1501–7.
31. Solanki G, Schauffler HH. Cost-sharing and the utilization of clinical preventive services. Am J Prev Med. 1999;17(2):127–33.
32. Freeman JD, Kadiyala S, Bell JF, Martin DP. The causal effect of health insurance on utilization and outcomes in adults a systematic review of US studies. Med care. 2008;46(10):1023–32.
33. Collins SR, Doty MM, Robertson R, Garber T. Help on the horizon: how the recession has left millions of workers without health insurance, and how health reform will bring relief. Issue Brief (Commonwealth Fund). 2011 Mar.

34. Institute of Medicine. Coverage matters: insurance and health care. Washington, DC: Institute of Medicine; 2001.

35. Powell-Griner E, Bolen J, Bland S. Health care coverage and use of preventive services among the near elderly in the United States. Am J Public Health. 1999;89(6):882–6.

36. Sudano Jr JJ, Baker DW. Intermittent lack of health insurance coverage and use of preventive services. Am J Public Health. 2003;93(1):130–7.

37. DeVoe JE, Fryer GE, Phillips R, Green L. Receipt of preventive care among adults: insurance status and usual source of care. Am J Public Health. 2003; 93(5):786–91.

38. Ward E, Halpern M, Schrag N, et al. Association of insurance with cancer care utilization and outcomes. CA Cancer J Clin. 2008;58(1):9–31.

39. Coverage of Certain Preventive Services Under the Affordable Care Act; Notice of proposed rulemaking, 25 Federal Register 78 (6 February 2013), pp. 8456–8476. http://webapps.dol.gov/FederalRegister/Pdf Display.aspx?DocId=26648. Accessed 14 Jun 2013.

40. Cohen JT, Neumann PJ, Weinstein MC. Does preventive care save money? Health economics and the presidential candidates. N Engl J Med. 2008;358(7):661–3.

41. Maciosek MV, Coffield AB, Edwards NM, Flottemesch TJ, Goodman MJ, Solberg LI. Priorities among effective clinical preventive services: results of a systematic review and analysis. Am J Prev Med. 2006;31(1):52–61.

42. Neumann PJ, Cohen JT. Cost savings and cost-effectiveness of clinical preventive care. The synthesis project. Research synthesis report. Tufts University School of Medicine, Boston, MA, 2009 Sep (18).

43. Russell LB. Prevention's potential for slowing the growth of medical spending. Washington, DC: National Coalition on Health Care; 2007.

44. Maciosek MV, Coffield AB, Flottemesch TJ, Edwards NM, Solberg LI. Greater use of preventive services in U.S. health care could save lives at little or no cost. Health Aff (Millwood). 2010;29(9):1656–60.

45. Frieden TR, Mostashari F. Health care as if health mattered. JAMA. 2008;299(8):950–2.

46. Russell LB. The role of prevention in health reform. N Engl J Med. 1993;329(5):352–4.

47. Woolf SH. The power of prevention and what it requires. JAMA. 2008;299(20):2437–9.

48. Goetzel RZ. Do prevention or treatment services save money? The wrong debate. Health Aff (Millwood). 2009;28(1):37–41.

49. Woolf SH. A closer look at the economic argument for disease prevention. JAMA. 2009;301(5):536–8.

50. Centers for Disease Control and Prevention (CDC). CDC works for you 24/7. http://www.cdc.gov/24-7/. Accessed 14 Jun 2013.

51. Centers for Disease Control and Prevention (CDC). CDC: the nation's prevention agency. Morb Mortal Wkly Rep. 1992;41(44):833.

52. Division of Parasitic Diseases. Malaria control in war areas (MCWA) (1942–1945). Atlanta: Centers for Disease Control and Prevention; 2004.

53. Parascandola J. From MCWA to CDC–origins of the centers for disease control and prevention. Public Health Rep. 1996;111(6):549–51.

54. Centers for Disease Control and Prevention (CDC). The CDC prevention guidelines database. http://won der.cdc.gov/wonder/prevguid/prevguid.html. Accessed 18 Oct 2012.

55. Centers for Disease Control and Prevention (CDC). Disease surveillance and monitoring. http://www.cdc. gov/24-7/CDCFastFacts/surveillance.html. Accessed 18 Oct 2012.

56. Centers for Disease Control and Prevention (CDC). Prevention research centers. http://www.cdc.gov/prc/. Accessed 18 Oct 2012.

57. Centers for Disease Control and Prevention (CDC). CDC data and statistics. http://www.cdc.gov/scien tific.htm. Accessed 18 Oct 2012.

58. Centers for Disease Control and Prevention (CDC). Behavioral risk factor surveillance system. http:// www.cdc.gov/BRFSS/. Accessed 18 Oct 2012.

59. Centers for Disease Control and Prevention (CDC). Emerging infectious diseases. http://wwwnc.cdc.gov/ eid/pages/about.htm. Accessed 18 Oct 2012.

60. Centers for Disease Control and Prevention (CDC). Morbidity and mortality weekly report – MMWR. http://www.cdc.gov/mmwr/. Accessed 19 Oct 2012.

61. Agency for Healthcare Research and Quality (AHRQ). Prevention and chronic care program. http://www.ahrq.gov/clinic/prevenix.htm. Accessed 29 July 2012.

62. Office of Disease Prevention and Health Promotion. U.S. Preventive Services Task Force. http://odphp. osophs.dhhs.gov/pubs/guidecps/uspstf.htm. Accessed 20 Aug 2012.

63. The Office of the Surgeon General. http://www.sur geongeneral.gov/index.html. Accessed 22 Aug 2012.

64. The Office of the Surgeon General. Duties of the surgeon general. http://www.surgeongeneral.gov/about/ duties/index.html. Accessed 22 Aug 2012.

65. The Office of the Surgeon General. The surgeon general's initiatives. http://www.surgeongeneral.gov/ini tiatives/index.html. Accessed 22 Aug 2012.

66. U.S. Public Health Service Commissioned Corps: America's Health Responders. http://www.usphs.gov/.

67. Satcher D. Surgeon general's column. Commissioned Corps Bulletin. 2001; Vol XV, No 12. http://ccmis. usphs.gov/ccbulletin/PDF_docs/dec01ccb.pdf Accessed 14 Jun 2013.

68. Galson SK. USPHS commissioned corps: a global emergency preparedness and response asset. Public Health Rep. 2009;124(5):622–3.

69. Office of Disease Prevention and Health Promotion. http://odphp.osophs.dhhs.gov/reports.asp. Accessed 10 Aug 2012.

70. Office of Disease Prevention and Health Promotion. Dietary guidelines for Americans. http://health.gov/dietaryguidelines/. Accessed 19 Oct 2012.

71. Office of Disease Prevention and Health Promotion. Health communication, health literacy, and e-Health. http://health.gov/communication/Default.asp. Accessed 18 Oct 2012.

72. Office of Disease Prevention and Health Promotion. Healthfinder.gov: quick guide to healthy living. http://www.healthfinder.gov/. Accessed 18 Oct 2012.

73. Office of Disease Prevention and Health Promotion. 2008 physical activity guidelines for Americans. http://health.gov/paguidelines/. Accessed 18 Oct 2012.

74. Office of Disease Prevention and Health Promotion. Healthy people: health communication and health IT topic area. http://health.gov/communication/healthy people/. Accessed 18 Oct 2012.

75. Office of Disease Prevention and Health Promotion. National health information center. http://www.health.gov/nhic/. Accessed 18 Oct 2012.

76. National Prevention, Health Promotion and Public Health Council. National prevention strategy. http://www.surgeongeneral.gov/initiatives/prevention/strategy/. Accessed 14 Jun 2013.

77. National Prevention, Health Promotion and Public Health Council. http://www.surgeongeneral.gov/initiatives/prevention/about/index.html. Accessed 14 Jun 2013.

78. Office of Disease Prevention and Health Promotion. What is healthy people? http://www.healthypeople.gov/about/whatis.htm. Accessed 18 Oct 2012.

79. Topics & Objectives Index - Healthy People. http://www.healthypeople.gov/2020/topicsobjectives2020/default.aspx. Accessed 18 Oct 2012.

80. State Health & Human Services Agencies. http://www.hhs.gov/recovery/statewebsites.html. Accessed 14 Jun 2013.

81. Association of State and Territorial Health Officials (ASTHO). http://www.statepublichealth.org/. Accessed 19 Oct 2012.

82. American Board of Preventive Medicine. What is preventive medicine. http://www.abprevmed.org/aboutus.cfm. Accessed 15 Aug 2012.

83. American Academy of Preventive Medicine (ACPM). Who we are… Leaders in science, practice, and policy of preventive medicine. Washington, DC.

The Rise of Comparative Effectiveness Research

Michael Hochman and Danny McCormick

Learning Objectives

After completing this chapter, the reader should be able to answer the following questions:

- Understand how the concept of comparative effectiveness research arose.
- Understand the definition of comparative effectiveness research.
- Understand the comparative effectiveness research priority areas identified by the Institute of Medicine.
- Understand the newly established Patient-Centered Outcomes Research Institute, which was created with the passage of the Patient Protection and Affordable Care Act.
- Understand the challenges for ensuring that comparative effectiveness research leads to improvements in the US health care system.

Introduction

In 2007, a critical study was published in the field of cardiology. The Clinical Outcomes Utilizing Revascularization and Aggressive Drug

Note: Several paragraphs of this chapter have been adapted with consent of the publisher from Hochman M, McCormick D. Comparative Effectiveness Research. In Kronenfeld J, Parmet W, Zezza M (eds): Debates on U.S. Health Care. Thousand Oaks, CA: SAGE Publications, Inc; 2012

M. Hochman, M.D. (✉)
AltaMed Health Services, 2040 Camfield Ave,
Los Angeles, CA 90040, USA
e-mail: meh1979@gmail.com

D. McCormick, M.D., M.P.H
Chief of Social and Community Medicine,
Cambridge Health Alliance, Harvard University
Medical School, Boston, MA, USA
e-mail: danny_mccormick@hms.harvard.edu

Evaluation trial – or COURAGE as it is more commonly known – compared the use of medications versus the immediate use of a surgical procedure called percutaneous coronary intervention (PCI) to open blocked arteries in patients with stable coronary blockages [1]. To the surprise of many, the trial found that immediate PCI was no better than medications in preventing heart attacks or death. While there was a small improvement in quality of life among patients assigned to the PCI group early in the follow-up period, the difference had disappeared after 3 years. Since COURAGE was a large and well-designed trial, most experts concluded following its publication that patients with stable coronary artery disease should receive a trial of medications before considering treatment with PCI.

COURAGE was notable not only because it provided important insight about a common and important clinical question, but it also demonstrated the value of so-called comparative effectiveness research (CER). In contrast to placebo-controlled studies, CER aims to help doctors use existing health care treatments and services more effectively by comparing different treatments, tests, and diagnostic strategies against each other.

Though the rationale for CER may seem intuitive, CER studies such as COURAGE are relatively uncommon, particularly in the USA, because a large portion of clinical research is commercially funded and intended to evaluate new products in an effort to secure approval from the Food and Drug Administration (FDA) to bring them to market rather than to help doctors use existing services more effectively.

The publication of COURAGE heralded calls for more CER from advocates for this type of research. Many of these advocates argued that CER not only had the potential to improve health outcomes by improving medical knowledge, but also that it might lead to more efficient care and perhaps would even lower health care costs. For example, CER might demonstrate that some expensive treatments or services are no better than less expensive alternatives, and thus might lead to a reduction in wasteful health care spending.

Before the CER movement could gain too much momentum, however, the COURAGE investigators announced some disturbing news. Based on an analysis of data from a large national cardiovascular disease registry, it appeared that COURAGE had not led to a meaningful change in clinical practice patterns – that is, the study results did not change how doctors treated patients with stable blockages in their arteries [2]. Prior to the publication of COURAGE, 43.5 % of US patients with stable coronary artery disease received a trial of optimal medical therapy before undergoing revascularization. After COURAGE, the number increased only very slightly to 44.7 %. What was going on?

Multiple factors likely explain COURAGE's lackluster impact. One potential reason is that doctors do not always stay up-to-date with the medical literature and may not be aware of new findings (or the current treatment guidelines).

Another possibility is that some doctors and patients may simply not have believed the findings. That revascularization would not improve outcomes in patients with blocked coronary arteries likely struck many as counterintuitive. Yet another possibility is that financial incentives caused some doctors, either consciously or subconsciously, to dismiss COURAGE's findings. Since cardiologists typically get reimbursed at higher rates for performing procedures such as PCI than they do for evaluation and management services such as providing optimal medical therapy, many would have had a strong financial incentive to provide immediate PCI for their patients despite the lack of clear benefit.

Overall, the story of COURAGE illustrates both the possibilities and challenges of conducting and funding comparative effectiveness research. In this chapter, we will describe these possibilities and challenges in more detail. In addition, we will explore how the evidence-based medicine movement evolved into a movement for comparative effectiveness research. Finally, we will discuss the newly created Patient-Centered Outcomes Research Institute (PCORI), which has been charged with building an improved CER infrastructure in the USA.

Definition of Comparative Effectiveness Research

Many physicians and health care professionals commonly assume that CER refers to studies that directly compare two or more active therapies. While many such studies would qualify as CER, the term actually refers to a much broader concept of research.

The Institute of Medicine (IOM) – a well-known, independent nonprofit organization that Congress frequently looks to for advice about medical topics – recently defined CER as: "The generation and synthesis of evidence that compares the benefits and harms of alternative methods to prevent, diagnose, treat, and monitor a clinical condition or to improve the delivery of care. The purpose of CER is to assist consumers, clinicians, purchasers, and policy makers to make informed decisions that will improve health care at both the individual and population levels" [3].

The IOM definition conveys that CER encompasses more than just head-to-head comparative studies of two (or more) treatments. For example, CER may involve comparisons of alternative diagnostic tests or strategies. It also may involve evaluations of different models of care delivery, payment strategies, or public health programs. In fact, CER does not necessarily even refer to studies that compare alternative health services. For example, many experts might classify a placebo-controlled trial designed to evaluate a widely used but yet untested medical treatment as CER. Although such a trial does not compare alternative services, the goal of such a study aligns with the CER mission of providing evidence about the use of an existing health care service (rather than a novel service).

Because CER refers to a concept rather than to a specific type of study, no single definition can clearly delineate what is CER and what is not [4]. In some cases, experts may even disagree. Perhaps a good way to think about CER is not as a specific type of study, but rather as any research aimed at helping health care workers, patients, third-party payers, and other stakeholders make more informed decisions about the use of existing clinical services of any kind. In contrast, non-CER studies may refer to research aimed at winning FDA approval or acceptance for new products or services, often with a commercial goal in mind. Later in this chapter, we will also provide more examples to help clarify the concept.

CER in the Context of the Evidence-Based Medicine Movement

While physicians have long tried to apply scientific principles to the practice of medicine, the concept that medical decision-making should largely be driven by the results of research – rather than expert opinion – has become widespread only in recent decades. In 1972, the respected Scottish epidemiologist Archie

Cochrane – for whom the Cochrane Collaboration is named – published a seminal book titled *Effectiveness and Efficiency: Random Reflections on Health Services* [5], which emphasized the critical importance of evaluating medical services before they become widely used. The book also underscored the need for so-called randomized trials – in which study subjects are randomly assigned to receive different treatments – for assessing the value of health care services. According to Cochrane, random assignment of patients increases the validity of a study's results by reducing the likelihood that unknown factors unrelated to the treatment under study are responsible for the findings (more on this to follow). The term "evidence-based medicine" was later coined in 1990 by Gordon Guyatt, a Canadian professor of Clinical Epidemiology and Biostatistics, and described in a famous paper published in the *Journal of the American Medical Association* [6].

During the 1990s and early 2000s, the concept of evidence-based medicine became increasingly popular. Medical training programs began teaching students and resident physicians to look to the literature for answers to questions, and professional organizations began producing evidence-based guidelines and evidence summaries to assist doctors in their decision-making. Additionally, the randomized trial became the clear gold standard by which the quality of evidence was measured, a belief that was greatly strengthened in 2002 with the publication of the Women's Health Initiative [7], a well-designed randomized trial that demonstrated significant harms from the use of postmenopausal hormone therapy. Results from the WHI contradicted previous data, based on non-randomized studies, suggesting that hormone therapy protected women from cardiovascular disease.

Just as the evidence-based medicine movement began to gain steam, however, some experts began questioning whether the existing research infrastructure was optimal for generating clinical evidence. Chief among these critiques, some of which we will delve into later in the chapter, are that:

- Randomized trials often do not adequately represent all types of patients. For example, a trial showing the benefits of a health education program among a highly educated group of patients may not be applicable to patients of lower socioeconomic status who might not have the reading skills to optimally benefit from the program. In addition, groups such as women, minorities, children, and the elderly have been disproportionately excluded from randomized trials, raising questions about whether services that work among white males also work in these other groups [8].

- As exemplified by the story of the COURAGE trial [2], medical providers often do not effectively implement new medical research findings. One widely cited study suggests that Americans receive only about half of the health care services that they should receive when they visit the doctor [9]. Another suggests that there is a lag of almost 20 years between the time that knowledge is generated through research and the time it is widely incorporated into clinical practice [10].
- Very little research has evaluated the cost/value of health care services [11].
- Few well-designed studies have evaluated public health interventions (e.g., school-based tobacco prevention programs) or health care delivery changes (e.g., the effects of different payment models on clinician practice), both of which could potentially improve health.
- Because clinical research receives considerable funding from commercial entities, it has disproportionately focused on evaluating novel commercial products so that these products might be considered for regulatory approval. Studies examining services such as lifestyle intervention programs and commonly performed procedures have received less attention [12].

The recognition of these shortcomings caused some to call for a shift in how clinical research should be conceived, generated, and applied. By the mid 2000s, these ideas gained increasing momentum and converged into a concept which many began calling CER. CER, these experts believed, was the next stage in the evidence-based medicine movement.

Clinical Research Funding

The funding structure for clinical research in the USA helps to explain some of the shortcomings of existing clinical research.

Much of the clinical research conducted in the USA is supported by commercial entities such as pharmaceutical companies and device makers. Many experts have raised concerns that commercially funded research may be biased in favor of products or services produced by the sponsors. Indeed, it is well documented that commercially funded research is considerably more likely than non-commercially funded research to generate favorable results [13], at least in part through the way such studies are designed [14].

Another less-appreciated concern with commercially funded research is its scope. Commercial entities – which have a fiduciary responsibility to generate profits – fund research primarily for the purpose of winning regulatory (FDA) approval for new products or to expand indications for existing products. One might expect that commercial entities would want to compare their new products against those of their competitors to show their products' superiority. But often it does not happen this way. Instead, commercially funded studies disproportionately compare new products against placebos [12]. Upon closer examination, this strategy makes commercial sense: in order to win approval for new products, companies frequently only need to prove that their products are better than nothing (a placebo) – which is often easier than showing that new products are better than existing products that have already been shown to be effective. Once the new products are approved, the companies can use marketing to gain market share, even if no one knows whether a new product is better or worse than existing products already in use.

In addition, commercial entities do not have incentives to fund studies aimed at helping health care practitioners use existing services more effectively. Why, for example, would a company fund a study evaluating a care coordination program or a public health program that does not involve the use of a commercial product? Why would a company fund a study to determine the optimal use of a treatment strategy among patients from an underrepresented minority group? Why would a company fund a study to evaluate a new diagnostic test in a "real-world" setting if the test has already won regulatory approval based on research conducted in a more favorable experimental setting?

Because most commercially funded research focuses on the development and approval of new products, the responsibility for funding CER most often falls to noncommercial entities (non-profits and governmental agencies). Because noncommercial research funding is limited, so is the amount of CER produced in the USA.

Comparative Effectiveness Research Priorities

To provide additional clarity about CER, in 2009 the IOM issued a report identifying some CER priority areas [3]. Because the IOM is well regarded by many policy makers and Congress, this report has generated considerable interest, and it has been a key reference for organizations that fund medical research. Table 7.1 lists examples of priority topics identified by the IOM report. The examples demonstrate the wide array of topics that the IOM considers to be part of CER, including studies that evaluate the effectiveness of diagnostic tests, those that test health system changes such as care coordination programs, and those that compare surgical vs. non-surgical treatments. The list also includes public health interventions as well as research aimed at determining which groups of patients are most likely to benefit from health care services, e.g., which medications are most effective in elderly patients or those with a particular genetic makeup.

As noted previously, while most CER involves a comparison of multiple tests or treatments, this is not always necessary. For example, the IOM listed the evaluation of a procedure called upper endoscopy in which a camera is inserted into the esophagus of patients with heartburn as a CER priority topic even though the comparison group for such an evaluation would likely include

Table 7.1 Examples of CER priority topics from the Institute of Medicine

Topics
"Compare the effectiveness of treatment strategies for [managing a common heart arrhythmia known as atrial fibrillation] …"
"Compare the effectiveness of primary prevention methods, such as exercise and balance training, versus clinical treatments in preventing falls in older adults …"
"Compare the effectiveness of [a procedure known as upper endoscopy in which a camera is inserted into the esophagus] for [evaluating] patients with [heartburn or reflux] …"
"Compare the effectiveness of different strategies of introducing [expensive new medications known as biologics] into the treatment algorithm for inflammatory diseases …"
"Compare the effectiveness of various strategies … to prevent obesity, hypertension, diabetes, and heart disease in at-risk populations such as the urban poor and American Indians …"
"Compare the effectiveness of management strategies for [early stage] prostate cancer …"
"Compare the effectiveness of comprehensive care coordination programs … in managing children and adults with severe chronic disease, especially in populations with known health disparities …"
"Compare the effectiveness of dissemination and translation techniques to facilitate the use of CER by patients, clinicians, payers, and others …"

Source: Data from Ref. [3]

patients not receiving any intervention. The IOM presumably classified this study as CER even though it does not involve the comparison of multiple different health care services because endoscopy is an existing and widely used service, and additional research is needed to clarify the appropriate use of endoscopy.

While the definition of CER has only been clearly articulated in recent years, numerous studies that would clearly be classified as CER have been previously conducted. Here are a few commonly cited examples:

- The seminal studies demonstrating that lumpectomy is as effective as total mastectomy in many women with breast cancer [15]
- Studies comparing different dieting strategies [16]
- The Antihypertensive and Lipid-Lowering Treatment to Prevent Heart Attack Trial

(ALLHAT) [17], which compared several commonly used blood pressure medications against each other

Comparative Effectiveness Research Initiatives

Congress has responded to the recent interest in CER by passing laws that create and fund two important federal initiatives to support this type of research in the years ahead: the American Recovery and Reinvestment Act and the Patient Protection and Affordable Care Act (PPACA). The purpose of these initiatives is to support CER since the existing systems for supporting such research appear to be insufficient.

The Recovery Act, which was signed into law in February 2009, provided $1.1 billion in funding for CER, $400 million of which was allocated to the US Department of Health and Human Services (a federal agency that oversees many publicly sponsored health and social programs), $400 million of which was allocated to the National Institutes of Health (a federal agency that sponsors medical research) [18], and $300 million of which was allocated to the Agency for Healthcare Research and Quality (a federal agency charged with promoting quality, safety, efficiency, and effectiveness of healthcare). These funds were used to support a variety of CER studies by researchers from around the USA (including academic institutions, nonprofit organizations, and for-profit companies). Most of these studies are ongoing.

The Recovery Act provided only a one-time infusion of CER funds, however. Congress made a longer term commitment to CER in 2010 when it passed the PPACA. The new law established the Patient-Centered Outcomes Research Institute (PCORI), an independent nonprofit organization similar to the National Academy of Sciences that will ultimately receive more than $500 million annually to support CER [19]. The PCORI – which has a Board of Governors chaired by Eugene Washington, the Dean of UCLA Medical School, as well as a Methodology Committee – will assume a prominent role in sponsoring

Table 7.2 Draft priorities for CER from PCORI

"Assessment of Prevention, Diagnosis, and Treatment Options. The research goal is to determine which option(s) work best for distinct populations with specific health problems"

"Improving Healthcare Systems. Focuses on ways to improve healthcare services, such as the coordination of care for patients with multiple chronic conditions"

"Communication and Dissemination. Looks at ways to provide information to patients so that they, in turn, can make informed healthcare decisions with clinicians"

"Addressing Disparities. Assures that research addresses the healthcare needs of all patient populations. This is needed as treatments may not work equally well for everyone"

"Accelerating Patient-Centered and Methodological Research. Includes patients and caregivers in the design of research that is quick, safe, and efficient"

Source: Data from Ref. [35]

clinical research in the USA. It will also work closely with the other main public agencies that fund clinical research in the USA, the National Institutes of Health and the Agency for Healthcare Research and Quality, to ensure a unified strategy for promoting clinic research in the USA. Since being formed, the PCORI has developed draft guidelines describing priorities for CER (Table 7.2). These guidelines are less specific but consistent with those from the IOM. The PCORI issued its first round of pilot grants to US clinical researchers in 2012.

Because of the new funding opportunities resulting from the Recovery Act and the ACA, there will likely be a considerable increase in investment in CER in the coming years.

Real-World Research

As noted previously, the early phases of the evidence-based medicine movement underscored the importance of randomized trials for evaluating health care services. In contrast to other types of research studies, patients in randomized trials are randomly assigned to different interventions. This random allocation reduces the chance that so-called confounding factors, i.e. factors other than the intervention under study, could be responsible for the results. These factors can potentially invalidate the findings of non-randomized studies. For example, a non-randomized study might show that patients who take a particular medication do better than those who do not, but it is difficult to ascertain whether the better outcomes are the result of that medication or whether they are due to another factor, for example, the fact that patients who opt to take the medication happen to be healthier than those who do not. In contrast, in a randomized trial, patients would be randomly assigned to either the medication or control group and would likely be very similar to each other. As a result, any difference in outcomes between the two groups would likely be attributable to the medication under study rather than another factor.

In recent years, however, some experts have criticized randomized trials because they must be conducted under experimental conditions that are often not representative of real-world situations. To address these concerns, the concept of "pragmatic trials" has emerged. In pragmatic trials, patients are randomized to alternative intervention arms; however, considerable efforts are made to ensure that the study is conducted in a way that is representative of a real-world setting. Specifically, pragmatic trials should involve interventions that are feasible in a broad range of settings, should involve a diverse patient population recruited from a wide array of practice settings, and should evaluate multiple health outcomes [20].

In addition, there has been a reexamination of the merits of non-randomized studies. Though non-randomized studies are potentially less reliable than randomized trials, some have argued that findings from non-randomized studies may be more relevant in some situations because these studies can be conducted under non-experimental conditions. In addition, researchers have developed advanced statistical methods, known as "multivariate analysis," to reduce the risk of confounding factors influencing study results. Key examples of these advanced methods are propensity scores and instrumental variables [21], the details of which are beyond the scope of this chapter. While concerns persist about the ability of even these newer techniques to properly control for confounding factors [22], some evidence suggests that observational study results are valid most of the time [23].

Thus far, the PCORI leadership has been very supportive of alternative research strategies aimed at addressing clinical questions in "real-world" situations [24], as well as evidence syntheses that aim to combine the results of randomized and non-randomized research to address clinical questions that are challenging to study [25]. Indeed, it may be the overall study quality that is most important rather than specific methodology that is used.

Research Dissemination and Implementation

As the story of COURAGE illustrates, research findings are not always disseminated and implemented in regular clinical practice. Other prominent examples of CER that have not yet been widely adopted in routine clinical practice include:

- Following publication of the ALLHAT trial – which showed that inexpensive thiazide diuretics are at least as effective as newer, more expensive drugs as first-line therapy for hypertension [17] – there was little change in the use of thiazides by US physicians [26].
- Many patients with another heart condition known as heart failure do not receive the appropriate medications.
- A substantial number of hospitals do not follow protocols that have been proven to reduce the risk of hospital-acquired infections.

The discordance between what the research shows and how clinicians practice raises important questions about the value of CER. If patients and health care providers do not follow the results, how can CER improve the health care system?

As noted in Table 7.1, the PCORI has listed research aimed at identifying better ways for disseminating and translating research findings into the clinical decision-making process a top priority of CER. There has also been growing interest in the use of clinical practice guidelines, which aim to summarize and synthesize research findings into easy-to-use recommendations that can aid in clinical decision-making. Quality organizations such as the National Center for

Quality Assurance are also developing tools to assess the extent to which evidence-based practices are followed. The hope is that this monitoring will facilitate quality improvement efforts that will lead to improved uptake of new findings.

Some experts also believe that the USA should look to other countries to get ideas for addressing concerns about research dissemination and implementation. In 1999, the United Kingdom established the National Institute for Clinical Excellence (now called the National Institute for Health and Clinical Excellence, or NICE), a governmental body charged with promoting the use of the best available evidence in clinical decision-making. With the aid of "independent committees of health professionals, academics, and industry and lay representatives" who are guided by data on clinical efficacy and cost as well as social values, NICE develops guidelines to aid clinicians in their decision-making, determines which services will be covered by the British National Health Service, and promotes implementation of "high-value medical innovations" [27]. Though the process is still being refined, early evidence suggests that NICE's efforts are leading to improvements in the quality and efficiency of the British health care system [28].

CER and Political Controversy

Despite the intuitive appeal of CER, the CER movement has also provoked political controversy. Some of these critiques have centered on concerns about the dissemination and implementation of CER findings. If clinicians and patients ignore the findings, some have argued, perhaps we should not invest in CER at all [29]. In addition, some have pointed out that although CER might provide useful information to aid in clinical decision-making, the resources for producing CER are more urgently needed in other areas (for example, by directly paying for health care services or for non-health care needs such as education).

Other concerns run deeper, however. Specifically, critics largely from the political right have charged that unfavorable CER results might provide "ammunition" for third-party payers to deny coverage for costly services or interfere with regulatory approval for new treatments and technologies. In addition, these critics fear that health care providers might avoid the use of costly services based on the results of cost-effectiveness data obtained from CER. The net effect, they argue, could be limits on access to new services for patients [30].

While these political critiques did not succeed in blocking the federal initiatives to expand CER funding, they did result in two notable changes. First, to emphasize the potential for CER to improve care for patients, political advocates began referring to CER as patient-centered outcomes research, and the organization charged with promoting CER in the USA was named the Patient-Centered Outcomes Research Institute. Second, and more importantly, the PPACA banned the PCORI from promoting any cost-effectiveness research.

Cost Effectiveness Research

CER may be used not only to determine which health care services are best for individual patients, but may also provide information about the relative costs of different health care strategies. Such information can guide policy makers and developers of medical practice guidelines in determining which services have the highest value.

As an example, imagine that strategy A is as effective as strategy B, but strategy A is less expensive. This information might allow physicians who are developing a treatment guideline to recommend strategy A over strategy B in guidelines. Similarly, policy makers at an insurance organization might decide to cover strategy A but not strategy B as first-line therapy. (Hopefully, however, strategy B would also be covered in patients who did not have an adequate response to treatment A, or in subgroups of patients in whom strategy B was known to be more effective.)

Cost-effectiveness data may also be helpful in circumstances in which a health care service is marginally effective but extremely expensive. As an example, a new treatment for advanced prostate cancer was recently found to extend life by an average of 4 months; however, the new treatment costs $93,000 [31]. A panel of medical experts might use such information to recommend that insurance organizations and Medicare not cover this treatment simply because the small benefit is not worth the cost.

As noted earlier in the ACA, Congress decided to ban the PCORI from funding research that uses a common method of cost analysis in which a monetary threshold is used to determine whether health care services are cost-effective – known as quality-adjusted life years (QALYs). While the language is ambiguous, many have interpreted it as meaning that the PCORI cannot fund any research involving cost analyses at all. In addition, the legislation states that the findings from CER "may not be construed as mandates, guidelines, or recommendations for payment, coverage, or treatment or used to deny coverage" [32].

Many advocates for CER have expressed vigorous objections to the above limitations. They argue that preventing the PCORI from promoting cost-effectiveness research could greatly limit the impact of CER for channeling resources to the highest value services [33, 34], particularly at a time when health care costs are spiraling at potentially unsustainable rates [35].

The Challenges Ahead

The new initiatives contained in the Recovery Act and PPACA represent important opportunities to improve the infrastructure for clinical research in the USA. The creation of the PCORI in particular provides a mechanism for ongoing support for CER in the years ahead. There remain important challenges for CER, however.

First, the PCORI will need to strike a balance of supporting research that is applicable in real-world settings but at the same time is valid. This will likely require a balance between traditional randomized trials, pragmatic trials, non-randomized studies, and evidence syntheses. It is likely that different study designs and methods will be optimal in different situations. Additionally, the PCORI will need to promote research in groups such as women, minorities, children, and the elderly that

historically have not been well represented in medical research.

Second, more effective mechanisms will need to be developed to disseminate and promote implementation of CER findings in a clear, useable, and timely format. In addition, clinicians will need tools such as easy-to-follow guidelines to better enable them to provide evidence-based services. Currently, both the theoretical underpinnings and the infrastructure for effective wide-scale dissemination and implementation of what works in medicine are only in their infancy.

Third, the PPACA states that CER findings "may not be construed as mandates, guidelines, or recommendations for payment, coverage, or treatment or used to deny coverage," a requirement that, if followed literally, could place substantial restraints on the ability of CER to change clinical practice.

Fourth, despite the limitations on the ability of PCORI to support CER involving costs, researchers and policy makers will need to find creative ways to use CER findings to channel resources to the highest value services. Even without the aid of explicit cost analyses, CER findings could provide key data for policy makers and other groups that need to make difficult decisions during times of resource shortages. Such decisions, however, should be made with input from the public in a transparent, equitable, and thoughtful manner.

References

1. Boden WE, O'Rourke RA, Teo KK, Hartigan PM, Maron DJ, Kostuk WJ, et al. Optimal medical therapy with or without PCI for stable coronary disease. N Engl J Med. 2007;356(15):1503–16.
2. Borden WB, Redberg RF, Mushlin AI, Dai D, Kaltenbach LA, Spertus JA. Patterns and intensity of medical therapy in patients undergoing percutaneous coronary intervention. JAMA. 2011;305:1882–9.
3. Institute of Medicine. Initial national priorities for comparative effectiveness research. Washington, DC: The National Academies Press; 2009.
4. Luce BR, Drummond M, Jönsson B, Neumann PJ, Schwartz JS, Siebert U, Sullivan SD. EBM, HTA, and CER: clearing the confusion. Milbank Q. 2010;88(2):256–76.

5. Cochrane AL. Effectiveness and efficiency: random reflections on health services. London: Hodder Arnold Publishers; 1999.

6. Evidence-Based Medicine Working Group. Evidence-based medicine. A new approach to teaching the practice of medicine. JAMA. 1992;268(17):2420–5.

7. Rossouw JE, Anderson GL, Prentice RL, LaCroix AZ, Kooperberg C, Stefanick ML, Jackson RD, Beresford SA, Howard BV, Johnson KC, Kotchen JM, Ockene J, Writing Group for the Women's Health Initiative Investigators. Risks and benefits of estrogen plus progestin in healthy postmenopausal women: principal results from the women's health initiative randomized controlled trial. JAMA. 2002;288(3):321–33.

8. Beech BM, Goodman M. Race & research: perspectives on minority participation in health studies. Washington, DC: American Public Health Association; 2004.

9. McGlynn EA, Asch SM, Adams J, Keesey J, Hicks J, DeCristofaro A, Kerr EA. The quality of health care delivered to adults in the United States. N Engl J Med. 2003;348(26):2635–45.

10. Contopoulos-Ioannidis DG, Alexiou GA, Gouvias TC, Ioannidis JP. Medicine. Life cycle of translational research for medical interventions. Science. 2008; 321(5894):1298–9.

11. American College of Physicians. Information on cost-effectiveness: an essential product of a national comparative effectiveness program. Ann Intern Med. 2008;148(12):956–61.

12. Hochman M, McCormick D. Characteristics of published comparative effectiveness studies of medications. JAMA. 2010;303(10):951–8.

13. Bekelman JE, Li Y, Gross CP. Scope and impact of financial conflicts of interest in biomedical research: a systematic review. JAMA. 2003;289(4):454–65.

14. Hochman M, McCormick D. Endpoint selection and relative (versus absolute) risk reporting in published medication trials. J Gen Intern Med. 2011;26(11):1246–52.

15. Fisher B, Anderson S, Bryant J, Margolese RG, Deutsch M, Fisher ER, Jeong JH, Wolmark N. Twenty-year follow-up of a randomized trial comparing total mastectomy, lumpectomy, and lumpectomy plus irradiation for the treatment of invasive breast cancer. N Engl J Med. 2002;347(16):1233–41.

16. Sacks FM, Bray GA, Carey VJ, Smith SR, Ryan DH, Anton SD, McManus K, Champagne CM, Bishop LM, Laranjo N, Leboff MS, Rood JC, de Jonge L, Greenway FL, Loria CM, Obarzanek E, Williamson DA. Comparison of weight-loss diets with different compositions of fat, protein, and carbohydrates. N Engl J Med. 2009;360:859–73.

17. ALLHAT Officers and Coordinators for the ALLHAT Collaborative Research Group. Major outcomes in high-risk hypertensive patients randomized to angiotensin-converting enzyme inhibitor or calcium channel blocker vs diuretic: the antihypertensive and lipid-lowering treatment to prevent heart attack trial (ALLHAT). JAMA. 2002;288(23):2981–97.

18. American Recovery and Reinvestment Act of 2009 (ARRA), Pub. L. No. 111–5, (Feb. 17, 2009).

19. Clancy C, Collins FS. Patient-centered outcomes research institute: the intersection of science and health care. Sci Trans Med. 2010;2(37):37cm18.

20. Tunis SR, Stryer DB, Clancy CM. Practical clinical trials: increasing the value of clinical research for decision making in clinical and health policy. JAMA. 2003;290(12):1624–32.

21. Concato J, Lawler EV, Lew RA, Gaziano JM, Aslan M, Huang GD. Observational methods in comparative effectiveness research. Am J Med. 2010;123(12 suppl 1):e16–23.

22. Dahabreh IJ, Sheldrick RC, Paulus JK, Chung M, Varvarigou V, Jafri H, Rassen JA, Trikalinos TA, Kitsios GD. Do observational studies using propensity score methods agree with randomized trials? A systematic comparison of studies on acute coronary syndromes. Eur Heart J. 2012;33(15):1893–901.

23. Concato J, Shah N, Horwitz RI. Randomized, controlled trials, observational studies, and the hierarchy of research designs. N Engl J Med. 2000;342(25):1887–92.

24. Methodology Committee of the Patient-Centered Outcomes Research Institute (PCORI). Methodological standards and patient-centeredness in comparative effectiveness research: the PCORI perspective. JAMA. 2012;307(15):1636–40.

25. Institute of Medicine Roundtable on Evidence-Based Medicine. Learning what works best: the nation's need for evidence of comparative effectiveness in healthcare. Washington, DC: Institute of Medicine; 2007.

26. Pollack A. The evidence gap: the minimal impact of a big hypertension study. The New York Times. 2008 Nov 28.

27. Chalkidou K. Comparative effectiveness review within the U.K.'s National Institute for Health and Clinical Excellence. Issue Brief (Commonw Fund). 2009;59:1–12.

28. Kerr DJ, Scott M. British lessons on health care reform. N Engl J Med. 2009;361(13):e21.

29. Brook RH. Possible outcomes of comparative effectiveness research. JAMA. 2009;302(2):194–5.

30. Garber AM, Tunis SR. Does comparative-effectiveness research threaten personalized medicine? N Engl J Med. 2009;360(19):1925–7.

31. Szabo L. FDA approves $93K prostate cancer vaccine. USA Today. 2010 Apr 30. http://www.usatoday.com/news/health/2010-04-30-prostatevaccine30_ST_N.htm

32. Neumann PJ, Weinstein MC. Legislating against use of cost-effectiveness information. N Engl J Med. 2010;363(16):1495–7.

33. Walley T. Translating comparative effectiveness research into clinical practice: the UK experience. Drugs. 2012;72(2):163–70.

34. Garber AM, Sox HC. The role of costs in comparative effectiveness research. Health Aff (Millwood). 2010;29(10):1805–11.

35. Chernew ME, Baicker K, Hsu J. The specter of financial armageddon – health care and federal debt in the United States. N Engl J Med. 2010;362:1166–8.

Health Information Technology: Clinical and Policy Context

8

Emily R. Maxson and Sachin H. Jain

Learning Objectives

After completing this chapter, the reader should be able to answer the following questions:
- Elucidate the benefits and challenges of health information technology (health IT) adoption.
- Provide the rationale behind the movement to transition from paper to electronic systems.
- Explain key policies and programs established in the American Recovery and Reinvestment Act's HITECH Act, including the Meaningful Use regulation to incentivize electronic health record adoption and integration.
- Detail the current status of health IT adoption in the United States.
- Postulate the next steps and future opportunities for policymakers in the field of health IT.

Introduction

Hospitals, physician offices, and health-care delivery systems lag far behind their counterparts in other sectors in the integration of technology to maximize service, quality, and efficiency. Physicians and policymakers have recognized the

E.R. Maxson, M.D. (✉)
Department of Internal Medicine, Brigham and Women's Hospital and Harvard Medical School, Boston, MA 02115, USA
e-mail: emaxson@partners.org

S.H. Jain, M.D., M.B.A.
Boston VA Medical Center, Harvard Medical School, and Merck and Company, Boston, MA 02115, USA
e-mail: shjain@gmail.com

need to transition from a predominantly paper-based health-care system to an electronic one, but the transition until recently had been slow and challenging.

Early supporters of Electronic Health Record (EHR) systems—and associated technologies including electronic prescribing, computerized physician order entry, and clinical registries—cited the potential to achieve improvements in quality of care, efficiency, and reliability of billing, but the systems required substantial up-front investments in time and capital [1–3].

Critics reported on several risks of poorly implemented EHRs including the possibility of new types of medication errors and clinical alert fatigue from misplaced or persistent clinical reminders [4, 5]. Perhaps because of these

M.K. Sethi and W.H. Frist (eds.), *An Introduction to Health Policy: A Primer for Physicians and Medical Students*, DOI 10.1007/978-1-4614-7735-8_8, © Springer Science+Business Media New York 2013

challenges—in addition to the substantial cultural and financial investment involved in transitioning to paperless practices—EHR adoption remained low for the first decade of the new millennium [6].

But policymakers understood that patient safety depends on more accessible and more timely information in the hands of physicians and that quality improvement relies on adequate measurements of baselines and progress towards stated goals. The vision of a paperless health-care system able to seamlessly and securely transmit information across multiple health-care institutions relies upon a more robust health information technology (health IT) infrastructure than the one the United States possessed. Important policy changes have facilitated progress.

This chapter provides the context for and details of recent landmark policy changes to facilitate health IT adoption and integration, including the unprecedented investment in health IT seen in the HITECH Act and Meaningful Use Incentive Program.

The Context: Promises and Pitfalls of Health IT

There is substantial debate over the benefits and risks of health IT, with many published studies in both categories [7]. Skeptics have questioned whether the technology merits substantial policy emphasis and investment. Several studies have documented dissatisfaction with electronic clinical alerts which use data to remind providers to take action ("alert fatigue"), and they have raised concern that electronic systems—while reducing some types of errors—introduce other ones.

There have been concerns over privacy breaches and the potential for decreased patient satisfaction [8, 9]. There is also mixed evidence regarding care process efficiency, with studies supporting increased and decreased provider efficiency depending on the process or metric studied [7]. Some physicians have also reported difficulty customizing EHRs to meet the needs of innovative practice models, which becomes ever more relevant as policymakers push towards health care and payment reform [10].

Though these concerns are legitimate and certainly merit policymakers' attention, a recent review of literature published from 2007 to 2010 demonstrated significant evidence supporting the expansion of health IT [7]. Of 154 studies ultimately reviewed in detail, 96 (62 %) were associated with improvement in one or more aspects of care (without decrements in care), and 142 (92 %) were completely positive or mixed positive. The mixed-positive studies each had a positive conclusion overall but documented at least one negative aspect of health IT. When individual outcomes were aggregated across all studies, the authors identified 240 out of 278 outcome measures (86 %) with at least mixed-positive outcomes. In addition, many of the studies deemed negative included caveats that poor outcomes could have been mitigated by more thoughtful system selections and health IT implementations.

Despite the weight of the evidence in favor of health IT for improved efficiency and patient care, EHR adoption was slow throughout the first decade of the twenty-first century [11]. Even as late as 2008, estimates of EHR adoption lagged at 17 % of all physicians and 20 % of primary care physicians [6]. This was an environment that was in some ways primed for the policy changes initiated in the United States in 2009.

The HITECH Act and the Meaningful Use Incentive Program

The drive to improve the health-care system's technical infrastructure has achieved bipartisan support. The George W. Bush administration articulated goals for improved health IT adoption in 2004, but it was not until 2009 that comprehensive policy was passed in Congress to fiscally and organizationally support health IT [12].

A sizeable component of the American Recovery and Reinvestment Act of 2009, the Health Information Technology for Economic and Clinical Health (HITECH) Act, dedicated $2 billion to policy and programming and $14 to $27 billion dollars in incentives to accelerate the adoption and integration of health IT [11, 13]; the range exists based on variable estimates of eventual health IT adoption.

The incentive component became known as the Medicare and Medicaid "Meaningful Use" program, founded on the idea that switching from paper to electronic health records is necessary but insufficient. In order to achieve improvement, systems must be thoughtfully implemented and "meaningfully used" [13].

Under the Medicare EHR Incentive Program, eligible professionals who demonstrate meaningful use of their health IT systems are entitled to up to $44,000 over 5 years, with additional moneys available to providers who serve in Health Professional Shortage Areas. Eligible hospitals and critical access hospitals can receive at least $2 million in incentives for achieving meaningful use. Importantly, physicians, hospitals, and critical access hospitals eligible for Medicare incentives will be subject to financial penalties in the form of reimbursement adjustments if they do not satisfy Meaningful Use requirements by 2015 [14].

The Medicaid EHR Incentive Program is federally supported but administered by select states and territories. Eligible professionals under this program can receive up to $63,750 over 6 years of participation. As in the Medicare Incentive Program, eligible hospitals and critical access hospitals may receive incentives starting at $2 million for satisfying Meaningful Use requirements. Unlike the Medicare program, there are no financial penalties for eligible providers and institutions which fail to meet Meaningful Use requirements [14].

Physicians in group practices are evaluated individually, and each individual may only receive one incentive payment per year regardless of his or her total number of practice sites. Professionals who are otherwise eligible but provide at least 90 % of services in a hospital emergency room or inpatient setting cannot receive incentive payments; these individuals are referred to as hospital-based and are ineligible for the program.

The categories of medical professionals eligible for Medicaid incentives include physicians, nurse practitioners, midwives, dentists, and certain physician assistants; these providers must also satisfy a Medicaid volume requirement (minimum 20 % Medicaid patient volume for pediatricians, noting that Children's Health Insurance Program patients do not count towards the volume criteria; minimum 30 % Medicaid patient volume for other practitioners).

Providers eligible for both programs must choose whether they will participate in the Medicare or Medicaid Incentive Programs and cannot receive payments from both. Hospitals eligible under the Medicare Incentive Program include hospitals paid under the Inpatient Prospective Payment System, Critical Access Hospitals, and Medicare Advantage-affiliated hospitals. Hospitals eligible under the Medicaid Incentive Program include hospitals with at least 10 % Medicaid patient volume and all children's hospitals, without regard to Medicaid patient volume. Hospitals eligible under both programs may receive incentives from both Medicare and Medicaid Meaningful Use Incentive Programs.

Eligibility for Meaningful Use Incentive Programs

The Meaningful Use regulation published July 2010 set forth metrics and goals that physicians and institutions must meet in order to qualify for the incentive payments and avoid future penalties [14].

First, health-care professionals and hospitals must meet eligibility requirements for either or both programs [14, 15]. Eligible professionals under the Medicare Incentive Program include physicians, dentists, podiatrists, optometrists, and chiropractors.

Meaningful Use Requirements

The Meaningful Use regulations defined three progressive stages to guide the distribution of incentive payments for Meaningful Use of EHRs.

Under Stage 1 of Meaningful Use, the eligible professionals detailed earlier must satisfy 15 Core Objectives and their choice of at least 5 additional objectives from a "Menu Set" of 10 more (Table 8.1) [14]. Several Core Objectives for eligible professionals require explanation and understanding of the basic functionalities of EHRs.

Table 8.1 Stage 1 meaningful use objectives

Core objectives for eligible professionals and hospitals (must satisfy ALL)	Menu set objectives for eligible professionals (must choose 5, including at least one public health measure)	Menu set objectives for hospitals (must choose 5, including at least one public health measure)
E-prescribe[a]	Perform drug-formulary checks	Perform drug-formulary checks
Utilize computerized physician order entry	Incorporate clinical lab test results as structured data	Incorporate clinical lab test results as structured data
Report ambulatory clinical quality measures to CMS/states	Generate lists of patients by specific conditions	Generate lists of patients by specific conditions
Implement ONE clinical decision support rule	Identify and provide patient-specific education resources to patient	Identify and provide patient-specific education resources to patient
Provide patient with electronic copy of their health information upon request	Reconcile medications electronically	Reconcile medications electronically
Provide clinical after visit summaries for patients	Provide a summary of care record for each transition of care/referrals	Provide a summary of care record for each transition of care/referrals
Utilize drug-drug and drug-allergy interaction checks	Send reminders to patients per patient preference for preventive/follow-up care	Record advanced directives for patients 65 years or older
Record patient demographic information	Provide patients with timely electronic access to their health information	Develop capability to provide electronic submission of reportable lab results to public health agencies *(public health measure)*
Maintain up to date problem list of current and active diagnoses	Develop capability to submit electronic data to immunization registries/systems *(public health measure)*	Develop capability to submit electronic data to immunization registries/systems *(public health measure)*
Maintain active medication list	Develop capability to provide electronic syndromic surveillance data to public health agencies (public health measure)	Develop capability to provide electronic syndromic surveillance data to public health agencies *(public health measure)*
Maintain active medication allergy list		
Record and chart changes in vital signs		
Record smoking status for patients 13 years and older		
Electronically exchange key clinical information among care providers and patient-authorized entities		
Protect electronic health information		

Source: Data from Ref. [14]

[a]E-prescribing is the only core measure that applies only to eligible professionals; hospitals need not satisfy this core requirement

The most fundamental of these is record keeping. Health-care professionals of all types can use an EHR to record clinical information and document the details of a clinical encounter. For example, a medical secretary may record the patient's demographic information upon intake, after which the medical assistant may then enter vital signs and record allergy information in the patient's electronic record. The physician may then document his or her progress note, including the patient's history of present illness, physical exam, assessment, and plan, and he or she will use the computer to request a specialist referral or order a medication. The nurse may finally document administration of the patient's flu shot before he leaves the office. This information is all password protected, encrypted, and stored so that it may be accessed only by the appropriate personnel.

Computerized physician order entry is the functionality that enables health-care physicians to directly enter orders for medications, labs, images, immunizations, or other procedures into the EHR system, which prompts other activities or provides necessary authorization to accomplish the task or treatment at hand. Electronic prescribing (also called e-prescribing or eRx) utilizes the computer to directly transmit a prescription to the pharmacy, safely and securely.

All of these functionalities are required for physicians to satisfy Stage 1 of Meaningful Use Objectives. The Core Objectives also include somewhat more advanced EHR functionalities: clinical decision supports and automated assessment and alerts for medication interactions and allergies. Clinical decision support tools utilize information stored in the patient's record to cue evidence-based reminders. For example, EHRs can be programmed to alert the physician if the patient is eligible and due for a certain vaccine or to prompt the appropriate lab order if a diabetic is overdue for a necessary test.

In order to qualify for Meaningful Use incentive payments, eligible professionals must also ensure their system checks for medication interactions and drug-allergy interactions; this EHR functionality then requests the physician to change the order or document rationale for overriding the alert.

An additional essential Core Objective for eligible professionals is to share key information electronically with appropriate physicians and other health-care providers, safely and securely.

The Menu Set of objectives for Stage 1 of Meaningful Use includes 10 additional metrics, of which eligible professionals must satisfy at least five, including one designated public health metric (Table 8.1).

The Stage 1 Meaningful Use requirements for hospitals are similar to those for eligible professionals, with a few notable exceptions. Hospitals are not required to electronically prescribe to satisfy Stage 1 of Meaningful Use. While hospitals, too, must choose 5 out of 10 available Menu Set Objectives, there are several objectives unique to eligible professionals and hospitals, respectively, that comprise slightly different Menu Sets for each group (Table 8.1).

Stage 2 of Meaningful Use will be implemented in 2014 and will require eligible professionals and hospitals to build on existing functionalities and achieve advanced capabilities such as safe and secure online access for patients to explore their own records facile and secure exchange of health information between authorized care providers.

Stage 3 of Meaningful Use is expected to be implemented in 2016. Though the regulations will be developed at a later date, Stage 3 is expected to require improvements in quality, safety, cost efficiency, and population health metrics [14].

Programmatic Assistance for Meaningful Use

In addition to the aforementioned funding for the Medicare and Medicaid Incentive Program, the American Recovery and Reinvestment Act's HITECH Act allotted $2 billion to the Office of the National Coordinator for Health Information Technology to develop and fund programs to support the achievement of Meaningful Use.

The keystone is the Regional Extension Center Program, which has established 60 local organizations tasked with the provision of onsite technical assistance to bring a cumulative 100,000 primary care physicians, physician assistants, and nurse practitioners across the United States to meaningful use of EHRs [16]. These Regional Extension Centers help local physicians understand Meaningful Use requirements, assist practices to adopt and integrate EHRs into their workflow, and work with office staff to maximize the use of their technologies for patient benefit.

The State Health Information Exchange Program has funded 56 states, territories, and state-designated entities to develop and enhance capacity for information exchange. These and other programs launched by ONC will support the Centers for Medicare and Medicaid Services Meaningful Use Incentive Program in the effort

Table 8.2 Programs to support meaningful use of health information technology

Program	Responsible organization	Funding	Purpose
Meaningful Use Incentive Program	CMS[a]	$14–27 billion	Provide financial incentives to ease Medicare and Medicaid providers' transition to meaningfully used EHRs
Regional Extension Center Program	ONC[b]	$677 million	Develop 60 regional technical assistance centers across the country to aid primary care providers in their transition to meaningfully used EHRs
State Health Information Exchange Cooperative Agreement Program	ONC	$547 million	Assist states and designated entities to develop infrastructure for electronic information exchange
Beacon Community Cooperative Agreement Program	ONC	$250 million	Fund 17 advanced communities to demonstrate the potential of health IT to enable improvements in quality, cost efficiency, and population health
Nationwide Health Information Exchange	ONC	N/A	Establish a set of standards, services, and policies that will govern and enable safe and secure electronic health information exchange

Source: Data from Ref. [14]
[a]CMS denotes Centers for Medicare and Medicaid Services
[b]ONC denotes Office of the National Coordinator for Health Information Technology

to modernize the US health-care system through the use of health information technology (Table 8.2). To better understand the role of government and state agencies in health care, please see Chap. 16.

Current Status and Future Considerations

As of November 2011, 52 % of all office-based physicians reported that they were planning on enrolling in the Medicare and Medicaid EHR Incentive Programs [6]. EHR usage has grown significantly over the last 3 years. The percentage of physicians who use EHRs has increased from 17 % to 34 %; the percent of primary care physicians who use EHRs has increased from 20 % to 39 % [6]. Nonetheless, substantial challenges remain.

Foremost among these is the development of a sustainable Nationwide Health Information Network (NHIN). Rather than a concrete, tangible system of servers, the NHIN is a set of standards, services, and policies that will govern and enable safe and secure electronic health information exchange [17]. Once standards are in place

that require systems to operate using the same languages, it will be easier to exchange coded information electronically and use information in decision-making. This will expand the utility of health IT beyond the typical duties of office practices to the public health sphere. Already some large health-care networks are using information culled from EHRs to survey for flu outbreaks and other epidemics of public concern, maintain immunization registries, and automate mandatory reporting of certain infections. While significant progress has been made towards the development of the NHIN—supported by the Office of the National Coordinator for Health Information Technology—the effort continues to remain in a fledgling state, with significant debate over the best pathway forward.

The caution in developing this and other advanced uses of health IT will be that new clinical systems, while more efficient, will bring additional, sometimes unintended challenges to the health-care system.

For example, one study found that implementation of electronic reporting of suspected Lyme disease led to overreporting (increased total number of reports submitted, but decreased percentage of true Lyme disease cases after investigation) [18]. Physicians will therefore need to develop more focused algorithms as they seek to approximate clinical decision-making.

Once the exchange of information has been streamlined, data within EHRs could potentially be used to facilitate comparative health effectiveness research and advance public health goals.

Conclusion

The vision of the United States health-care system driven by health IT is one that is able to seamlessly and securely transfer patient information electronically, better equipping health-care providers and physicians with the information they need at the point of care. It is one that takes advantage of advancements in technology to provide timely reminders to assist physicians in meeting best-practice goals. Ultimately, it is a health-care system that can achieve and sustain improvements in health-care quality, cost efficiency, and population health.

Policymakers in the future will need to consider additional steps necessary to assist meaningful users to achieve even more from their EHR systems. They will also need to consider revising the current reimbursement system to reward efficiencies gained through health information technology rather than simply rewarding the volume of services delivered. Progress has been made—in the direction of Accountable Care Organizations and bundled payment models—but we still have far to go.

For our part, physicians will need to rise to the challenge, accepting the difficulties of EHR implementation and workflow redesign and embracing opportunities to improve care.

References

1. Shekelle PG, Morton SC, Keeler EB. Costs and benefits of health information technology. Evid Rep Technol Assess (Full Rep). 2006;132:1–71.
2. Chaudhry B, Wang J, Wu S, Maglione M, Mojica W, Roth E, et al. Systematic review: impact of health information technology on quality, efficiency, and costs of medical care. Ann Intern Med. 2006;144:742–52.
3. Wang SJ, Middleton B, Prosser LA, Bardon CG, Spurr CD, Carchidi PJ, et al. A cost-benefit analysis of electronic medical records in primary care. Am J Med. 2003;114:397–403.
4. Koppel R, Metlay JP, Cohen A, Abaluck B, Localio AR, Kimmel SE, et al. Role of computerized physician order entry systems in facilitating medication errors. JAMA. 2005;293:1197–203.
5. van der Sijs H, van Gelder T, Vulto A, Berg M, Aarts J. Understanding handling of drug safety alerts: a simulation study. Int J Med Inform. 2010;79:361–9.
6. Hsiao CJ, Hing E, Socey TC, Cai B. Electronic health record systems and intent to apply for meaningful use incentives among office-based physician practices: United States, 2001–2011. NCHS Data Brief. 2011; 79:1–8.
7. Beeuwkes Buntin M, Burke MF, Hoaglin MC, Blumenthal D. The benefits of health information technology: a review of the recent literature shows predominantly positive results. Health Aff. 2011;30(3):464–71.
8. Myers J, Frieden TR, Bherwani KM, Henning KJ. Ethics in public health research: privacy and public health at risk: public health confidentiality in the digital age. Am J Public Health. 2008;98(5):793–801.
9. Zickmund SL, Hess R, Bryce CL, McTigue K, Olshansky E, Fitzgerald K, et al. Interest in the use of computerized patient portals: role of the provider-patient relationship. J Gen Intern Med. 2008;23 Suppl 1:20–6.
10. Fernandopulle R, Patel N. How the electronic health record did not measure up to the demands of our medical home practice. Health Aff (Millwood). 2010;29(4):622–8.
11. Blumenthal D. Launching HITECH. N Engl J Med. 2010;362(5):382–5.
12. Bush GW. Remarks by the president at the American Association of Community Colleges Annual Convention. Minneapolis; 2004 April 26.
13. Blumenthal D, Tavenner M. The "Meaningful Use" regulation for electronic health records. N Engl J Med. 2010;363:501–4.
14. Centers for Medicare and Medicaid Services. 42 CFR Parts 412, 413, 422 et al. Medicare and medicaid programs; electronic health record incentive program; final rule. Fed Regist [serial on the Internet]. 2010 Jul 28 [cited 2012 June 19]. http://edocket.access.gpo.gov/2010/pdf/2010-17207.pdf
15. Medicaid Provider Scope and Eligibility. 42 CFR 495.304 2010 Oct 1 [cited 2012 June 19]. http://www.gpo.gov:80/fdsys/pkg/CFR-2010-title42-vol5/xml/CFR-2010-title42-vol5-sec495-304.xml
16. Maxson E, Jain S, Kendall M, et al. The regional extension center program: helping physicians meaningfully use health information technology. Ann Intern Med. 2010;153:666–70.
17. Rishel W, Riehl V, Blanton C. Summary of the NHIN prototype architecture contracts. Washington, DC: U.S. Department of Health and Human Services; 2007.
18. Centers for Disease Control and Prevention. Effect of electronic lab- oratory reporting on the burden of Lyme disease surveillance—New Jersey, 2001–2006. MMWR Morb Mortal Wkly Rep. 2008;57(2):42–5.

Prescription Drug and Pharmaceutical Policy

9

Phillip A. Choi and Walid F. Gellad

Learning Objectives

After completing this chapter, the reader should be able to answer the following questions:

- Understand the scope of prescription drug use in the United States.
- Know how drugs are developed, approved, and brought to market for use by patients in the United States.
- Understand the difference between brand and generic medications.
- Understand how drugs are paid for by patients and other entities.
- Understand the role of pharmacy benefit managers (PBMs) and the components of pharmacy benefit design.
- Identify recent pharmaceutical policy issues involving off-label prescribing, conflicts of interest, biologics and biosimilars, and personalized medicine.

P.A. Choi, B.S.
University of Pittsburgh School of Medicine,
Pittsburgh, PA 15213, USA
e-mail: choi.phillip@medstudent.pitt.edu

W.F. Gellad, M.D., M.P.H. (✉)
Center for Health Equity Research and Promotion,
VA Pittsburgh Healthcare System and University of
Pittsburgh, Pittsburgh, PA 15206, USA
e-mail: walid.gellad@va.gov

How Are Drugs Used: Epidemiology of Prescription Drugs

Role of Prescription Drugs in Health Care

Prescription drugs play a key role in modern health care. They provide a substantial public health benefit to populations with access to them. Treatment for many diseases has been improved dramatically by improved pharmaceuticals, including HIV/AIDS, acid reflux disease, diabetes, coronary heart disease, and cancer. Prescription drugs have played a large role in cutting the mortality of heart disease and stroke by half from 1970 to 2000 through reducing risk factors such as hypertension and hyperlipidemia [1].

M.K. Sethi and W.H. Frist (eds.), *An Introduction to Health Policy: A Primer for Physicians and Medical Students*, 101
DOI 10.1007/978-1-4614-7735-8_9, © Springer Science+Business Media New York 2013

Table 9.1 Number of filled prescriptions per capita, stratified by age, in 2011

Patient age	Prescriptions per capita
80+	36.7
70–79	28.8
65–69	20.8
60–64	22.2
50–59	19.8
26–49	8.2
19–25	4.2
0–18	3.4
Total	11.3

Source: Data from Ref. [4]

The number of prescriptions written for patients in the USA has been steadily rising. Between 1999 and 2009, the total number of dispensed prescriptions increased from 2.8 billion to 3.9 billion, an increase of 39 % [2, 3]. In 2011, over 4 billion prescriptions were dispensed in the United States, or 11.3 prescriptions per person (Table 9.1) [4, 5]. Whereas slightly more than half of the US population under age 55 had a prescription expense in 2009, more than 91 % of those over age 65 had an expense [6]. The US population is projected to increase steadily from 310 million in 2010 to 439 million in 2050, and the number of US residents over the age of 65 will more than double from 40 million in 2010 to 88 million due to the baby boom and increased longevity [7, 8]. These factors ensure continual increases in the number of prescriptions written and dispensed for the foreseeable future.

Spending on Prescription Drugs

In 2011, the United States spent approximately $320 billion on pharmaceuticals, with $49 billion paid out of pocket by patients [4, 5]. Spending on pharmaceuticals accounted for only 10 % of total health-care spending in 2010, yet it has become a major policy issue because of high out-of-pocket costs for patients and the acceleration in spending that occurred starting in the mid-1990s, with growth of 114 % between 2000 and 2010 compared to 83 % growth for health-care spending overall [9]. Increased use of prescription drugs,

development of patent-protected drugs for common conditions (e.g., atorvastatin (Lipitor) for high cholesterol), increases in prices, increased cost for developing new drugs, and an explosive increase in direct-to-consumer advertising fueled the increase in pharmaceutical expenditures [2, 3]. Growth in prescription drug spending has since slowed due to changes in pharmaceutical benefit design, fewer new drugs, expired patents for some blockbuster drugs, and increased use of generic drugs [10]. Yet, more than a quarter of non-elderly patients allocate more than 50 % of their out-of-pocket health-care spending to paying for prescription drugs [10]. This burden is especially high for patients with public insurance and low income.

Billions of dollars are still spent on individual drugs in the USA, giving them "blockbuster" status. For example, in 2010, total spending on Lipitor, the most commonly used statin medication for cholesterol control, was $7.2 billion [11]. Other blockbuster drugs in 2010 included esomeprazole (Nexium) ($6.3 billion), clopidogrel (Plavix) ($6.1 billion), and fluticasone/salmeterol (Advair Diskus) ($4.7 billion).

Research and Development of Drugs and the FDA Approval Process

Bringing a Drug to Market

Developing a drug is a complex multistep, multi-year process involving academia, private industry, and the federal government. Novel chemical entities are developed and screened for pharmacological activity by pharmaceutical companies or universities partnered with pharmaceutical companies. Prominent medical schools, such as Harvard Medical School and the University of California, San Francisco, have recently developed partnerships with pharmaceutical companies, such as Pfizer and Sanofi, to develop drugs in multimillion-dollar collaborations [12].

Clinical trials test the safety and efficacy of new compounds in humans. Prior to clinical testing, pharmaceutical companies will submit an Investigational New Drug (IND) application to the FDA, which is needed to ship the drug across state lines for clinical testing. An IND is composed of information from preclinical studies, which includes animal pharmacology and toxicology studies, manufacturing information pertaining to composition, stability, and other physical and chemical properties. Clinical trials are carried out in three phases prior to approval and a post-marketing phase if deemed necessary by the FDA [13]:

- *Phase 1 trials* are carried out with a small group (20–80) of healthy volunteers to determine a safe dosing range, identify side effects, and evaluate safety.
- *Phase 2 trials* use a larger group of people (100–300) to determine safety and efficacy.
- *Phase 3 trials* are the last step in clinical testing prior to submission to the FDA for drug approval and typically consist of randomized controlled trials. A large group of people are administered the drug, and information is gathered regarding efficacy, safety, and advantages over current treatments.
- *Phase 4 trials* are post-marketing studies that provide additional information on the drug's risks, benefits, and optimal use and are sometimes required as part of the FDA approval process.

Prior to approval, a prescription label must be developed by the manufacturer. The label is the documentation that will provide physicians and patients with information on the indications, contraindications, dosing, side effects, pharmacodynamics, pharmacokinetics, and the clinical trials leading to approval [14]. Once the New Drug Application (NDA) has been approved, the manufacturer is able to market and sell the drug.

Cost and Risk of Bringing a Drug to Market

The process of discovering and developing a drug is an expensive and risky one. Estimates of the cost to bring a drug to market vary according to the study as well as the type of drug being developed. However, recent studies estimate the out-of-pocket costs of developing a drug to be well over $800 million with capitalized costs over $1.8 billion per drug [15–17]. Out-of-pocket cost is the amount of money spent by the company during the time period developing the drug. Capitalized cost is out-of-pocket cost plus the return on investment that could have been expected if that same money had been used elsewhere.

In addition to being expensive, drug development is risky and requires a significant time investment. One study estimates that it takes between 11 and 13 years to discover a drug and bring it to market [17], and another found that 24.3 potential drugs must be discovered in preclinical testing to produce a single FDA-approved drug [17].

Orphan Drugs

Orphan drugs are defined as drugs and biologics "for the safe and effective treatment, diagnosis, or prevention of rare diseases/disorders that affect fewer than 200,000 people in the U.S., or that affect more than 200,000 persons but are not expected to recover the costs of developing and marketing a drug" [18–21]. The orphan drug designation was added in 1983 through the Orphan Drug Act with the goal of stimulating research and development of pharmaceuticals for diseases that affected relatively few patients and thus did not command the attention of pharmaceutical companies like other, much more widespread diseases [22]. Numerous incentives such as tax credits for clinical trials, an exclusive right to market the drug for the approved indication for 7 years, and federal grants helped make developing these orphan drugs attractive to manufacturers.

Brand Versus Generic Drugs

Brand-name drugs can be protected from copying by other manufacturers through two different methods: patent protection and market exclusivity [23–25]. Patent protection is conferred by the United States Patent and Trademark Office and lasts for 20 years [23–26]. Pharmaceutical companies will typically file patents for new drugs prior to clinical studies/after discovery; this creates variability in the length of time they are able to sell the drug with patent protection. Market exclusivity is an exclusive right to market the drug and is granted by the FDA. Market exclusivity begins from the moment the drug is approved by the FDA. For normal drugs, this period is 5 years. Orphan drugs receive 7 years of market exclusivity. The overall effect of patent protection and market exclusivity is that no other manufacturer can sell a drug using the same active ingredient as the protected drug during the time of protection. During this protected time period, the drug is categorized as a single-source brand-name drug [27].

Generic drugs contain the same active ingredient as their brand-name counterparts and must have the same strength, purity, dosage, stability, safety, quality, and route of administration [23–25]. However, the inactive ingredients may be different between the brand and generic versions of a drug. Generic drugs are typically manufactured by companies other than the one that developed the brand-name drug. They must also go through an FDA approval process, but instead of an NDA, the manufacturers must submit an Abbreviated New Drug Application (ANDA). ANDAs were introduced in 1984 by the Hatch-Waxman Act to streamline the process of generic drug approvals by not requiring the new manufacturer to repeat all the costly and lengthy preclinical and clinical trials that are needed for NDAs. In addition to a faster approval process, the Hatch-Waxman Act also conferred market exclusivity to the new generics for 180 days after approval, providing an incentive for companies to bring generics to the market. Once approved, the drug is now a multisource drug with brand and generic versions [27].

Generic drugs provide significant savings to both individuals and the health-care system. In 2010, generic medications saved the US health-care system over $157 billion, according to the Generic Pharmaceutical Association [28], and represented 80 % of all prescriptions dispensed in 2011 [4, 5]. Use of generic drugs grew by more than 40 % between 2004 and 2011 [29]. State laws mandating generic substitution at the point of sale, present in many but not all states, have helped increase the use of generics and reduced spending on drugs [30].

From Machine to Mouth: The Pharmaceutical Supply Chain

Once drugs are approved for use by the FDA, how do they reach patients? The pharmaceutical supply chain contains numerous players that coordinate with each other to ensure development, manufacture, transport, and payment for drugs. This section is modeled on the Kaiser Family Foundation's comprehensive "Follow the Pill" report and will focus on the flow of drugs from manufacturers to consumers [31]. The complex interactions between entities in payment for pharmaceuticals are beyond the scope of this chapter, but are addressed in detail in the Kaiser Family Foundation report, and readers are encouraged to reference this document.

Manufacturers

Manufacturers are the start of the pharmaceutical supply chain. They can either be brand-name manufacturers or generic manufacturers. Most physicians and consumers are aware of brand-name manufacturers such as Pfizer, Merck, and Novartis, but are not familiar with generic manufacturers such as Mylan, Roxane, and Barr. The pharmaceutical manufacturing industry is comprised of relatively few, large global corporations that hold the majority of market share [31]. In 2011, the 10 largest pharmaceutical companies had US sales of $164.1 billion and 51 % of market share [32]. Generic manufacturers make less in sales, but can be comparable to brand-name manufacturers in number of prescriptions dispensed [31]. Once drugs are manufactured, they are sold to other intermediaries in the pharmaceutical supply chain. Drugs are most commonly sold to wholesaler distributors. Manufacturers will also sell drugs directly to retail pharmacies, mail-order pharmacies, specialty pharmacies, hospital chains, health plans, and government purchasers. Drugs typically do not go from manufacturers directly to consumers.

Wholesale Distributors

Wholesale distributors act as the link between pharmaceutical manufacturers and other entities that will distribute drugs to consumers. These other entities include pharmacies, hospitals, nursing homes, and other smaller medical facilities. Some wholesale distributors sell to a broad range of organizations, while others will specialize in either selling a certain type of drug, such as biologics, or selling to a certain type of client, such as nursing homes. In addition to simply purchasing drugs from pharmaceutical manufacturers and reselling them to other entities further along the supply chain, wholesale distributors also participate in drug repackaging (repackaging drugs into smaller containers for sale), reimbursement support, and drug buyback programs (programs in which wholesale distributors and manufacturers buy drugs back from pharmacies, which reduces the risk taken on by pharmacies when they stock drugs) [31].

The pharmaceutical wholesale distribution industry is highly consolidated due to pressures to lower costs through economies of scale. The number of wholesalers declined from more than 200 in 1975 to less than 50 in 2000 [31]. Currently, the top three wholesale distributors, McKesson, Cardinal Health, and AmerisourceBergen, control over 85 % of the wholesale market [33]. In 2011, the big three wholesale distributors had approximately $291.6 billion in sales [33].

Pharmacies

Pharmacies are often the final physical step in the pharmaceutical supply chain before drugs reach the outpatient consumer. Pharmacies purchase drugs from wholesale distributors or manufacturers and dispense them to patients with prescriptions. In addition to dispensing drugs, pharmacies play a key role in the exchange of information

between payers and suppliers such as drug manufacturers, health plans, pharmacy benefit managers, employers, and the government. When a prescription is being filled, the pharmacy will typically check for drug interactions with other prescriptions and check whether the drug is on the health plan's formulary and for generic alternatives. The pharmacy is also a key point for recording information about the use of pharmaceuticals for demographic purposes.

Pharmacies exist in many different forms such as retail pharmacies (chain or independent), mail-order pharmacies (includes Internet-based services), supermarket pharmacies, long-term care pharmacies, and specialty pharmacies (Table 9.2) [4, 5]. Retail pharmacies are the most commonly used type of pharmacy in the USA. The top three chains in the USA are Walgreens, CVS, and Rite Aid [34]. In retail pharmacies, prescriptions are brought in by patients, called in by doctor's offices, sent electronically, and dispensed for patients to pick up. Mail-order pharmacies receive orders by mail, fax, or electronically and ship prescriptions to patients. Mail-order pharmacies tend to fill prescriptions for a 90-day supply of drugs instead of the usual 30-day supply and focus on chronic conditions that require maintenance medication. Mail-order pharmacies represent a small portion of the pharmacy market but also the fastest growing segment. Long-term care pharmacies provide specialized services for nursing homes. Four chains provide the majority of prescription drugs to nursing homes: Omnicare, PharMerica, NeighborCare, and Kindred Healthcare [31].

Pharmacy Benefit Managers

Although typically not a part of the physical supply chain providing drugs to consumers, pharmacy benefit managers (PBMs) play a key role in controlling and regulating the flow of drugs through the supply chain. PBMs manage prescription drug benefits for employers, health plans, and other organizations that provide health-care benefits. Some of the largest PBMs in the country include the recently merged Express Scripts – Medco Health Solutions, CVS Caremark, and

Table 9.2 Distribution of prescriptions dispensed in the United States, 2011

Channel	Prescriptions dispensed (millions)	Percentage	Examples
Total	4,024	100	
Retail total	3,695	91.8	
Chain stores	2,212	54.9	CVS, Walgreens, Rite Aid
Independent	740	18.3	Spartan Pharmacy, Sullivan's Pharmacy, Rxtra Care Pharmacy
Food stores	483	12.0	Kroger, Safeway, Wal-Mart
Mail service	260	6.5	McKesson, Walgreens, Aetna
Long-term care	329	8.2	HCR ManorCare, Golden Living, Kindred Healthcare

Source: Data from Ref. [4, 5]

ICORE Healthcare [35, 36]. The PBM industry currently brings in revenues of over $227 billion and employs more than 125,000 people [37].

The stated aims of a number of PBM functions are driving down health-care costs and improving patient outcomes. PBMs use tiered formularies to encourage consumers to use lower-cost, therapeutically equivalent drugs and negotiate lower prices with manufacturers. PBMs can negotiate rebates with manufacturers on behalf of the consumers and payers associated with the PBM. PBMs administer programs designed to aid in disease management and improve medication adherence for patients in order to improve health outcomes and proper utilization of drugs.

PBMs also provide services that improve the efficiency of the delivery of drugs to consumers. PBMs negotiate with pharmacies to create a network of pharmacies from which patients in a health plan can get their prescriptions dispensed. These agreements between PBMs and pharmacies typically lower prescription drug prices. This generally creates convenience for consumers by giving them many choices of where to fill their prescriptions. However, this may force patients to switch pharmacies if their preferred pharmacy is not a part of the network. PBMs also often operate their own mail-order pharmacy service, which, like most mail-order pharmacies, are especially targeted to patients with chronic disease. In addition to providing convenience to patients, mail-order pharmacies also give PBMs an opportunity to lower costs by encouraging switches to generic or lower-cost, therapeutically equivalent drugs and enforcing formulary compliance.

More detail on the role of PBMs and formularies will be discussed in a later section.

Prescribers

Prescribers are the gatekeepers of the pharmaceutical supply chain for patients. Prescribing privileges are defined at the state level. All physicians (M.D. and D.O.) can prescribe any drug given they are properly licensed. Practitioners such as veterinarians and dentists have prescribing powers for drugs relevant to their fields. Physician assistants are able to prescribe drugs under supervision of a physician, although their ability to prescribe controlled substances is limited and varies by state [38–40]. Similarly, nurse practitioners hold prescribing authority in certain states with variation on their ability to prescribe controlled substances. A recent movement by psychologists to gain prescribing authority has resulted in limited prescribing privileges for psychologists in New Mexico and Louisiana, with efforts ongoing in other states [41].

Pharmacy Benefit Design

Defining Pharmacy Benefit Design

Pharmacy benefit design refers to the way in which prescription drugs are covered in insurance plans, how much of a medication a patient can receive, and how much members will pay for each drug [42]. PBMs or the insurance plan itself will

Table 9.3 Pharmacy benefit design definitions

Term	Definition
Formulary	List of drugs covered by an insurance plan or PBM
(Formulary) tier	In a tiered formulary, drugs are placed on certain levels (or tiers), with a set copay/coinsurance for each tier based on availability of generics or therapeutically equivalent therapies within the class
Step therapy	Requirement to use lower-cost (usually therapeutically equivalent) drugs before using higher-cost drugs
	Requirement to prescribe therapies in a predetermined order to patients
Prior authorization	Requirement that physician get approval to prescribe a drug before the prescription is filled
Quantity limit	Limits on the number of pills a patient can receive at one time and the number of refills they can obtain

Source: Data from Ref. [42]

design the pharmacy benefit primarily to reduce health-care costs through substitution of expensive brand-name drugs with generic or lower-cost, therapeutically equivalent drugs. The elements of pharmacy benefit design include tiered formularies and various utilization management tools including step therapy, prior authorization, and quantity limits (Table 9.3) [42].

Formularies

When choosing a course of treatment for a patient, physicians must consult with plan guidelines to determine whether a particular drug is on the formulary for that plan. A formulary is a list of drugs that are covered by the insurance plan [42]. The drugs within a formulary are typically separated into tiers. There are typically three tiers with increasing out-of-pocket expenses for higher tier drugs. The first tier consists of generic drugs ($5–10 copay), the second tier is preferred brand-name drugs ($20–30 copay), and the third tier is non-preferred brand-name drugs ($50 or more copay) [42]. Selection of brand-name drugs as "preferred" or "non-preferred" (and thus placement on tiers) is often based in part on negotiations between the PBM and manufacturers/distributors. Brand-name drugs for which the PBM is able to achieve favorable savings will typically be put onto the second tier, and those for which the PBM does not achieve favorable costs will be put onto the non-preferred tier to discourage patient use. The clinical effectiveness

of the drug also plays a role in tier placement. There may also be a fourth tier for self-injectable drugs and biologics due to their high cost compared to other pharmaceuticals [43].

Utilization Management Tools

When selecting a drug, the physician must check whether the plan has step therapy requirements, the drug requires prior authorization, or quantity limits exist for the drug. Step therapy consists of guidelines for treatment that begin with low-cost drugs and ramp up to more expensive drugs if the lower-cost drugs fail. For example, a health plan may require patients with acid reflux disease to use histamine-2 (H2) inhibitors before they are allowed to use proton pump inhibitors (PPIs) [43]. In addition to step therapy guidelines, physicians must consider which drugs require prior authorization. High-cost branded drugs may require that the plan give prior authorization to the physician before they are able to prescribe the drug to the patient. Prior authorization implies conditional coverage of a drug because the PBM will only cover the drug if certain requirements (such as step therapy) are met. Quantity limits usually specify how much of a drug a patient can receive for each prescription and how often a prescription may be refilled [42].

PBMs attempt to drive down health-care costs in a number of ways. Due to the large number of prescriptions they handle and the influence they have on drug use through formulary management,

PBMs can negotiate with pharmaceutical manufacturers for rebates on large quantities of drugs. These rebates can range between 5 % and 25 % and are usually paid by manufacturers 6–12 months after a prescription is filled [44]. A portion of these rebates are passed on to consumers. Enforcing generic substitution through tiered formularies also drives down cost. One study by the U.S. Government Accountability Office found that PBMs are able to negotiate 18 % lower costs compared to those plans without a PBM [45].

How Are Drugs Paid for?

In previous sections, we have reviewed how drugs are used, how they are developed and approved for use, and how they move from manufacturers to patients. The issue of how drugs are paid for is complicated and convoluted, like much of the payment systems in health care. Nonetheless, a basic understanding of drug pricing and payment, which follows, is necessary in order to fully comprehend why many patients have such difficulty paying for prescription drugs. For a more complete and comprehensive economic description of how drugs are priced, see the working paper by Ernst Berndt and Joseph Newhouse from the National Bureau of Economic Research from 2010 [46].

On average, prices for brand-name medications are 35–55 % lower in other industrialized countries compared to the USA [47]. These other countries, like Canada and most of Western Europe, regulate, or set, the prices for drugs, rather than letting the market set them. The oft-used, but controversial, justification for higher US prices is the need to cover the costs of research and development of new drugs [48].

Rather than one specific price for each drug product, there are actually a number of different prices that determine the ultimate cost of an individual product. The most well known is the Average Wholesale Price (AWP), a benchmark used by Medicaid and other programs to set payment rates for medications. The AWP was meant to reflect the average "list" price at which wholesalers sell drugs to retail pharmacies, in contrast to the Average Manufacturer Price (AMP), which is the average price paid by wholesalers to manufacturers for drugs, after discounts. In recent years, the AWP has come under intense scrutiny, because of evidence that the organizations that publish the AWPs colluded to increase published prices (which in turn increased reimbursement to pharmacies under programs like Medicaid that rely on the AWP [49, 50]). Wholesalers and retail pharmacies negotiate a set of rebates and discounts based on the volume of drugs they are able to sell, which changes the actual price paid for each medication; these rebates and discounts are proprietary and not publically available. Thus, in the typical scenario, wholesalers purchase medications from manufacturers and sell them to retail pharmacies for a profit, and retail pharmacies then sell them to consumers for a profit, some of which is determined by a fixed dispensing fee paid by the insurer for each medication dispensed, and some based on the difference between the cost for procuring the drug and the reimbursed cost for the drug. Wholesalers and retail pharmacy dispensing fees account for about a quarter of a prescription's retail price, by one estimation, with the manufacturer's price accounting for the rest [51]. This scenario is different for large pharmacy chains that might have their own wholesale and distribution networks or for large mail-order pharmacies that purchase directly from the manufacturer.

Most patients actually think about the price of their drug based on the copayment or coinsurance they have to pay after filling a drug at the pharmacy, which is quite removed from the prices discussed previously. These copayments vary from $5–10 for generic medications (or $4 for specific generics from Wal-Mart and other large retailers) to $50 or higher for third and fourth tier brand-name drugs [52]. These copayments are fixed for specific drugs, much like copayments for office visits are fixed. A coinsurance payment, on the other hand, is a percentage of the overall cost for a medication that a patient pays; for example, if a patient buys a medication priced at $100 and they face 20 % coinsurance, they would owe $20.

While the prices of brand-name drugs have been steadily rising, the increased use of generics has recently held down the overall amount that most patients have to pay out-of-pocket for prescription drugs [10]. There are examples, however, of very high out-of-pocket costs for specialty drugs for conditions like arthritis, ulcerative colitis, and cancer as health plans institute coinsurances for these medications, which can cost tens of thousands of dollars a year [53]. These high costs are critically important, since not only do they add financial pressures to patient's lives (in some cases, causing them difficulty in buying basic necessities like food), but research has clearly shown that increased cost sharing leads to reduced initiation of pharmaceutical treatment and worse adherence among those who have already started treatment [54, 55].

The amount that remains to be paid after patients have paid their copayment or coinsurance is variable, depending on the specific insurer and the prices they have negotiated with each of the players described above (PBMs, Pharmacies, Manufacturers). Private insurers paid almost half of all prescription expenditures in 2008, with the government picking up over a third of expenditures.

Medicare and Medicaid are the two largest government payers of prescription drugs. Medicare began prescription coverage (Medicare Part D) in 2006 for older adults and those younger than 65 who qualify for Medicare based on disability (see Chap. 2). Part D coverage has led to lower out-of-pocket costs, improved adherence to medications, and potentially improvements in health [56–59]. Nonetheless, the Part D benefit is strongly criticized because of the presence of a gap in coverage known as the "donut hole," which subjects beneficiaries to thousands of dollars in uncovered prescription expenses after an initial coverage period. The health reform law of 2010 began closing the "donut hole" by initially offering discounts on drugs in 2011 (50 % on brands, 7 % on generics), and by 2020 the gap will be eliminated. For further discussion of the donut hole, please see Chap. 19. Medicaid, the federal-state partnership that provides health insurance to low income Americans, accounts for about a quarter of government spending on prescription drugs; this proportion changed substantially in 2006 when Medicare replaced Medicaid as the main source of drug coverage for the dual eligibles (those eligible for both Medicare and Medicaid). The Department of Veterans Affairs and the Department of Defense are two other government payers of prescription drugs, although they obtain much lower prices for their drugs [60].

Selected Pharmaceutical Policy Issues

Off-Label Use

Off-label prescribing is when a medication is prescribed for an indication or patient population other than what is approved by the FDA [61]. Off-label use is important because it gives physicians an opportunity to innovate in clinical practice [62]. Physicians prescribe drugs off-label with the rationale that the effects of that drug will carry over to milder forms of the approved indication, related conditions, or distinct conditions with symptom overlap [62]. For example, the use of SSRIs for anxiety and ACE inhibitors for congestive heart failure began off-label [63]. Now, both are the standard of care for their respective diseases. Likewise, numerous standards of care in oncology, pediatrics, and obstetrics are based on off-label prescribing [61]. However, there has been much debate over the role of pharmaceutical companies in off-label use and whether physicians are prescribing drugs off-label without enough evidence.

Physicians have the ability to prescribe any drug to any patient if they believe it will benefit them. On the other hand, the FDA limits the marketing of drugs by pharmaceutical companies to only the approved indications [64]. Pharmaceutical companies have a very strong economic incentive to encourage off-label use of their drugs because it can significantly expand the market of the drug. For example, approximately 90 % of Neurontin's over $2.7 billion of sales in 2004 were for off-label use in diabetic neuropathy [65, 66]. From 1995 to 2008, off-label use of antipsychotics such as quetiapine, risperidone, and haloperidol rose in the USA from 4.4 million treatment visits to 9.0 million treatment visits [63].

The marketing practices of pharmaceutical companies can contribute to physician miseducation regarding the off-label use of drugs. Scientific evidence supporting off-label use can range from adequately studied to completely nonexistent [67]. In one study, a little over half of physicians surveyed were able to pick out correct pairs of drugs and their FDA-approved indications [68]. Another study found that 73 % of off-label prescribing had little or no scientific support [69]. There is also evidence indicating that research for off-label drug use, especially when funded by pharmaceutical companies, may be incorrectly reported and of questionable value [70]. Uneducated or unsupported off-label prescribing can be harmful because it may erode the public expectation that drugs will be safe and effective; increase health-care costs; cause manufacturers to pursue FDA approval for indications with cheaper clinical trials that can then be used for off-label promotion of the drug; and promote a culture that ignores evidence-based guidelines [62].

The FDA has pursued legal action against pharmaceutical companies in an effort to cut down on off-label marketing of drugs to physicians. The FDA has used the False Claims Act to prosecute marketing by pharmaceutical companies of off-label uses of drugs. Pfizer paid a $430 million settlement in 2003 for off-label marketing of Neurontin [65]. Recently, GlaxoSmithKline paid $3 billion for off-label marketing of nine drugs including Paxil, Wellbutrin, and Avandia [49]. Eli Lilly, Bristol Myers Squibb, Pfizer, and AstraZeneca have reached settlements worth more than $2.7 billion regarding the off-label marketing of antipsychotics to physicians for use in pediatric populations [71]. Due to the tension between the medical necessity of off-label prescribing and the desire of pharmaceutical companies to expand their markets, it is likely that more of these settlements will be seen in the future.

Conflicts of Interest

According to the Institute of Medicine, conflicts of interest are "circumstances that create a risk that professional judgments or actions regarding a primary interest will be unduly influenced by a secondary interest" [72]. The primary interests of physicians include providing patients with the best treatment possible and conducting high-quality, ethical research. Financial interests are the most scrutinized secondary interest, but other interests such as professional advancement and showing favor to friends, family, students, and colleagues are also secondary interests [72]. Conflicts of interest in academic medical centers have traditionally been associated with small gifts, free meals, funding for continuing medical education, speakers bureaus, ghostwriting, and consulting and research contracts [73]. Substantial efforts have been made to reduce exposure of trainees to these conflicts of interest, but many practices that could cause a conflict of interest among clinicians, researchers, and administrators still exist [74]. This section will focus on conflicts of interest involving patient care and research activities.

Two practices in patient care that have received attention for leading to conflicts of interest are free samples of prescription drugs and physician detailing. Free prescription drug samples are defended by pharmaceutical companies as a safety net that allows those with inadequate pharmaceutical benefits and little money to get the drugs they need. In 2004, $16.4 billion worth of free prescriptions were given out as samples [75]. However, a recent study showed that wealthier patients and those with continuous health insurance were more likely to receive samples than poorer patients and those who were uninsured for some or all of the year [76, 77]. The authors concluded that drug samples are not a safety net, but instead a marketing tool used to introduce patients to the latest prescription drugs. Patients who receive samples often have higher prescription drug costs than patients who do not [78]. One study found that frequently distributed drug samples for pediatric populations include one schedule 2 substance and four with black box warnings for serious side effects [76, 77]. Although the scientific literature indicates free samples ultimately do not improve the health of patients or bring down their health-care costs on a large scale, it is nonetheless possible that individual patients can benefit from samples in certain circumstances, either by saving on copayments or receiving a medication immediately without need to go to a pharmacy.

Physician detailing is a practice in which pharmaceutical sales representatives meet with physicians and highlight, or "detail", the uses and benefits of a drug [72]. One study estimates that $20.4 billion was spent on physician detailing in 2004 [79]. Physician detailing has been positively correlated with increased prescribing of a drug in numerous studies [72]. In a study of detailing for Neurontin, visits were found to be short (two-thirds of visits were less than 5 minutes long) but effective because 46 % of physicians planned to prescribe Neurontin more frequently as a result of the detailing [80].

There are many potential sources of a conflict of interest in research for physicians. Developing new innovations in medical treatment requires cooperation between industry and academia. Over half of all funding for biomedical research in the United States comes from industry [81]. When carrying out clinical trials funded by industry, a physician may relinquish the ability to control the design of the trial, access to data collected from the trial, or even the ability to write the manuscript [72]. This last practice, where a company writes the manuscript and the physician simply adds their name to it, is known as ghost writing. Another potential fear is that physicians will be driven by incentives such as financial benefits and professional advancement to continue studies that harm patients. Studies have consistently found that clinical trials funded by industry are much more likely than studies not funded by industry to have results favorable to industry in terms of drug efficacy and safety [72].

Efforts are being made by academic institutions and other organizations to reduce potential sources for conflicts of interest. Disclosure of financial relationships is one of the key elements to identifying and managing conflict of interest for physicians. Almost all medical journals require that physicians disclose any financial ties they have to industry. Medical schools typically require that physicians disclose financial ties to industry as well. When clinical trials are carried out in an academic setting, steps such as independent monitoring of the research project, internal or external data safety monitoring, or disclosing significant financial ties with industry to patients may be taken to manage the conflict of interest. Many medical schools require that investigators eliminate their financial interest in the company funding the trial.

Prescription Drug Abuse

Prescription drug abuse is a major problem in the United States that has coincided with a rise in the prescription of opioids for pain treatment. The CDC calls prescription drug abuse the "fastest growing drug problem in the United States" [82]. Unintentional overdose deaths increased by 124 % between 1999 and 2007 in the United States [83]. In 2007, over 11,000 people died from opioid overdose, more than cocaine and heroin combined [84]. In 2009, 15,597 people died from overdose of opioid analgesics [18–21]. A greater emphasis on treating patient pain has resulted in a huge increase in the amount of opioids prescribed to patients. Sales of oxycodone and methadone nearly quadrupled between 1997 and 2002 [84]. Sales of all opioids per person in the United States increased by 402 % between 1997 and 2007 [85]. One interesting effect of prescription opioid abuse is that rural states that previously did not have severe drug abuse issues, such as West Virginia, Utah, and Kentucky, have been hit hardest by the prescription drug abuse epidemic [82, 84]. The relatively easy accessibility of opioids in pharmacies has caused drug abuse problems in areas that previously did not have problems with illegal drugs.

Opioids and other potentially dangerous prescription drugs are regulated by the Drug Enforcement Agency (DEA) under the Controlled Substances Act (1970). Scheduled drugs (those that have the potential for abuse) are divided into five schedules of decreasing potential for abuse (Table 9.4). Schedule I drugs have a high potential for abuse, have no accepted medical use, and cannot be prescribed (1970). Schedules II through V can all be prescribed to patients. Physicians

Table 9.4 Examples of scheduled drugs

Schedule	Examples
I	Heroin, lysergic acid diethylamide (LSD), mescaline, marijuana, methaqualone
II	Oxycodone/OxyContin, methylphenidate, morphine
III	Hydrocodone, Tylenol w/codeine, buprenorphine, anabolic steroids, ketamine
IV	Clonazepam, Zolpidem, Modafinil, Midazolam
V	Robitussin w/codeine

Source: Data from [86, 87]

may only prescribe scheduled substances after registering with the DEA, and renewal of registration is required every 3 years [39, 40, 49, 50].

Physicians are in the difficult position of trying to balance the legitimate need for pain control in patients and preventing prescription drug abuse [84, 88]. One intervention used to prevent prescription drug abuse is a prescription drug monitoring program (PDMP). PDMPs collect data on dispensing of any controlled substance and make that information available for prescribers to see [38]. The goal of these programs is to enable physicians to make better informed decisions regarding whether a patient legitimately needs a drug or may be abusing or diverting the drug [38, 89]. According to the DEA, 37 states currently have operational PDMPs, and 11 states are putting PDMPs into place [38].

The latest effort to curb abuse of opioid analgesics is a recently approved FDA program called the Risk Evaluation and Mitigation Strategy (REMS) [18–21]. Approved in mid-2012, REMS applies to extended-release and long-acting prescription opioids such as OxyContin, Kadian, and Dolophine [18–21]. There are two components to REMS: a prescriber component and a patient component. The prescriber component is an optional educational program that will aid prescribers in determining when patients need opioids, whether adjustments in pain control need to be made, whether they are abusing opioids, and how to discontinue opioid prescriptions for patients that no longer need them [18–21]. Likewise, the patient component involves educating patients on how to use opioids safely, prevent and recognize overdose in themselves and others,

and dispose of extra drugs [18–21]. There was substantial debate over how far the REMS should go in regulating and tracking use of opioids [84, 90, 91]. It is unclear whether the REMS will ultimately be successful in slowing the abuse of opioids in the United States.

Medication Adherence

Nonadherence to medical treatment is a major problem in every health-care system. Adherence is defined as "the extent to which patients take medications as prescribed by their health care providers" [92]. The WHO estimates that adherence to treatment for chronic diseases in developed countries is approximately 50 % [93]. In many cases, adherence drops significantly in the first 6 months of treatment for chronic disease [92, 94–96]. In the USA, poor adherence leads to significantly worse health outcomes and costs the country between $100 and $300 billion in direct and indirect health-care costs annually [92, 97].

Medication adherence has taken on increased policy importance in the last few years, primarily because of the development of quality measures for medication use that include adherence measurement (Pharmacy Quality Alliance). With passage of the health reform law of 2010, Medicare Advantage plans will receive quality-based payments beginning in 2012 based on ratings that are publically reported (the "Star Ratings") [98]. Three of the 53 metrics used to calculate these ratings are measures of medication adherence for statins, oral diabetes, and hypertension medications. After statistical weights are applied, these three measures account for 11 % of the overall Star Rating for Medicare Advantage plans in 2012, thus taking on incredible financial, and thus policy, importance [99].

Interventions to improve adherence have had mixed results. One meta-analysis found that adherence was only increased 4–11 % for most interventions. Simplifying dosing regimens, improving patient health literacy, communicating the benefits and side effects of drugs, and expanding hours of operation have been shown to increase adherence [92]. Electronic reminder systems such as text messages, telemonitoring, and automated electronic monitoring devices are generally ineffective when used alone [100]. In person interventions such as counseling, family therapy, psychological therapy, crisis intervention, and manual telephone follow-up can be combined with electronic approaches to improve adherence, but they are costly, complex, and difficult to scale [92, 97]. In addition, gains in adherence have not proven to be sustainable for long periods of time [100]. Research is ongoing to develop new ways to overcome the many barriers leading to nonadherence.

Innovation

Despite continuous debate over whether individual drugs are safe and effective and debate over the best way to deliver drugs to patients, pharmaceuticals slowly but surely improve public health. The future of pharmaceuticals is an exciting one. The small molecule compounds that have been the mainstay of pharmaceutical therapy are slowly being enhanced with synthetic biological compounds. The increased availability of patient genetic information has the potential to provide patients with individualized therapies. New electronic technologies are streamlining and improving the safety of providing patients with drugs. In the following sections, we provide a brief overview of the first two areas of innovation. See Chap. 8 for a further discussion of emerging health information technology.

Biologics and Biosimilars

Broadly speaking, the FDA defines biological medicinal products as including "vaccines, blood and blood components, allergenics, somatic cells, gene therapy, tissues, and recombinant therapeutic proteins" [101]. "Biologics" are a subclass of biological medicinal products that are created by recombinant DNA technology. The European Agency for the Evaluation of Medicinal Products defines biologics as "products containing biotechnology-derived proteins as active substances" [102]. In contrast to conventional small molecule pharmaceuticals such as aspirin or fluoxetine, biologics are carbohydrates, proteins, nucleic acids, complex mixtures of any of these three, cells, or tissues [101]. Biologics are much more sensitive to manufacturing conditions than conventional pharmaceuticals and contain much more uncertainty in terms of structure and exact characterization [101]. The practices of rheumatology and oncology have been revolutionized by the development of monoclonal antibodies such as etanercept, adalimumab, and trastuzumab [18–21]. However, biologics can be extremely costly. For example, imiglucerase for Gaucher's diseases costs $200,000 per year [103].

The potential benefits that patients can receive from biologics and their high cost have spurred biopharmaceutical companies and regulatory agencies to push development and approval of "generic biologics" [104]. However, due to the inherent differences between pharmaceuticals produced with chemical methods (conventional drugs) and biological methods (biologics), there is much debate over how to regulate "follow-on" biologics. The term given to these follow-on biologics is biosimilars. Biosimilars are not called generic biologics because they are often manufactured using different processes from the original and have some differences in regard to structure and function (generic conventional drugs have identical active ingredients) [105]. Due to the size and complexity of biopharmaceuticals, biosimilars are not exactly identical to their biologic counterparts and may have decreased efficacy or safety (typically due to immunogenicity issues) [105]. In 2009, Congress passed the Biologics Price Competition and Innovation Act (BCPI) in order to create an abbreviated pathway for biosimilars [104]. However, the inherent differences between biologics and biosimilars require a substantial amount of testing data that keeps the approval process costly and lengthy, potentially offering no advantage over submitting a new Biologics License Product [103]. The FDA has yet to approve a drug through the biosimilars pathway.

Numerous other issues exist with biosimilars. One difficulty for biosimilars is that they do not provide the same level of cost savings as generic drugs do. Biosimilar products usually cost 25–30 % less than biologics instead of 80 % less like conventional drugs [103]. Also, biosimilars cannot be switched for their brand-name biologics without a prescriber order or unless the products are shown to be interchangeable [23–25]. Two products are interchangeable only if they can be expected to produce the same clinical result in any given patient and the risk of adverse effects or decreased efficacy is not any less when alternating between the two drugs compared to using only one drug [23–25]. These standards have been imposed because biosimilars have caused adverse immune reactions not seen in the original biologic [105]. Ongoing research and debate regarding how to make the benefits of biologic drugs available to patients at a reasonable cost without unnecessary risks will be required.

Personalized Medicine

In 2003, the Human Genome Project was completed after 13 years to great fanfare [106]. Researchers and physicians believed that a new age of personalized medicine with genomics informing medical decisions would soon follow. Patients would be able to receive treatments with a high possibility of working and avoid unnecessary disappointment and cost with treatments that were doomed from the beginning due to their genetic makeup. While such certainty is not yet a reality, there are already genetic tests that are used to help determine treatment plans for patients with certain conditions. Gene variants of cytochrome 2C9 (CYP2C9) and vitamin K epoxide reductase complex 1 (VKORC1) in combination with observable physical data such as age, height, and weight can be used to calculate warfarin dosages for patients. Targeted therapies are used frequently in the treatment of cancer to only use drugs in patients with gene variants that will allow the drug to be effective. Some examples include trastuzumab for HER2-positive metastatic breast cancer, imatinib for Philadelphia chromosome-positive chronic myeloid leukemia, and epidermal growth factor inhibitor for non-small cell lung cancer [107]. As of 2010, pharmacogenomic information was available on about 10 % of FDA-approved drug labels [108].

There is also optimism for using genetic information to aid in drug development. Genetic testing may help researchers to identify subpopulations at high risk for side effects [109]. These subpopulations could be excluded from clinical trials, the drugs could be shown to be efficacious and safe in all other patients, and the drugs could be approved along with a diagnostic test for the genes that predispose to side effects [109]. Ideally, this personalized approach would help open up the drug development pipeline. Promising drugs from the past that were shelved during clinical trials due to adverse events could be revisited to see whether a certain gene mutation or group of mutations predisposed patients to serious side effects [108].

Despite the great promise of genomics and personalized medicine, questions and concerns exist over how to implement it properly. It is currently unclear what level of evidence should be required before a genetic test is used to inform clinical decisions. Are randomized controlled trials necessary to validate a test or can retrospective or prospective observational studies be used instead? What kind of clinical end points are appropriate for determining whether a test provides predictive value? Commentators have also raised concerns over whether genetic testing will truly be able to decrease costs and improve outcomes [110]. There has also been concern regarding the use of genetic information in a discriminatory manner by employers, insurance companies, and others. Congress partially addressed this question through the Genetic Information Nondiscrimination Act of 2008 which prevents employers and health insurers from considering genetic information when making decisions regarding individuals or requesting that they get genetic testing [111]. As genetic testing become more ubiquitous, there is likely to be more discussion on how the information should be used.

References

1. Wood AJJ. A proposal for radical changes in the drug-approval process. N Engl J Med. 2006;355(6):618–23.
2. Kaiser Family Foundation: Prescription drug trends. http://kaiserfamilyfoundation.files.wordpress.com/2013/01/3057-08.pdf (2010). Accessed 28 July 2012.
3. Kaiser Family Foundation. Prescription drug costs background brief. 2010. http://www.kaiseredu.org/Issue-Modules/Prescription-Drug-Costs/Background-Brief.aspx, Accessed 28 July 2012.
4. IMS Institute for Healthcare Informatics. Channel distribution by U.S. dispensed prescriptions. 2012. http://www.imshealth.com/deployedfiles/ims/Global/Content/Corporate/Press%20Room/Top-Line%20Market%20Data%20&%20Trends/2011%20Top-line%20Market%20Data/Channels_by_RX.pdf, Accessed 28 July 2012.
5. IMS Institute for Healthcare Informatics: The use of medicines in the United States: review of 2011. http://www.imshealth.com/ims/Global/Content/Insights/IMS%20Institute%20for%20Healthcare%20Informatics/IHII_Medicines_in_U.S_Report_2011.pdf (2012). Accessed 28 July 2012.
6. AHRQ. Prescription medicines – mean and median expenses per person with expense and distribution of expenses by source of payment: United States, 2009. http://meps.ahrq.gov/mepsweb/data_stats/tables_compendia_hh_interactive.jsp?_SERVICE=MEPSSocket0&_PROGRAM=MEPSPGM.TC.SAS&File=HCFY2009&Table=HCFY2009_PLEXP_A&VAR1=AGE&VAR2=SEX&VAR3=RACETH5C&VAR4=INSURCOV&VAR5=POVCAT09&VAR6=MSA&VAR7=REGION&VAR8=HEALTH&VARO1=4+17+44+64&VARO2=1&VARO3=1&VARO4=1&VARO5=1&VARO6=1&VARO7=1&VARO8=1&_Debug= (2009). Accessed 29 August 2012.
7. United States Census Bureau. 2008 national population projections. 2008. http://www.census.gov/population/www/projections/2008projections.html Accessed 3 August 2012
8. Centers for Disease Control and Prevention. Life tables. 2011. http://www.cdc.gov/nchs/products/life_tables.htm#life Accessed 24 August 2012.
9. Kaiser Family Foundation: Health care costs: a primer. http://kaiserfamilyfoundation.files.wordpress.com/2013/01/7670-03.pdf (2012). Accessed 28 July 2012.
10. Gellad WF, Donohue JM, et al. The financial burden from prescription drugs has declined recently for the nonelderly, although it is still high for many. Health Aff. 2012;31(2):408–16.
11. IMS Institute for Healthcare Informatics: The use of medicines in the United States: review of 2010. http://www.imshealth.com/deployedfiles/imshealth/Global/Content/IMS%20Institute/Static%20File/IHII_UseOfMed_report.pdf (2011). Accessed 19 Aug 2012.
12. Armstrong D. Pfizer Sees Harvard Collaboration as spark for new drugs. 2012. http://www.bloomberg.com/news/2012-06-15/pfizer-sees-harvard-collaboration-as-spark-for-new-drugs.html Accessed 20 Aug 2012.
13. NIH. Understanding clinical trials. 2007. http://clinicaltrials.gov/ct2/info/understand Accessed 29 July 2012.
14. FDA. How drugs are developed and approved. 2010. http://www.fda.gov/Drugs/DevelopmentApprovalProcess/HowDrugsareDevelopedandApproved/default.htm Accessed 1 Sep 2012.
15. DiMasi JA, Hansen RW, et al. The price of innovation: new estimates of drug development costs. J Health Econ. 2003;22(2):151–85.
16. Adams CP, Brantner VV. Estimating the cost of new drug development: is it really $802 million? Health Aff. 2006;25(2):420–8.
17. Paul SM, Mytelka DS, et al. How to improve R&D productivity: the pharmaceutical industry's grand challenge. Nat Rev Drug Discov. 2010;9(3):203–14.
18. FDA. Developing products for rare diseases & conditions. 2012. http://www.fda.gov/ForIndustry/DevelopingProductsforRareDiseasesConditions/default.htm Accessed 1 Sep 2012
19. FDA. Questions and answers: FDA approves a Risk Evaluation and Mitigation Strategy (REMS) for Extended-Release and Long-Acting (ER/LA) opioid analgesics. 2012. http://www.fda.gov/Drugs/DrugSafety/InformationbyDrugClass/ucm309742.htm, Accessed 9 Jan 2013
20. FDA. Risk Evaluation and Mitigation Strategy (REMS) for Extended-Release and Long-Acting opioids. 2012. http://www.fda.gov/drugs/drugsafety/informationbydrugclass/ucm163647.htm Accessed 9 Jan 2013.
21. FDA. The road to the biotech revolution – highlights of 100 years of biologics regulation. 2012. http://www.fda.gov/AboutFDA/WhatWeDo/History/FOrgsHistory/CBER/ucm135758.htm, Accessed 25 Aug 2013.

22. Kesselheim AS. Using market-exclusivity incentives to promote pharmaceutical innovation. N Engl J Med. 2010;363(19):1855–62.

23. FDA. Frequently asked questions on patents and exclusivity. 2011. http://www.fda.gov/Drugs/DevelopmentApprovalProcess/ucm079031.htm, Accessed 9 Jan 2013.

24. FDA. Generic drugs: questions and answers. 2011. http://www.fda.gov/Drugs/ResourcesForYou/Consumers/QuestionsAnswers/ucm100100.htm, Accessed 9 Jan 2013

25. FDA. Information for consumers (biosimilars). 2011. http://www.fda.gov/Drugs/Development ApprovalProcess/HowDrugsareDevelopedand Approved/ApprovalApplications/Therapeutic BiologicApplications/Biosimilars/ucm241718.htm. Accessed 1 Jan 2013

26. United States Patent and Trademark Office. Patents. 2012. http://www.uspto.gov/inventors/patents.jsp, Accessed 24 Aug 2013

27. OIS. Generic drug utilization in State Medicaid programs. http://oig.hhs.gov/oei/reports/oei-05-05-00360.pdf (2006). Accessed 19 Aug 2012.

28. Generic Pharmaceutical Association: Savings: an economic analysis of generic drug usage in the U.S. http://www.gphaonline.org/media//cms/IMSStudy Aug2012WEB.pdf (2011). Accessed 29 July 2012.

29. ASPE HHS: Expanding the use of generic drugs. http://aspe.hhs.gov/sp/reports/2010/genericdrugs/ib.shtml (2010). Accessed 30 Aug 2012.

30. Shrank WH, Choudhry NK, et al. State generic substitution laws can lower drug outlays under Medicaid. Health Aff. 2010;29(7):1383–90.

31. Kaiser Family Foundation: Follow the pill: understanding the U.S. commercial pharmaceutical supply chain. http://kaiserfamilyfoundation.files.wordpress.com/2013/01/follow-the-pill-understanding-the-u-s-commercial-pharmaceutical-supply-chain-report.pdf (2005). Accessed 19 Aug 2012.

32. PharmExec. Pharm Exec 50: growth from the bottom up. 2012. http://www.pharmexec.com/pharmexec/article/articleDetail.jsp?id=773562&pageID=1&sk=&date=, Accessed 29 Aug 2013.

33. Modern Distribution Management. Trends and top distributors in the pharmaceuticals sector. 2012. http://www.mdm.com/2012_pharmaceuticals_mdm-market-leaders, Accessed 19 Aug 2013

34. Pembroke Consulting: The 2011–2012 economic report on retail and specialty pharmacies. http://www.drugchannels.net/2012/01/2011-12-economic-report-on-retail-and.html (2012). Accessed 30 Aug 2012.

35. Pharmacy Benefit Management Institute. PBM market share. 2010. http://www.pbmi.com/PBMmarketshare1.asp, Accessed 20 Aug 2012

36. Berry E. 2 of 3 largest PBMs combine. 2012. http://www.ama-assn.org/amednews/2012/04/16/bisb0416.htm, Accessed 20 Aug 2013.

37. IBISWorld. Pharmacy benefit management in the US: market research report. 2012. http://www.ibisworld.com/industry/pharmacy-benefit-management.html, Accessed 24 Aug 2012.

38. DEA. Office of Diversion Control. State prescription drug monitoring programs. 2011. http://www.deadiversion.usdoj.gov/faq/rx_monitor.htm, Accessed 7 Aug 2012.

39. DEA. Office of Diversion Control. Mid-level practitioners authorization by state. 2012. http://www.deadiversion.usdoj.gov/drugreg/practioners/mlp_by_state.pdf, Accessed 19 Aug 2013.

40. DEA. Office of Diversion Control. Questions & answers. 2012. http://www.deadiversion.usdoj.gov/drugreg/faq.htm, Accessed 7 Aug 2013

41. American Psychological Association. Can psychologists prescribe medications for their patients? 2012. http://www.apa.org/support/about/psych/prescribe.aspx#answer, Accessed 19 Aug 2012.

42. PBM Plus Inc: Pharmacy benefit design considerations. http://www.pbmplus.com/docs/pharmacy_benefit_design.pdf (2008). Accessed 4 Aug 2012.

43. Malkin JD, Goldman DP, et al. The changing face of pharmacy benefit design. Health Aff. 2004;23(1):194–9.

44. California Healthcare Foundation: Navigating the pharmacy benefits marketplace. http://www.chcf.org/~/media/MEDIA%20LIBRARY%20Files/PDF/N/PDF%20NavPharmBenefits.pdf (2003). Accessed 26 Aug 2012.

45. GAO: Effects of using pharmacy benefit managers on health plans, enrollees, and pharmacies. http://www.gao.gov/new.items/d03196.pdf (2003). Accessed 4 Aug 2012.

46. Berndt, ER, Newhouse, JP.: Pricing and reimbursement in US pharmaceutical markets. National Bureau of Economic Research. http://www.nber.org/papers/w16297 (2010). Accessed 3 Sept 2012.

47. Frank RG. Prescription-drug prices. N Engl J Med. 2004;351(14):1375–7.

48. Scherer FM. Price controls and global pharmaceutical progress. Health Aff. 2009;28(1):w161–4.

49. Department of Justice: McKesson Corp. Pays U.S. more than $190 million to resolve false claims act accusations. http://www.justice.gov/opa/pr/2012/April/12-civ-539.html (2012). Accessed 3 Sept 2012.

50. Department of Justice. GlaxoSmithKline to plead guilty and pay $3 billion to resolve fraud allegations and failure to report safety data. 2012. http://www.justice.gov/opa/pr/2012/July/12-civ-842.html, Accessed 5 Aug 2012.

51. Frank RG. Prescription drug prices: why do some pay more than others do? Health Aff. 2001;20(2):115–28.

52. Zhang Y, Zhou L, et al. Potential savings from greater use of $4 generic drugs. Arch Intern Med. 2011;171(5):468.

53. Pollack, A. States seek curb on patient bills for costly drugs. The New York Times. http://www.nytimes.com/2012/04/13/health/states-seek-to-curb-exorbitant-drug-costs-incurred-by-patients.html?pagewanted=all (2012). Accessed 3 Sept 2012.

54. Gellad W, Haas J, et al. Race/ethnicity and nonadherence to prescription medications among seniors:

results of a national study. J Gen Intern Med. 2007;22(11):1572–8.

55. Goldman DP, Joyce GF, Zheng Y. Prescription drug cost sharing: associations with medication and medical utilization and spending and health. JAMA. 2007;298(1):61–9.

56. Madden JM, Graves AJ, et al. Cost-related medication nonadherence and spending on basic needs following implementation of Medicare Part D. JAMA. 2008;299(16):1922–8.

57. Zhang Y, Donohue JM, et al. The effect of Medicare Part D on drug and medical spending. N Engl J Med. 2009;361(1):52–61.

58. McWilliams JM, Zaslavsky AM, Huskamp HA. Implementation of Medicare Part D and nondrug medical spending for elderly adults with limited prior drug coverage. JAMA. 2011;306(4): 402–9.

59. Polinski JM, Donohue JM, et al. Medicare Part D's effect on the under-and overuse of medications: a systematic review. J Am Geriatr Soc. 2011;59(10):1922–33.

60. Gellad W, Schneeweiss S, et al. What if the federal government negotiated pharmaceutical prices for seniors? An estimate of national savings. J Gen Intern Med. 2008;23(9):1435–40.

61. Roebuck MC, Liberman JN. Impact of pharmacy benefit design on prescription drug utilization: a fixed effects analysis of plan sponsor data. Health Serv Res. 2008;44(3):988–1009.

62. Stafford RS. Regulating off-label drug use— rethinking the role of the FDA. N Engl J Med. 2008;358(14):1427–9.

63. Alexander GC, Gallagher SA, et al. Increasing off-label use of antipsychotic medications in the United States, 1995–2008. Pharmacoepidemiol Drug Saf. 2011;20(2):177–84.

64. (1962). Kefauver-Harris Drug Amendments Public Law 87–781. 21 U.S.C. 352(n).

65. Armstrong D, Zimmerman R. Pfizer to settle Medicaid-fraud case. 2004. http://online.wsj.com/article/0,,SB108440099145209983,00.html, Accessed 26 Aug 2012.

66. Pfizer: Annual review 2004. http://www.pfizer.com/investors/financial_reports/financial_reports_annualreview_2004.jsp (2005). Accessed 25 Aug 2012.

67. Avorn J, Kesselheim A. A hemorrhage of off-label use. Ann Intern Med. 2011;154(8):566–7.

68. Chen DT, Wynia MK, et al. U.S. physician knowledge of the FDA-approved indications and evidence base for commonly prescribed drugs: results of a national survey. Pharmacoepidemiol Drug Saf. 2009;18(11):1094–100.

69. Radley DC, Finkelstein SN, Stafford RS. Off-label prescribing among office-based physicians. Arch Intern Med. 2006;166(9):1021–6.

70. Vedula SS, Bero L, et al. Outcome reporting in industry – sponsored trials of gabapentin for off-label use. N Engl J Med. 2009;361(20):1963–71.

71. Szalavitz, M.: Why are so many foster care children taking antipsychotics? Time. http://healthland.time.com/2011/11/29/why-are-so-many-foster-care-children-taking-antipsychotics/ (2011). Accessed 20 Aug 2012.

72. IOM: Conflict of interest in medical research, education, and practice. http://www.iom.edu/Reports/2009/Conflict-of-Interest-in-Medical-Research-Education-and-Practice.aspx (2009). Accessed 7 Aug 2012.

73. Brennan TA, Rothman DJ, Blank L, et al. Health industry practices that create conflicts of interest: a policy proposal for academic medical centers. JAMA. 2006;295(4):429–33.

74. AMSA. Conflict of interest policies at academic medical centers. 2012. http://www.amsascorecard.org/, Accessed 25 Aug 2012

75. Donohue JM, Cevasco M, Rosenthal MB. A decade of direct-to-consumer advertising of prescription drugs. N Engl J Med. 2007;357(7):673–81.

76. Cutrona SL, Woolhandler S, et al. Free drug samples in the United States: characteristics of pediatric recipients and safety concerns. Pediatrics. 2008;122(4):736–42.

77. Cutrona SL, Woolhandler S, et al. Characteristics of recipients of free prescription drug samples: a nationally representative analysis. Am J Public Health. 2008;98(2):284–9.

78. Alexander GC, Zhang J, et al. Characteristics of patients receiving pharmaceutical samples and association between sample receipt and out-of-pocket prescription costs. Med Care. 2008;46(4):394–402.

79. Gagnon MA, Lexchin J. The cost of pushing pills: a new estimate of pharmaceutical promotion expenditures in the United States. PLoS Med. 2008;5(1):e1.

80. Steinman MA, Harper GM, et al. Characteristics and impact of drug detailing for gabapentin. PLoS Med. 2007;4(4):e134.

81. Moses H, Dorsey ER, et al. Financial anatomy of biomedical research. JAMA. 2005;294(11):1333–42.

82. CDC. CDC grand rounds: prescription drug overdoses – a U.S. epidemic. 2012. http://www.cdc.gov/mmwr/preview/mmwrhtml/mm6101a3.htm, Accessed 7 Aug 2012

83. Bohnert AS, Valenstein M, Bair MJ, Ganoczy D, McCarthy JF, Ilgen MA, Blow FC. Association between opioid prescribing patterns and opioid overdose-related deaths. JAMA. 2011;305(13):1315–21.

84. Okie S. A flood of opioids, a rising tide of deaths. N Engl J Med. 2010;363(21):1981–5.

85. Manchikanti L, Fellows B, Ailinani H, Pampati V. Therapeutic use, abuse, and nonmedical use of opioids: a ten-year perspective. Pain Physician. 2010;13:401–35.

86. (1970). Controlled Substances Act - schedules of controlled substances. 21 U.S.C. United States, http://www.deadiversion.usdoj.gov/21cfr/cfr/2108cfrt.htm.

87. (1970). Controlled Substances Act Public Law 91–513. U.S.C.

88. Perrone J, Nelson LS. Medication reconciliation for controlled substances—an "ideal" prescription-drug monitoring program. N Engl J Med. 2012;366(25):2341–3.

89. Gugelmann HM, Perrone J. Can prescription drug monitoring programs help limit opioid abuse? JAMA. 2011;306(20):2258–9.

90. Goozner M. Oncologists want FDA to rethink REMS. J Natl Cancer Inst. 2010;102(23):1748–51.

91. Nelson LS, Perrone J. Curbing the opioid epidemic in the United States: the risk evaluation and mitigation strategy (REMS). JAMA. 2012;308(5):457–8.

92. Osterberg L, Blaschke T. Adherence to medication. N Engl J Med. 2005;353(5):487–97.

93. WHO: Adherence to long-term therapies. http://whqlibdoc.who.int/publications/2003/9241545992.pdf (2003). Accessed 8 Aug 2012.

94. Haynes RB, McDonald HP, Garg AX. Helping patients follow prescribed treatment: clinical applications. JAMA. 2002;288(22):2880–3.

95. Jackevicius CA, Mamdani M, Tu JV. Adherence with statin therapy in elderly patients with and without acute coronary syndromes. JAMA. 2002;288(4):462–7.

96. Cramer J, Rosenheck R, et al. Medication compliance feedback and monitoring in a clinical trial: predictors and outcomes. Value Health. 2003;6(5):566–73.

97. Bosworth HB, Granger BB, Mendys P, Brindis R, Burkholder R, Czajkowski SM, et al. Medication adherence: a call for action. Am Heart J. 2011;162(3):412–24.

98. Kaiser Family Foundation: Reaching for the stars: quality ratings of Medicare advantage plans, 2011. http://kaiserfamilyfoundation.files.wordpress.com/2013/01/8151.pdf (2011). Accessed 4 Sept 2012.

99. McKethan A, Benner J, et al. Seizing the opportunity to improve medication adherence. Health Aff. 2012 Aug 28. http://healthaffairs.org/blog/2012/08/28/seizing-the-opportunity-to-improve-medication-adherence/, Accessed 4 Sep 2012.

100. Granger BB, Bosworth HB. Medication adherence: emerging use of technology. Curr Opin Cardiol. 2011;26(4):279–87.

101. FDA. What are "biologics" questions and answers. 2009. http://www.fda.gov/AboutFDA/CentersOffices/OfficeofMedicalProductsandTobacco/CBER/ucm133077.htm, Accessed 9 Jan 2012.

102. Committee for Medicinal Products for Human Use: Guideline on similar biological medicinal products, European Medicines Agency. http://www.ema.europa.eu/docs/en_GB/document_library/Scientific_guideline/2009/09/WC500003517.pdf (2005). Accessed 30 Aug 2012.

103. Engelberg AB, Kesselheim AS, et al. Balancing innovation, access, and profits—market exclusivity for biologics. N Engl J Med. 2009;361(20):1917–19.

104. Kozlowski S, Woodcock J, et al. Developing the nation's biosimilars program. N Engl J Med. 2011;365(5):385–8.

105. Roger S, Mikhail A. Biosimilars: opportunity or cause for concern? J Pharm Pharm Sci. 2007;10(3):5.

106. DOE. Human genome project information. 2012. http://www.ornl.gov/sci/techresources/Human_Genome/home.shtml, Accessed 11 Aug 2013.

107. Lesko LJ. Personalized medicine: elusive dream or imminent reality? Clin Pharmacol Ther. 2007;81(6):807–16.

108. Hamburg MA, Collins FS. The path to personalized medicine. N Engl J Med. 2010;363(4):301–4.

109. Evans WE, Relling MV. Moving towards individualized medicine with pharmacogenomics. Nature. 2004;429(6990):464–8.

110. Burke W, Psaty BM. Personalized medicine in the era of genomics. JAMA. 2007;298(14):1682–4.

111. Hudson KL, Holohan MK, et al. Keeping pace with the times—the Genetic Information Nondiscrimination Act of 2008. N Engl J Med. 2008;358(25):2661–3.

Health Disparities

10

Neil M. Issar and Manish K. Sethi

> **Learning Objectives**
> *After completing this chapter, the reader should be able to answer the following questions*:
> - When did health disparities become a focus of research?
> - How is the term "health disparities" defined?
> - How are health disparities and the factors that affect health disparities measured?
> - What are some examples of health disparities associated with race/ethnicity?
> - What are some examples of health disparities associated with socioeconomic status?
> - What are some examples of health disparities associated with education?
> - What are some examples of health disparities associated with a lack of health insurance?
> - What are some examples of health disparities associated with geography and living conditions?
> - What are some examples of health disparities associated with disability?
> - How are health disparities being addressed?

N.M. Issar, B.S.
Vanderbilt University Medical Center,
Vanderbilt University School of Medicine,
Nashville, TN 37232, USA
e-mail: neil.issar@vanderbilt.edu

M.K. Sethi, M.D. (✉)
Director of the Vanderbilt Orthopaedic Institute Center
for Health Policy, Assistant Professor of Orthopaedic
Trauma Surgery, Department of Orthopaedic Surgery
and Rehabilitation, Vanderbilt University School of
Medicine, Nashville, TN 37232, USA
e-mail: manish.sethi@vanderbilt.edu

Introduction

Disparities in health across different social groups have always existed, and the Healthy People initiative of the US Department of Health and Human Services (DHHS) has aimed to eliminate health disparities among different segments of the US population (defined in terms of income, education, insurance status, race/ethnicity, residence, disability, etc.) since the 1970s. However, global research efforts were first truly galvanized in 1980 by the publication of a report commissioned by the Department of Health and Social Security in the United Kingdom, entitled "Inequalities in Health" [1]. The term "inequalities," more commonly referred to as "disparities" in the United States, was used to characterize the poor relative health of socially and economically deprived populations [2]. Since then, health disparities have been considered a matter for concern, both nationally and internationally.

In 1985, DHHS Secretary Margaret Heckler released the Secretary's Task Force Report on Black and Minority Health, which documented excess deaths from cancer, cardiovascular diseases, diabetes, chemical dependency, homicide, unintentional injuries, and infant mortality experienced by minority populations and focused attention on significant gaps in health status between whites and minorities [3]. The report also revealed decades of neglect in seeking solutions and thrust the health of minorities and other disadvantaged groups back onto the national agenda. The Task Force report spurred the DHHS in 1986 to establish the Office of Minority Health (OMH), which was designated with the responsibility to implement the report's recommendations.

In 1988, the Centers for Disease Control and Prevention (CDC) created the Office of the Associate Director for Minority Health, which then became the CDC's Office of Minority Health in 2002. In 2005, the CDC strengthened its commitment to promote health and quality of life and to eliminate health disparities for vulnerable populations by forming the Office of Minority Health and Health Disparities (OMHD), which subsequently became the National Center on Minority Health and Health Disparities (NCMHD).

The more recent passage of the Health Care and Education Reconciliation Act of 2010 authorized the transition of NCMHD to become the National Institute on Minority Health and Health Disparities, expanding its mission to planning, reviewing, coordinating, and evaluating all minority health and health disparities research activities conducted and supported by the NIH institutes and associated centers.

The Health Care and Education Reconciliation Act also supports the goals of the aforementioned Healthy People initiative. This initiative serves as the US government's strategic management instrument by identifying preventable threats to health and setting the country's agenda for the prevention of disease and reduction of mortality. The first edition of health objectives for racial and ethnic minority populations was initiated in Healthy People 2000. The elimination of health disparities became an official objective in Healthy People 2010. The next iteration, Healthy People 2020, seeks to eliminate preventable disease, disability, injury, and premature death; achieve health equity, eliminate disparities, and improve the health of all groups; create social and physical environments that promote good health for all; and promote healthy development and healthy behaviors across every stage of life.

Definitions

Although the 1980 report by United Kingdom's Department of Health and Social Security had a specific characterization of the term "inequalities," used interchangeably with the term "disparities," research over the last three decades has substantially muddled the term's definition. In addition, how one defines "health disparities" can have important policy implications with practical consequences. It can determine not only which measurements are monitored by national, state, and local governments and international agencies, but also which activities will receive support from resources allocated to address the disparities.

One of the earliest concise definitions of health disparities was articulated by Professor Margaret Whitehead in the 1990s as "differences in health that are not only unnecessary and avoidable but, in addition, are considered unfair and unjust." She wrote that "equity in health implies that everyone should ideally have a fair opportunity to attain their full health potential and, more pragmatically, that no one should be disadvantaged from achieving this potential, if it can be avoided" [4, 5]. Whitehead further defined equity in healthcare "as equal access to available care for equal need, equal utilization for equal need, and equal quality of care for all" [5]. Thus, while Whitehead did not specifically use the term "disadvantaged" in her definition of health disparities, it is clear from her definition of health equity that she was referring to disparities or differences that adversely affected disadvantaged groups of individuals. To demonstrate this, she used examples of differences in children's life expectancies according to their parents' social class or in adults' life expectancies according to their own social class, as well as differences in a range of health indicators by residence in urban versus rural settings or in slums versus affluent areas within the same city [4]. Consequently, socioeconomic status is a factor that has consistently been linked with health disparities.

The definition further evolved when the 1995–1998 WHO initiative on Equity in Health and Health Care defined equity in health as "minimizing avoidable disparities in health and its determinants – including but not limited to healthcare – between groups of people who have different levels of underlying social advantage or privilege." These social advantages were implied to include different levels of power, wealth, or prestige due to positions in society relative to other groups of individuals, but could also include gender, ethnicity, age, and other differences [4].

Braveman and Gruskin further defined equity in health as the absence of systematic disparities in health (or in the major social determinants of health) between groups with different levels of underlying social advantage/disadvantage such as wealth, power, or prestige [4]. Inequities or disparities in health systematically put groups of people who are already socially disadvantaged (for example, by virtue of being poor, female, and/or members of a disenfranchised racial, ethnic, or religious group) at further disadvantage with respect to their health.

The aforementioned 2010 iteration of the Healthy People initiative indicated that health disparities included "differences by gender, race/ethnicity, education, income, disability, geographic location, or sexual orientation." As mentioned previously, this initiative focuses predominantly on racial/ethnic disparities due to the magnitude, pervasiveness, and persistence or widening of these gaps.

Dr. Paula Braveman subsequently proposed a more comprehensive definition of a health disparity as being a particular type of difference in health or in the most important influences on health that could potentially be shaped by policies. She states that it is a difference in which disadvantaged social groups (such as the poor, racial/ethnic minorities, women, or other groups that have persistently experienced social disadvantage or discrimination) systematically experience worse health or greater health risks than more advantaged groups [4].

In general, health disparities are systematic and avoidable health differences according to race/ethnicity, skin color, religion, or nationality; socioeconomic resources or position (reflected by, e.g., income, wealth, education, or occupation); gender, sexual orientation, gender identity; age, geography, disability, illness, political, or other affiliation; or other characteristics associated (though not necessarily causally linked) with discrimination or marginalization.

However, these definitions ultimately elicit debates around the world about the scope and measurement of health disparities, and there is still controversy as to whether definitions of health disparities should imply injustice or simply reflect differences in health outcomes, and whether or not they should be limited to associations with race and ethnicity. This chapter will view health disparities as a more inclusive term, analyzing disparities across a number of social standards and criteria, including race/ethnicity, socioeconomic status, level of education, health insurance, geography, physical environment, and disability status.

Before delving into the analysis of these disparities, it is important to point out a distinction elucidated by Adler and Rehkopf [6]. They distinguish between a health difference, which results from inherent biological distinctions, and a health disparity, which results predominantly from the social factors listed earlier. For example, the fact that only women are subject to ovarian cancer and men to prostate cancer would constitute a health difference and not a disparity. However, there may be a disparity in the death rates from these diseases if there is different allocation of resources for research and healthcare to one of these cancers over the other.

In addition, while genetics affect the disparities for some diseases, the effect is negligible in many cases. For example, African-Americans have higher rates of hypertension than European Americans, which may be attributable to a higher genetic vulnerability in the former group. However, this can be contested by the fact that the prevalence of hypertension among blacks is lower in Caribbean countries than in the United States and lower still among blacks in Africa. In fact, hypertension rates in Africa are equivalent to or lower than rates among whites in the USA [7]. This suggests that the higher rates of hypertension among African-Americans in the USA are more likely due to social factors than to underlying genetic vulnerability.

Thus, while health disparities may be affected by both biological differences and social factors, this chapter's focus on the latter is for two reasons: not only is the effect of social factors greater in almost all cases, but these factors are also largely avoidable and/or reversible.

Measuring Health Disparities

There are various ways of measuring and/or quantifying health disparities. When only two populations of individuals are compared, a rate ratio is most commonly calculated to measure a particular disparity. For example, in the United States, the annual rate of infant mortality among African-American babies (14.4 per 1,000 live births) is more than two times the rate among European American babies (5.7 per 1,000 live births) [4]. Two groups can also be compared by calculating a rate difference (typically defined as the absolute difference in rates). For example, the rate difference in infant mortality between African-Americans and European Americans is approximately 8 per 1,000 live births. Both absolute and relative differences can be meaningful [4].

Socioeconomic status may be measured based on level of education, occupational characteristics, income and expenditures, accumulated wealth, health insurance, and/or residence in geographic areas or physical environments with particular social or economic conditions. More complex statistical measurements such as population attributable risk can be used to quantify the magnitude of socioeconomic inequalities of health.

Economic inequality in particular can be measured using the Gini coefficient. Braveman explains this measure as one that reflects the overall difference between the observed distribution of economic resources (such as income) in a given society and a theoretical situation in which everyone has exactly the same economic resources. Some researchers have examined how income inequalities in certain geographic areas (using the Gini coefficient or similar measures) are associated with aggregate levels of health experienced by people residing in those areas [8, 9].

Finally, the index of dissimilarity (ID) has been proposed by some authors to measure the overall magnitude of disparities across diverse kinds of groups (such as those separated by race/ethnicity or socioeconomic status). The ID for a given health indicator sums the differences between rates in each subgroup and the overall population rate, expressing the total as a percentage of the overall population rate.

Thus, there are a number of statistical measurements that have been used or produced to quantify various forms of disparity. This chapter will tend to use simpler methods of quantification, with a greater emphasis on providing a broad range of examples of disparities instead of exhaustive statistical calculations.

Race and Ethnicity

Two major foci of disparities research in the USA are race and ethnicity. The 2000 US Census indicated that 34.6 million Americans identified as black or African-American, 10.2 million people as Asian or Asian-American, and 35.3 million people as Hispanic or Latino of any race [10]. Correspondingly, the 2006–2008 American Community Survey revealed that 38.6 % of the US population identified their race as nonwhite black or African-American (12.3 %), nonwhite Hispanic or Latino (15.1 %), or nonwhite other (11.2 %) [3]. More recently, the 2010 US Census suggested that the growth of blacks, Asians, and Hispanics is accelerating and that minorities will comprise a majority of the country's total population as early as 2042, when Hispanics will comprise 24 %, blacks 15 %, and Asians 8 % [11]. For instance, the Hispanic population increased by 15.2 million between 2000 and 2010, accounting for over half of the 27.3 million increase in the total population of the United States [12]. Thus, it is reasonable to expect that immigrants across all aforementioned ethnic groups will account for most of the population growth in the coming decades, further increasing the racial/ethnic heterogeneity of the US population and augmenting the importance of focusing on health disparities associated with race and ethnicity.

In general, race and ethnicity can be markers of poverty, preexisting conditions, and/or decreased access to health systems [13]. This is reflected in medical conditions such as sepsis, asthma, and cancer, as well as in insurance status and various other health-related measures. For example, sepsis is currently the tenth leading cause of death overall in the United States and represents a healthcare burden of nearly $17 billion [14]. Studies have shown that nonwhites are nearly twice as likely as whites to develop sepsis, with higher infection rates and a higher risk of acute organ dysfunction in blacks in particular [15]. Many of these studies may be confounded by the fact that black patients with sepsis had a greater likelihood of having HIV infection, diabetes mellitus, obesity, burns, and/or chronic kidney disease; however, this too represents a serious health disparity. In addition, more than 44 million Americans lack health insurance, and hospitalized black patients are more than three times as likely as white patients to be uninsured, resulting in limited access to preventive health services [14]. This disparity rises to nearly four times for black patients with sepsis [16].

Children of minorities are similarly affected by disparities in health. For example, Wegienka and colleagues noted racial disparities in allergic disease-related outcomes in children as early as 2 years of age, with black children being more likely than white children to have a positive skin prick test, an elevated allergic specific IgE, and atopic dermatitis [17]. These disparities could not be explained by family income, maternal education, parents' marital status, family housing payment,

prenatal exposure to indoor pets, living with a smoker, breastfeeding, or a host of other factors.

It makes sense then that asthma also disproportionately affects minority and disadvantaged children, including residents of federally assisted housing. An explanation for this disparity is that racial and ethnic minority and low-income children are more likely to live in substandard housing with greater exposure to allergens and higher asthma sensitization rates due to crowding, pest infestations, poor ventilation, deteriorated carpeting, excessive moisture and dampness, and/or structural deficits [11, 18]. Because environmental conditions in the home can exacerbate asthma symptoms, housing interventions to combat this disparity could include home assessment for asthma triggers (e.g., environmental tobacco smoke, dust mites, outdoor air pollution, cockroach allergen, pets, mold, and wood smoke), provision of products and services to reduce exposure to asthma triggers (e.g., mattress cases and chemical methods to reduce dust mites), and asthma education on identification of asthma triggers and how to reduce exposure [19]. A more detailed discussion of methods to reduce and eliminate disparities in general occurs later in this chapter.

More generally, Schuster and colleagues studied 5,119 public school fifth-graders and their parents in three US metropolitan areas and noted significant differences between black children and white children for 16 health-related measures, many of which are contributors to youth morbidity and mortality [20]. There were also significant differences between Latino children and white children for 12 of the 16 measures. For example, they found that 20 % of black children and 11 % of Latino children had witnessed a threat or injury with a gun, while only 5 % of white children had witnessed such an event. In addition, white children performed vigorous exercise on a greater number of days per week than black and Latino children. Black children also had higher levels of cigarette use, obesity, peer victimization, and discrimination and lower levels of consistent bike helmet use and psychological/physical quality of life than white children [20].

Blacks (or African-Americans) and Hispanics (or Latinos) are not the only racial/ethnic groups affected by disparity in health. For example, data from the Racial and Ethnic Approaches to Community Health (REACH) 2010 Risk Factor Survey demonstrated a high prevalence of self-reported cardiovascular disease, hypertension, high cholesterol, and diabetes with American Indian men and women having the highest median prevalence of obesity at 39.2 % and 37.5 %, respectively, compared with only 2.9 % and 3.6 % of Asian/Pacific Islander men and women, respectively [21]. Similarly, cigarette smoking was common in American Indian communities, with a median of 42.2 % for men and 36.7 % for women [21].

Ethnic minority and medically underserved populations also suffer disproportionate burdens of cancer, and the disparity appears to be growing. By 2050, it is estimated that the number of new cancer cases among Asian-Americans and Pacific Islanders will increase by 132 %, compared to a 31 % increase for whites. In addition, Asian-Americans and Pacific Islanders are the groups with the lowest cancer screening rate of all ethnic groups, and several of their subgroups have a higher percentage of late-stage diagnoses [22]. Moreover, it has been postulated that unequal distribution of funding for hospitals caring for minorities results in a lower quality of cancer care available to minority patients. A 2009 study of quality of care and surgical mortality after breast or colon cancer surgery found that lower quality care was a major determinant of disparities in outcome between minority populations and those who belong to the dominant culture [22].

Many have attempted to explain the prominent disparities associated with race or ethnicity. For example, Link and Phelan, as well as other researchers, have proposed that racism, in particular institutional racism (defined as the presence of societal structures that systematically constrain the opportunities of groups on the basis of their race or ethnicity), plays a prominent role in the persistence of health disparities associated with race or ethnicity [23–26]. Through racism, race becomes linked to socioeconomic status,

which in turn affects health outcomes and access to high-quality healthcare.

Another body of research, led by Dr. Arline T. Geronimus, posits that "weathering" of the body under persistent adversity (i.e., the increased wear and tear induced by stressful experiences that overuse and dysregulate pathways normally used for adaptation to threat) reflects an acceleration of normal aging processes [27–29]. Dr. Geronimus proposes that this process is also assailed by disparities. For example, African-Americans experience earlier deteriorations of health in a cumulative fashion, leading to progressively larger health disparities with age and a life expectancy that is 4–6 years less than for whites [30].

Shonkoff and colleagues also propose that influences in childhood can affect the regulation of biological systems [31] and that this is a major contributor to disparities affecting adults of different races and ethnicities in later life. For example, a fetus in an intrauterine environment characterized by poor nutrition may undergo energy-sparing metabolic changes that are designed to be adaptive in a postnatal environment of food scarcity. While these metabolic changes may be beneficial in the short run, problems can arise later in life when the initially adaptive advantage turns out to be nonadaptive. The early childhood environment will then be characterized by energy abundance, a carbohydrate-rich diet, and a sedentary lifestyle. This can result in an increased risk of obesity and other metabolic disorders [32, 33].

Disparities such as the ones outlined here also affect subgroups defined by social factors other than race or ethnicity. Studies have shown that other subgroups significantly and adversely affected include individuals with low socioeconomic status and residents of the southeastern United States and the Appalachians [21]. Similarly, individuals with less than a high school education tend to have a higher burden of cardiovascular disease and related risk factors regardless of race/ethnicity [21]. Consequently, disparities associated with socioeconomic status, geographic location, education, and the like merit discussion.

Socioeconomic Status

The correlation between low socioeconomic status and poor health outcomes is well studied and perhaps one of the most well appreciated. For example, poor living conditions early in life (e.g., inadequate nutrition, constraints on fetal and infant growth, and recurrent infections) are known to be associated with increased rates of cardiovascular, respiratory, and psychiatric diseases in adulthood [34–37].

Dr. Braveman and Dr. Susan Egerter have also shown that American adults living in poverty are more than five times as likely to report being in fair or poor health as adults with incomes at least four times the federal poverty level. The income-health relationship is not restricted to the poor [38]. Studies of Americans at all income levels reveal inferior health outcomes when compared to Americans at higher income levels.

Income is one of the most common markers of socioeconomic status, and its importance to health might not be surprising to some. However, the magnitude of the relationship is not always appreciated. For example, Woolf and coworkers calculated that 25 % of all deaths in Virginia between 1996 and 2002 would have been averted if the mortality rates of the five most affluent counties and cities had applied statewide [39]. Even more striking is that Muennig and colleagues estimated that living on incomes less than 200 % of the federal poverty level claimed more than 400 million quality-adjusted life years between 1997 and 2002 [40]. This means that poverty had a larger effect than tobacco use and obesity. Thus, income, like race/ethnicity, has a striking association with health outcomes and is a significant part of the web of social and economic conditions that affect health.

Education

Education has also been used as a marker of socioeconomic status, and disparities associated with level of education have been widely researched. Ma and coworkers calculated age-standardized

death rates and their average annual percent change for all cause and major causes (cancer, heart disease, stroke, diabetes, accidents) from 1993 through 2007 for individuals aged 25–64 years. They used education as a marker of socioeconomic status and found that all-cause mortality rate decreased annually by 1.5 % in men and 0.7 % in women (likely reflecting progress in prevention and treatment of major medical conditions causing death) [41]. However, the mortality improvement was mainly concentrated in the most educated populations. Those with the least education experienced either less progress or a worsening trend in mortality. For example, mortality in women with 12 or less years of education increased by 0.9 % from 1993 to 2007 [41].

Another study compared 31 developing countries regarding the likelihood of attending four or more antenatal care visits. The likelihood of this activity was 2.89 times higher for women with complete primary education than for those less educated [42]. Individuals with more education have also been shown to respond more cautiously when confronted with potentially harmful pharmaceutical advertising than those in less educated groups [43]. Moreover, education is significantly related to awareness of smoking cessation programs and access to medical information [44]. Furthermore, in schizophrenia, individuals with more formal education have better cognitive training response and adherence to treatment [45]. In fact, Elo and Preston reported that every additional year in educational attainment reduces the likelihood of dying by 1–3 %. This impact on life expectancy by education is true for every demographic group and has been persistent, if not increasing, since the study by Elo and Preston was published [46]. Thus, it is clear that education is another significant part of the web of social and economic conditions contributing to health disparities.

Health Insurance

In the United States, insurance is an independent factor affecting health outcomes and healthcare, as the high cost of health insurance matters for uninsured non-elderly adults and children, whether healthy or disabled, above or below the poverty level. Consequently, lack of health insurance is a major barrier to accessing preventive, diagnostic, or therapeutic health services. Due to the relationship between employment, income, and insurance, members of racial and ethnic minority groups who have suffered discrimination with respect to educational, economic, and immigration opportunities are more likely to be uninsured, particularly if they have limited proficiency in English [47].

In general, compared to those who are insured, individuals who lack health insurance are 3.9 times more likely to not obtain needed care (35 % vs. 9 %), 3.25 times more likely to not fill a prescription because of cost (13 % vs. 4 %), 4.7 times more likely to have no regular source of care (42 % vs. 9 %), and 3.1 times more likely to postpone care because of cost (47 % vs. 15 %) [48]. The uninsured are also more likely to be Hispanic and noncitizens (as many noncitizens are employed in low-wage jobs without health benefits and are ineligible for public coverage in most states) [49], die earlier and have poorer health status, be diagnosed at later stages of disease, and get less treatment than those with insurance. They are also sicker when hospitalized and are more likely to die during their stay [47]. In addition, both uninsured adults and children are much more likely to be low income than their insured counterparts. Among uninsured non-elderly adults, nearly 60 % have family incomes below 200 % of the federal poverty level, as do nearly 70 % of uninsured children [49]. In fact, in 2004, the high cost of health insurance was the primary reason for being uninsured across population subgroups defined by age, race/ethnicity, health status, family structure, employment, and income. High cost as a reason for being uninsured was particularly prevalent among older adults and older children, Hispanic individuals, noncitizens, and those who had been uninsured for longer periods of time [49]. Thus, a lack of health insurance is inexorably tied to health disparities associated with the aforementioned social factors such as race/ethnicity and socioeconomic status.

Geography and Living Conditions

Adler and Rehkopf point out that place of birth is a critical and frequently ignored component of socioeconomic and racial/ethnic disparities [6]. For most health outcomes, foreign-born individuals have lower rates of disease than individuals born in the USA, and they live on average 3.4 years longer—a number that has been increasing over the past three decades. The gap is the largest for native-born vs. immigrant blacks and Hispanics [6]. There are also significant health disparities between countries—life expectancy at birth in Zambia (41.2 years) is half that of Japan (82.4 years)—and within countries other than the United States [49]. Within the Scottish city of Glasgow, there is a 28-year gap in life expectancy between the wealthiest and poorest areas; among the poorest, male life expectancy is 8 years less than the average life expectancy in India. Similarly, the gap in life expectancy between men in Washington, DC, and in suburban Maryland is approximately 17 years [50].

Like location of birth, location of residence is also a commonly discounted component of disparities in healthcare and health outcomes. This has been demonstrated by the phenomenon of "small area variation" in rates of healthcare utilization. For example, the *Dartmouth Atlas of Health Care* used large samples of Medicare enrollees to measure such disparities across 306 Hospital Referral Regions (HRR) in the United States. Even after controlling for differences in underlying health status across regions, there was clear evidence of persistent and large differences in treatment patterns, even in adjacent areas. In addition to disparities in treatment patterns, there were also substantial variations in health outcomes by region [51]. Research has also documented race-specific and gender-specific variations at the county or state level in overall mortality rates, disease-specific mortality rates, and healthcare treatment. For example, Schneider and colleagues classified coronary artery bypass graft (CABG) surgery and percutaneous transluminal coronary angioplasty (PTCA) on a sample of Medicare beneficiaries who had all undergone coronary angiography. The sample was drawn from over 173 hospitals, and each individual's treatment was classified as being appropriate, uncertain, or inappropriate. The authors found that there was substantial variation between states in the inappropriate use of both CABG and PTCA. For PTCA, inappropriate rates were 24 % in California, 14 % in Pennsylvania, 8 % in Georgia, and 12 % in Alabama [52].

Similarly, Chandra found that 85 % of all black acute myocardial infarction (AMI) patients were treated by only 1,000 hospitals, whereas only 40 % of all white AMI patients were treated at these same hospitals. In fact, almost 3,000 hospitals in the United States treated no black AMI patients [53]. Because blacks and whites seem to go to different hospitals for AMI care, these differences may play an important role in racial disparities in outcomes for heart attacks. Another study by Barnato and colleagues found that within hospitals there were actually no black-white disparities in the use of effective medical treatments, such as aspirin and beta-blockers during hospitalization. But there were differences in the use of these treatments *between* hospitals [54]. These regional differences in treatment and utilization have clear implications for the percentage of racial minorities receiving appropriate healthcare.

It is important to note that the measurement of regional variation in healthcare utilization is difficult for many reasons, outlined by Chandra and Skinner [51]. First, a great deal of statistical power is necessary to measure utilization at the local level; even a sample of 50,000 observations quickly loses power when the data are separated by region and used to focus on specific diseases. Small sample sizes and inadequate statistical power can generate false area variation by mere random noise in measured average rates. Second, the problem of migration to hospitals must be considered. For example, Boston hospitals typically accept referrals from all over the New England area, and if these patients were counted, it might appear falsely that Boston residents were at elevated risk of hospitalization. Finally, one needs a sample that is not subject to selectivity bias. For example, the sample of Medicaid patients or of managed care patients is not likely

to be representative of the general population as Medicaid patients can become eligible due to serious illness, while managed care patients are likely to be healthier than the general population.

Besides geographic location, racial and ethnic minorities also live disproportionately in physical environments that lack the resources necessary to generate and sustain health. It has been shown, for example, that segregated African-American neighborhoods are often characterized by substandard housing, high levels of abandoned buildings, larger numbers of commercial and industrial facilities, and inadequate municipal services and amenities, including police and fire protection [6]. Physical locations also vary in exposure to toxins, pathogens, and carcinogens. The environment may present differential risks from chemical substances (e.g., lead paint), respiratory irritants (e.g., diesel fumes), litter, and noise. In addition, crowding, substandard housing, elevated noise levels, and elevated exposure to noxious pollutants and allergens (e.g., lead, smog, particulates, and dust mites) are all common in poor, segregated communities and have all been shown to adversely affect health. In many urban areas, the physical environment may constrain exercise. Neighborhoods that lack safe recreational spaces and in which residents have concerns about their personal safety also discourage individuals from participating in physical activity [6].

Where one lives may also limit access to healthy foods. Many large commercial enterprises avoid segregated urban areas; as a result, the available services are typically fewer in quantity, poorer in quality, and often higher in price than those available in less-segregated urban areas. The absence of stores with reasonably priced fresh fruits and vegetables may discourage individuals from including these foods in their daily diet. The consumption of healthy foods has been shown to be positively associated with their availability [55], and the availability of healthful products in grocery stores varies across zip codes. For example, Horowitz and coworkers demonstrated the remarkable disparity in healthy food access for patients with diabetes in New York's largely white and wealthy Upper East Side and the largely black and Latino East Harlem community nearby [56]. Differential access by race and ethnicity to full-service supermarkets [57], parks [58, 59], and other basic amenities has also been demonstrated. Thus, the high cost and poor quality of food choices in segregated neighborhoods can lead to worse nutrition and poorer associated health outcomes.

Residential segregation may also explain racial differences in other health outcomes that have strong environmental components such as homicide and drug abuse. African-Americans are much more likely than whites to be victims of all types of crime, including homicide, demonstrated by the fact that out of the 15 leading causes of death in the United States, the black-white gap is largest for homicide [60]. Additionally, a national study revealed that elevated rates of cocaine use by blacks and Hispanics could be mostly explained by neighborhood clusters [61]. Thus, living in certain neighborhoods places individuals at increased risks from tobacco, alcohol, drugs, and violence.

Not only does living in certain environments and states impact healthcare utilization and health outcomes, but healthcare costs also vary by geography, and this disparity has been growing over the past two decades. Between 1992 and 2006, overall Medicare spending rose by 3.5 % annually, but per capita inflation-adjusted spending in Miami grew at an annual rate of 5.0 %, as compared with just 2.3 % in Salem, Oregon, and 2.4 % in San Francisco. In dollar terms, the growth in per capita Medicare expenditures between 1992 and 2006 in Miami ($8,085) was nearly equal to the level of 2006 expenditures in San Francisco ($8,331) [62]. Even marginal differences in per capita spending can have large differences in overall regional expenditure. For example, per capita spending in East Long Island was $2,500 more than in San Francisco, which translates into approximately $1 billion additional annual Medicare spending from this region alone [62]. As it has already been shown that there is a disparity in healthcare utilization by different races/ethnicities between states, a difference in healthcare costs in these states only widens the racial disparity.

Disability

Costs associated with disabilities are more than $300 billion per year. Yet, individuals living with disabilities remain a critically underserved population, and there is significant evidence that disability is an independent factor affecting health disparities. A particularly vulnerable subgroup is women with disabilities who are also raising children. Kim and coworkers analyzed data on 28,629 women with and without disabilities who are raising children. They found that women with disabilities were less likely to have a partner or spouse, reported lower incomes and education levels, and were older. Women with disabilities raising children also reported significantly lower health-related quality of life including poor general health, frequent mental distress, and frequent poor physical health. In addition, they had higher prevalence of chronic health conditions (e.g., arthritis, cardiovascular diseases, diabetes, asthma, high blood pressure, high cholesterol, and obesity), higher prevalence of adverse health behaviors (e.g., smoking and lack of exercise), greater financial barriers to healthcare, and a greater lack of social and emotional support. These disparities remained even after controlling for age, education, income, and relationship status [63]. The results of this study are crucial as strong associations have been shown between increasing numbers of traumatic childhood events (which occur with higher frequency in children with mothers with disabilities) with greater prevalence of a wide array of health impairments, including coronary artery disease, chronic pulmonary disease, cancer, alcoholism, depression, and drug abuse [64, 65], as well as overlapping mental health problems [66–68], teen pregnancies [69], and cardiovascular risk factors such as obesity, physical inactivity, and smoking [70]. While this study demonstrates the health disparities associated with disability status alone, there is a wealth of research that also shows widespread associations between disability, having low income and education, and being a racial minority, all of which have already been shown to contribute to health disparities.

Addressing Health Disparities

As previously discussed, the DHHS Healthy People initiative is one of the most prominent efforts to reduce and ultimately eliminate health disparities. One of the two overarching goals of Healthy People 2010 is "to eliminate health disparities among different segments of the population," after defining health disparities as differences that occur by gender, race/ethnicity, education, income, disability, living in rural localities, or sexual orientation [71]. A similar goal to achieving health equity and eliminating health disparities was proposed by the Health and Human Services Secretary's Advisory Committee (SAC) for Healthy People 2020. Similarly, the director general of the World Health Organization established the Commission on Social Determinants of Health (CSDH) in 2005 to achieve analogous aims. Specifically, the CSDH produced recommendations to promote health equity based on three principles of action: improve the circumstances in which people are born, grow, live, work, and age; tackle the inequitable distribution of power, money, and resources (the structural drivers of conditions of daily life); and measure the problem, evaluate the action, and expand the knowledge base [50]. The CSDH call for action on social determinants of health also applies to differences between ethnic groups. This is especially important as it has been estimated that nearly 900,000 deaths could have been averted in the USA between 1991 and 2000 if mortality rates between white and black individuals had been equalized [50].

We previously outlined various definitions of the term "health disparities," and this is imperative as effective public policies require clear and contextually relevant operational definitions to support the development of objectives and specific targets, determine priorities for use of limited resources, and assess progress. The need for clear definitions is also compelling given the lack of progress toward reducing racial/ethnic and socioeconomic disparities in medical care [72] and health [73, 74] over the past few decades.

Dr. Meredith Minkler discusses two interrelated concepts relevant to eliminating health disparities: distributive justice and procedural justice. The former term, widely used in environmental justice work, typically refers to the need to rectify disproportionate exposure to pollutants and other environmental hazards in low-income communities and communities segregated by race/ethnicity. However, distributive justice also can relate to the disproportionate lack of access to resources or assets, such as safe recreation areas and stores selling high-quality and affordable fresh fruits and vegetables. Finally, eliminating health disparities requires the promotion of procedural justice, defined as equitable processes through which low-income communities, rural residents, and other marginalized groups can gain a seat at the table and have a voice in decision-making and policy implementation [75].

Research has also shown that provider-patient communication is another factor linked to patient satisfaction, compliance with medical instructions, and health outcomes. Thus, poorer health outcomes may result when sociocultural differences between patients and providers are not reconciled in the clinical encounter. More broadly, there is evidence that patient-centered care and cultural competence may be important in improving quality and eliminating racial/ethnic healthcare disparities [76]. Given the role of federal, state, and local governments in managing and financing healthcare delivery (see Chap. 16), especially for vulnerable or disadvantaged populations, cultural competence may be a method of increasing access to quality care for all patient populations. As minorities may have difficulty getting appropriate, timely, high-quality care because of linguistic and cultural barriers, cultural competence could change our "one size fits all" healthcare system to one that is more responsive to the needs of an increasingly diverse patient population, which, in turn, would help reduce health disparities associated with culture, race, and ethnicity.

Physician organizations are another crucial cog that must be actively engaged, as they are in a unique position to implement policies and programs to reduce/eliminate disparities. Peek and coworkers showed that despite the national priority to eliminate health disparities, greater than half of national physician organizations are doing little to address the problem. In fact, many physician organizations have inadvertently contributed to health disparities by promoting racial and ethnic bias in healthcare delivery through actions such as excluding racial and ethnic minority physicians from physician organizations and segregating minority patients and providers into health systems with inadequate resources [77].

Shonkoff and colleagues astutely point out that despite the unassailable association between social class (and other markers of disadvantage) and differences in health, we still lack unanimity regarding the precise causal mechanisms linking adversity to health status [31]. Some critics have suggested that there be greater focus on inequalities in service utilization and differential treatment by the healthcare system. Others have called for greater attention to the role of broader social and economic influences on health, although the task of translating this perspective into concrete policy initiatives has generated more rhetoric than action. Either way, educating medical professionals regarding the aforementioned differences and effective policy remedies, which is the purpose of this chapter, is an integral first step in reducing and ultimately eliminating health disparities.

Conclusion

Disparities in health have been a focus of intensive research for the last three to four decades, with the US DHHS Healthy People initiative being an exemplar of efforts to eliminate health disparities. These efforts have been aided by increasingly enhanced definitions of "health disparities," with many researchers viewing the term as an inclusive one involving disparities associated with race/ethnicity, socioeconomic status, education, health insurance, geography, physical environment, disability status, and other criteria. As demonstrated in this chapter, disparities are indeed associated with all of these social factors, with many of the disparities directly affecting health outcomes and the risk of incurring detrimental health conditions.

Overall, understanding and attempting to reduce health disparities are critical endeavors with policy implications and practical health consequences. These endeavors must be led by medical students and healthcare practitioners alike, as we are all in a distinct position to implement policies and programs to reduce and ultimately eliminate health disparities.

References

1. Black D, Morris J, Smith C, et al. Inequalities in health: report of a research working group. London: Department of Health and Social Security; 1980.
2. Starfield B, Gervas J, Mangin D. Clinical care and health disparities. Annu Rev Public Health. 2012;33:89–106.
3. Thomas SB, Quinn SC, Butler J, et al. Toward a fourth generation of disparities research to achieve health equity. Annu Rev Public Health. 2011;32:399–416.
4. Braveman P. Health disparities and health equity: concepts and measurement. Annu Rev Public Health. 2006;27:167–94.
5. Whitehead M. The concepts and principles of equity in health. Int J Health Serv. 1992;22:429–45.
6. Adler NE, Rehkopf DH. US disparities in health: descriptions, causes, and mechanisms. Annu Rev Public Health. 2008;29:235–52.
7. Cooper R, Rotimi C, Ataman S, et al. The prevalence of hypertension in seven populations of West African origin. Am J Public Health. 1997;87(2):160–8.
8. Kaplan GA, Pamuk ER, Lynch JW, et al. Inequality in income and mortality in the United States: analysis of mortality and potential pathways. BMJ. 1996;312: 999–1005.
9. Kennedy BP, Kawachi I, Prothrow-Stith D. Income distribution and mortality: cross sectional ecological study of the Robin Hood index in the United States. BMJ. 1996;312:1004–7.
10. Brondolo E, Gallo LC, Myers HF. Race, racism and health: disparities, mechanisms, and interventions. J Behav Med. 2009;32:1–8.
11. Carter-Pokras OD, Offutt-Powell TN, Kaufman JS, et al. Epidemiology, policy, and racial/ethnic minority health disparities. Ann Epidemiol. 2012;22:446–55.
12. US Census Bureau. Population distribution and change: 2000 to 2010. 2010 Census Briefs, 2011. Retrieved from http://www.census.gov/prod/cen2010/briefs/c2010br-01.pdf
13. Vogel RT. Update and review of racial disparities in sepsis. Surg Infect. 2012;13(4):1–6.
14. Hodgkin KE, Moss M. The epidemiology of sepsis. Curr Pharm Des. 2008;14:1833–9.
15. Mayr FB, Yende S, Linde-Zwirble WT, et al. Infection rate and acute organ dysfunction risk as explanations for racial differences in severe sepsis. JAMA. 2010; 303:2495–503.

16. Berkowitz DM, Martin GS. Disparities in sepsis: what do we understand? Crit Care Med. 2007;35:958–60.

17. Wegienka G, Havstad S, Joseph CLM, et al. Racial disparities in allergic outcomes in African Americans emerge as early as age 2 years. Clin Exp Allergy. 2012;42:909–17.

18. Northridge J, Ramirez OF, Stringone JA. The role of housing type and housing quality in urban children with asthma. J Urban Health. 2010;87:211–24.

19. Krieger JW, Takaro TK, Rabkin JC. Breathing easier in Seattle: addressing asthma disparities through healthier housing. In: Williams RA, editor. Healthcare disparities at the crossroads with healthcare reform. New York: Springer; 2011. p. 359–85.

20. Schuster MA, Elliott MN, Kanouse DE, et al. Racial and ethnic health disparities among fifth-graders in three cities. NEJM. 2012;367:735–45.

21. Mensah GA, Mokdah AH, Ford ES, et al. State of disparities in cardiovascular health in the United States. Circulation. 2005;111:1233–41.

22. Kagawa-Singer M, Valdez Dadia A, Yu MC, et al. Cancer, culture, and health disparities: time to chart a new course? CA Cancer J Clin. 2010;60:12–39.

23. Diez Roux AV. Conceptual approaches to the study of health disparities. Annu Rev Public Health. 2012;33: 41–58.

24. Link BG, Phelan J. Social conditions as fundamental causes of disease. J Health Soc Behav. 1995;35(Extra Issue):80–94.

25. Link BG, Phelan J. Understanding sociodemographic differences in health – the role of fundamental social causes. Am J Public Health. 1996;86:471–3.

26. Phelan JC, Link BG, Tehranifar P. Social conditions as fundamental causes of health inequalities: theory, evidence, and policy implications. J Health Soc Behav. 2010;51(Suppl):S28–40.

27. Geronimus AT. The weathering hypothesis and the health of African-American women and infants: evidence and speculations. Ethn Dis. 1992;2(3):207–21.

28. Geronimus AT. Black/white differences in the relationship of maternal age to birthweight: a population-based test of the weathering hypothesis. Soc Sci Med. 1996;42(4):589–97.

29. Geronimus AT, Hicken M, Keene D, et al. "Weathering" and age patterns of allostatic load scores among blacks and whites in the United States. Am J Public Health. 2006;96(5):826–33.

30. Harper S, Lynch J, Burris S, et al. Trends in the black-white life expectancy gap in the United States, 1983–2003. JAMA. 2007;297(11):1224–32.

31. Shonkoff JP, Boyce WT, McEwen BS. Neuroscience, molecular biology, and the childhood roots of health disparities. JAMA. 2009;301(21):2252–9.

32. Worthman CM, Kuzara J. Life history and the early origins of health differentials. Am J Hum Biol. 2005;17(1):95–112.

33. Gillman MW. Developmental origins of health and disease. NEJM. 2005;353(17):1848–50.

34. Barker DJ, Osmond C, Forsen TJ, et al. Trajectories of growth among children who have coronary events as adults. NEJM. 2005;353(17):1802–9.

35. Barker DJ, Osmond C, Simmonds SJ, et al. The relation of small head circumference and thinness at birth to death from cardiovascular disease in adult life. BMJ. 1993;306(6875):422–6.

36. Barker DJ, Winter PD, Osmond C, et al. Weight in infancy and death from ischaemic heart disease. Lancet. 1989;2(8663):577–80.

37. Nomura Y, Wickramaratne PJ, Pilowsky DJ, et al. Low birth weight and risk of affective disorders and selected medical illness in offspring at high and low risk for depression. Comp Pyschiatry. 2007;48(5):470–8.

38. Braveman PA, Cubbin C, Egerter S, et al. Socioeconomic disparities in health in the United States: what the patterns tell us. Am J Public Health. 2010;100(S1):S186–96.

39. Woolf SH, Jones RM, Johnson RE, et al. Avertable deaths associated with household income in Virginia. Am J Public Health. 2010;100(4):750–5.

40. Muennig P, Fiscella K, Tancredi D, et al. The relative health burden of selected social and behavioral risk factors in the United States: implications for policy. Am J Public Health. 2010;100(9):1758–64.

41. Ma J, Xu J, Anderson RN, et al. Widening educational disparities in premature death rates in twenty six states in the United States, 1993–2007. PLoS One. 2012;7(7):e41560.

42. Ahmed S, Creanga AA, Gillespie DG, et al. Economic status, education, and empowerment: implications for maternal health service utilization in developing countries. PLoS One. 2010;5(6):e11190.

43. Hoek J, Maubach N. Consumers' knowledge, perceptions, and responsiveness to direct-to-consumer advertising of prescription medicines. N Z Med J. 2007;120:U2425.

44. Kaufman A, Augustson E, Davis K, et al. Awareness and use of tobacco quitlines: evidence from the Health Information National Trends Survey. J Health Commun. 2010;15(S3):264–78.

45. Twamley EW, Burton CZ, Vella L. Compensatory cognitive training for psychosis: who benefits? Who stays in treatment? Schizophr Bull. 2011;37(S2): S55–62.

46. Elo IT, Preston SH. Educational differentials in mortality: United States 1979–1985. Soc Sci Med. 1996; 42(1):47–57.

47. Richardson LD, Norris M. Access to health and health care: how race and ethnicity matter. Mount Sinai J Med. 2010;77:166–77.

48. Kaiser Family Foundation Commission on Medicaid and the Uninsured. The uninsured: a primer. Menlo Park: Henry J. Kaiser Family Foundation; 2006.

49. Graves JA, Long SK. "Why do people lack health insurance?" in shifting ground: changes in employer sponsored insurance. Cover the Uninsured Week Research Report, 2006.

50. Marmot MG, Bell R. Action on health disparities in the United States: commission on social determinants of health. JAMA. 2009;301(11):1169–71.

51. Chandra A, Skinner J. Geography and Racial Health Disparities. National bureau of economic research, 2003; Working paper 9513.

52. Schneider EC, Leape LL, Weissman JS, et al. Racial differences in cardiac revascularization rates: does "Overuse" explain higher rates among white patients? Ann Intern Med. 2001;135(5):328–37.

53. Chandra A. Who you are and where you live: race and the geography of healthcare. Med Care. 2009;47(2): 135–7.

54. Barnato AE, Lucas FL, Staiger D, et al. Hospital-level racial disparities in acute myocardial infarction treatment and outcomes. Circulation. 2005;43:308–19.

55. Cheadle A, Psaty BM, Curry S, et al. Community-level comparisons between the grocery store environment and individual dietary practices. Prev Med. 1991;20:250–61.

56. Horowitz C, Colson KA, Hebert PL, et al. Barriers to buying healthy foods for people with diabetes: evidence of environmental disparities. Am J Public Health. 2004;94(9):1549–54.

57. Morland K, Wing S, Diez RA. The contextual effect of the local food environment on residents' diets: the atherosclerosis risk in communities study. Am J Public Health. 2002;92(11):1761–8.

58. Frumkin H. Guest editorial: health, equity, and the built environment. Environ Health Perspect. 2005; 113(5):A290–1.

59. Wolch J, Wilson JP, Fehrenback J. Parks and park funding in Los Angeles: an equity mapping analysis. Urban Geogr. 2006;26(2):4–35.

60. Williams DR, Collins CA. Racial residential segregation: a fundamental cause of racial disparities in health. Public Health Rep. 2001;116:404–15.

61. Lillie-Blanton M, Martinez RM, Taylor AK, et al. Latina and African American women: continuing disparities in health. Int H Health Serv. 1993;23:555–81.

62. Fisher ES, Bynum JP, Skinner JS. Slowing the growth of health care costs – lessons from regional variation. NEJM. 2009;360(9):849–52.

63. Kim M, Kim HJ, Hong S, et al. Health disparities among childrearing women with disabilities. Matern Child Health J. 2012 Aug 24. [Epub ahead of print].

64. Felitti VJ, Anda RF, Nordenberg D, et al. Relationship of childhood abuse and household dysfunction to many of the leading causes of death in adults: the adverse childhood experiences (ACE) study. Am J Prev Med. 1998;14(4):245–58.

65. Edwards VJ, Holden GW, Felitti VJ, et al. Relationship between multiple forms of childhood maltreatment and adult mental health in community respondents: results from the adverse childhood experiences study. Am J Psychiatry. 2003;160(8):1453–60.

66. Anda RF, Felitti VJ, Bremner JD, et al. The enduring effects of abuse and related adverse experiences in childhood: a convergence of evidence from neurobiology and epidemiology. Eur Arch Psychiatry Clin Neurosci. 2006;256(3):174–86.

67. Horwitz AV, Widom CS, McLaughlin J, et al. The impact of childhood abuse and neglect on adult mental health: a prospective study. J Health Soc Behav. 2001;42(2):184–201.

68. Schilling EA, Aseltine RH, Gore S. Adverse childhood experiences and mental health in young adults: a longitudinal survey. BMC Public Health. 2007;7:30.

69. Hillis SD, Anda RF, Dube SR, et al. The association between adverse childhood experiences and adolescent pregnancy, long-term psychosocial consequences, and fetal death. Pediatrics. 2004;113(2): 320–7.

70. Dong M, Giles WH, Felitti VJ, et al. Insights into causal pathways for ischemic heart disease: adverse childhood experiences study. Circulation. 2004; 110(13):1761–6.

71. Braveman PA, Kumanyika S, Fielding J, et al. Health disparities and health equity: the issue is justice. Am J Public Health. 2011;101(S1):S149–55.

72. Woelker R. Decades of work to reduce disparities in health care produce limited success. JAMA. 2008; 299(12):1411–13.

73. Singh GK, Siahpush M. Widening socioeconomic inequalities in US life expectancy, 1980–2000. Int J Epidemiol. 2006;35(4):969–79.

74. Singh GK, Kogan MD. Widening socioeconomic disparities in US childhood mortality, 1969–2000. Am J Public Health. 2007;97(9):1658–65.

75. Minkler M. Linking science and policy through community-based participatory research to study and address health disparities. Am J Public Health. 2010;100(S1):S81–7.

76. Betancourt JR, Green AR, Carillo JE, et al. Cultural competence and health care disparities: key perspectives and trends. Health Aff. 2005;24(2):499–505.

77. Peek ME, Wilson SC, Bussy-Jones J, et al. A study of national physician organizations' efforts to reduce racial and ethnic health disparities in the United States. Acad Med. 2012;87(6):694–700.

The Economics of Health Care

11

David A. Rosman and Jordan C. Apfeld

Learning Objectives

After completing this chapter, the reader should be able to answer the following questions:

- The size and structure of the health insurance market in the United States
- Health care as an economic good and be able to track where the money comes from in the health-care industry
- What factors and dynamics drive the costs for health services in America's insurance-based system
- How rising demand and the misalignment of risks and incentives have been part of the cause of rising health-care costs in the United States
- New cost-reduction and quality-improvement strategies being implemented in America today

Current Size and Structure of the US Health-Care Market

US Health-Care Market: The Size

A study in *Health Affairs* demonstrates that the United States spent more on health care in 2000 than any other country in the Organisation for Economic Co-operation and Development (OECD) [1]. In 2010, total national health expenditures reached $2.6 trillion [2], which was over 17 % of GDP [3]; this percentage is the highest to date in America because the rise in health-care costs has outpaced inflation since 1970. In fact, in 1970, shortly after Medicare/Medicaid was created, health-care expenditures had comprised a mere 7.2 % of GDP. In 2008, our per-capita health expenditure was $7,538, which was $2,500 more than the next highest per-capita expenditure of Norway [4].

However, after 2000, cost increases have lessened, from 9.5 % in 2002 to 3.9 % in 2010 [5]. Many attribute this to America's economic struggles, especially considering the 2007–2008 financial crisis. Essentially, fewer available dollars to spend would mean less demand for health care, which would also mean minimal price inflation.

D.A. Rosman, M.D., M.B.A. (✉)
Department of Abdominal Imaging, Massachusetts
General Hospital, Boston, MA 02144, USA
e-mail: drosman@partners.org

J.C. Apfeld, B.A.
Vanderbilt Orthopedic Institute Center for Health
Policy, Vanderbilt University Medical School,
Nashville, TN 37232, USA
e-mail: jordan.c.apfeld@vanderbilt.edu

M.K. Sethi and W.H. Frist (eds.), *An Introduction to Health Policy: A Primer for Physicians and Medical Students*,   133
DOI 10.1007/978-1-4614-7735-8_11, © Springer Science+Business Media New York 2013

Detractors of this theory contend that medicine is recession proof and that the slow leveling of costs is a genuine achievement in cost containment [6].

Health-care prices are also much higher in America than in any other country, in addition to the fact that costs of US medical care are the highest in the world [1]. The other 19 most wealthy countries (by GDP) pay less than half what the USA does for health care, and they also have added 6 more years of life expectancy than the USA (since 1970) [7]. Some assert that these statistics show that the US system is both the most costly and the most inefficient health-care system in the world. Others argue that the life expectancy in the USA reflects poor preventive health and the widespread obesity epidemic rather than the inefficiencies of the system. Regardless, our medical system is still the most advanced in the world, so it is now necessary for us to understand its structure in order to take the next steps—decreasing costs and improving quality.

US Health-Care Market: Characteristics

In understanding American health policy, it is instructive to view adverse health episodes as a "costly risk." Health episodes vary greatly in both rates of incidence (risk) and price of medical service (cost). But, in general, a patient will rarely encounter a certain condition, disease, injury, or health attack, but when he or she does, it is very costly. This idea is key to comprehending the market for health care.

Health as a "Good"

In health-care economics, "health care" is a "good" unlike anything else we regularly experience in the American economy. First of all, it is a derived good, as the demand for health care is really a demand for positive health or health outcomes. People want to be in a state of good health, and modern medicine has become the predominant vehicle through which to remain healthy in the United States.

Health care is often consumed like a good, granting relatively direct satisfaction, depending on the outcome of the medical care. The "utility" of getting treatment for a sudden life-threatening heart attack is extremely high because people want to survive to have a long life, but also because patients want to live with minimal pain, discomfort, or disability. When a person becomes injured or grows ill, the utility for curative or palliative care is suddenly very high, whereas it would have been nonexistent before. Consequently, there is a sudden very high demand for care, and that demand is relatively "inelastic," meaning people will probably purchase care even if the price rises. However, they will be less inclined to do so if they are paying out-of-pocket, as opposed to getting insurance to pay for it.

Health care can alternatively be built up like an investment in the long term. Depending on factors like lifestyle, exercise, diet, hereditary characteristics, and preventative care (especially relevant here), a young child will add or subtract from a certain amount of "health capital" over a lifetime. More health capital means a person will be healthier and will possess relatively less risk of becoming ill or injured. In America today, patients (and sometimes physicians) tend to focus on the short term, so they will not see tremendous value/utility in seeking preventative medicine because the results of this care only manifest in the long term. Consequently, demand for preventative medicine is more elastic than demand for curative medicine; people are more willing to forego preventative measures.

The aggregate supply of health-care provision is based on the combined decisions of many providers and can fluctuate based on specialty, regional trends, and health-care legislation, and in response to health-care consumers. However, the total supply of health care is so complex and institutionalized that it will change slowly over time. Aggregate supply of medical care is inelastic in the short term, which means that providers get accustomed to providing any amount of care at a given price and patient/consumer behavior will not be able to change this price. Supply will slowly expand over time, but it can also change suddenly depending on the type of consumer or insurer (meaning supply is also more elastic); this will be explained in detail in the following sections.

A Rational Basis for Health Insurance

It is worth noting that human beings put an extraordinary utility/value on their lives. In most developed countries, the "right to health" can be extrapolated to mean that everyone needs and deserves health care. In the United States, we declare the inalienable right to "life, liberty, and pursuit of happiness" [8]. Indirectly, modern American policy has evolved to guarantee access to health care for every citizen—or at least it aspires to provide for everyone. While public programs like Medicare/Medicaid are well-established ways to guarantee care today in America, the original and most common way to do so has been through health-care insurance.

The purchase of insurance is a *rational* decision by consumer/patients to ensure they can access and afford medical care. It is a *rational* way for third-party insurance companies to make money. And it is a *rational* way for providers to ensure and increase their business. Insurance is rationally advantageous for these three main entities involved in private medical care. This is because it "insures" against two critical problems in the market for health: uncertainty and asymmetric information.

Health, as well as health care, is intrinsically *uncertain*; properly dealing with uncertainty is, in many ways, a critical component in becoming a talented medical professional. Both the patient and the provider have little or no idea when sickness will strike. Therefore, it is difficult for the patient to plan for health-care access ahead of time. In the event that the ill can afford the proper care, there is no guarantee for ideal, certain outcomes from that treatment. Medicine is one of the most scientific disciplines, but does not always have predictable outcomes. The uncertainty about when and if the patient/consumer will need care, *plus* the uncertainty about the effectiveness and value of care, means that the health-care market is far from efficient.

The provision of health care also has intrinsic *information asymmetries*. Both providers and patients possess their own knowledge, which is often unavailable to the other party. Physicians have substantially more knowledge about health conditions than do patients, and they often charge for this expertise as a commodity. Sometimes doctors even "decommodify" themselves, saying we are "the best at joint replacements" or "we have the lowest infection rate" or "we will see you the fastest"—claims that patients might not completely understand. It is also difficult for doctors and insurers to decide on an upfront cost for care, as patients might withhold information about comorbidities or medical history. With this gap in knowledge and ambiguity in market price, there is a deadweight loss in market efficiency; there is a less-than-optimal provision of medical care.

Health uncertainty means that providers may not be paid for treatment except when disaster strikes, and at that time patients may not be able to pay for the expensive care. Here, at the point of service, supply and demand might not match up and purchased health care is foregone. In addition, patients do not possess "full and relevant information" about what treatment they require (as the doctors do), and they might withhold information from the doctor about their illness or ability to pay. Consequently, lack of information means that doctors are less likely to provide services and patients are less likely to seek it.

With the *risks of uncertainty* and the *risks of information asymmetry*, the market loses potential business and people need more care. Currently, the general health of Americans is getting worse, medical treatments are becoming more sophisticated, and therefore medical treatment and technology are getting more costly. These trends only exacerbate the risks that lead to a health-care market shortfall. Insurance is an economically rational, communal, and customary way to address both of these risks. Third-party insurance allows patients/customers to pool both minor and severe health risks, paying a little every month in order to avoid paying a lot when someone falls ill.

Additionally, insurance companies are one entity that might act as an arbiter between provider and patient. When people pool risk under the auspices of insurance corporations that possess more health-care expertise, two things happen. One, the company can negotiate on behalf of both provider and patient to determine a fair market price for services rendered. Two, the pooling of medical care for many under one insurance umbrella consolidates service and encourages business. Business in batches leads to less ambiguity in point-of-service health-care dealings.

Insurance offers a rational benefit to patients by making service more approachable and affordable; it offers a rational benefit to providers by bringing and facilitating more business than they would otherwise see. For patients, if the marginal cost of buying insurance is less than or equal to the actual benefits above, they will opt to purchase that insurance. Obviously, this does not always occur. Sometimes people will *perceive* fewer benefits from health insurance; for example, a 25-year-old might place his or her risk of being in an accident or getting cancer at "zero," when the *actual* risk is higher. Therefore, people (rationally or irrationally) withhold from buying insurance if the perceived benefit is lower than the actual cost of coverage.

The rising costs of medical care have made insurance less affordable and more important for patients/consumers. In order to understand these rising costs, we must first track how payments flow from patient to provider, usually facilitated by insurance.

US Health-Care Market: The Structure

As demonstrated earlier, the health-care market is both imperfect and complex. As demonstrated in every chapter of this book, health-care systems use an amalgam of payment structures, organizations, acronyms, and terminology. However, it is critical to note that underneath the labyrinth that is insured care, the health-care market revolves around the purchase of a good. Even if insurance obscures the actual flow of money, ultimately it follows that payment for this good goes from a consumer (the patient) to a seller (the provider). Keep this in mind as we trace where this money comes from and where this money goes to.

Where Does the Money Come from?
Payment Terminology

In order to understand where the money comes from, we should know a few terms. "Premiums" are the fees paid by patients (or on behalf of patients) to insurance providers with the expectation that the insurer pays for X amount of necessary medical care in the future. "Coinsurance" is the requirement for patients to share in the costs of medical care, usually a given percentage, sometimes through a "co-pay" for visits to the doctor, medical procedures, or pharmaceuticals. A "deductible" is the amount of expenses that must be paid "out-of pocket" before the third-party insurer will pay for medical expenses [9].

At the point of service, two distinctions are useful. One distinction is between "preventive care," which are anticipatory measures to deter negative health outcomes in the future, and "curative care," which is medical treatment of an illness, disease, or injury. Another distinction is between "charge" and "payment." While providers may have a common charge per visit or procedure, not all medical services are paid back in full. If there is payment for a procedure, sometimes third parties have an agreed-upon discount, which decouples the charge from the payment. However, the uninsured will always pay the full charge, or someone will have to pay that charge on their behalf.

Individual Private Insurance

The most straightforward mode of coverage in the United States is individual private insurance. This insurance group is often referred to as the "non-group." The American health-care system offers elective private insurance but does not require it. Patients who wish to insure against adverse health episodes pay a certain monthly premium, so that in the event of sickness, the insurance company will pay on their behalf. Many conditions are attached to an insurance deal—only certain procedures are covered, procedures are not necessarily covered in full, and the amount of coverage can be tiered according to price.

Effect on Prices

Individual consumers of private health insurance tend to pay more than those in small- and large-group employer-sponsored plans. Insurance corporations will generally not budge on premium levels on a person-to-person basis, since most of their business comes from the small- and large-group insurance market and because there is too much adverse risk in taking on individual customers.

Employer-Based Private Insurance

As mentioned in the previous chapters, 49 % of Americans obtain health insurance coverage through their employers—employer-sponsored insurance (ESI) [10]. Within a large company, numerous plans might be offered to all employees. In a very basic sense, a company steps in to pay some or all of an employee's premiums; more often than not, the worker will have to contribute a share of the premiums, coinsurance, and deductible.

Effect on Prices

Because their insurance is subsidized, employees generally pay less for their employer-sponsored plans than individuals do for private plans. By purchasing insurance en masse, a company can also lessen the overall price that is paid per unit for health insurance—essentially buying it wholesale. However, even if this does happen, total per-capita health expenditures for employee coverage are usually higher than the non-group market [11], because employees/employers will buy more insurance than individuals.

There are many reasons for this. First of all, employers get federal tax deductions for all health insurance they provide. In a 2008 report, the Congressional Research Service released a report arguing that employers will readily replace wages with more tax-free health insurance coverage, and therefore, employees will seek out more coverage than they otherwise would [12]. Especially due to higher-income people and families, tax deductions cause a significant over-purchase of insurance, which can increase health-care prices and make insurance less accessible to the poor and uninsured.

Medicare/Medicaid

In addition to the subsidy given for the previously mentioned tax exclusion, one of the US government's key roles in health care is to subsidize

health insurance for those who cannot access or afford coverage. Medicare offers defined federal benefits to patients under 65 years old: hospital care (Medicare Part A), necessary medical services and physician coverage (Part B), private network plans (Part C), and outpatient prescription drug assistance (Part D). Medicare patients on average cover half of their total health-care costs, paying for supplemental insurance, uncovered services, and coinsurance [13].

The Medicaid program is "means tested" and offered to poor children, their low-income parents, and people with certain disabilities [14]. In contrast to Medicare, Medicaid is managed predominantly at the state level, with funding from federal and state governments. Through fee-for-service or managed care programs approved by the US government, Medicaid covers more services than Medicare, including long-term care and comprehensive services for needy children.

Effect on Prices

Beneficiaries of both Medicare and Medicaid have to share the costs of medical care, some more than others. However, these public programs make their contributions directly to providers and not to patients (who contribute coinsurance), with many implications for health care costs. Because these programs are so expansive, they can bargain with providers for discounted health-care prices or even mandate the value of certain services [15]. While this approach can lower overall long-term health-care prices, physicians shift these costs to commercial insurance plans, and those patients see their premiums rise as a result [16]. As government's share of health-care expenditures continues to rise, public spending will continue to be a powerful policy-making and cost-bending tool.

Out-of-Pocket Payers

Many consumers opt out of health-care insurance. From the approach of rational economic theory, these people perceive the marginal cost of having insurance to be more than the marginal benefit. Out-of-pocket payers owe nothing until they seek elective or urgent medical care. Then they will pay full market price to the provider for whatever services are given. If they cannot pay the full value of services, the patient, provider reimbursement office, and any necessary government regulators or laws will decide on a proper patient contribution rate.

Without insurance, patients risk very sudden, exorbitant health-care costs, which shock their own finances in the short term and government finances in the long term. The costs of nonpayment by the patient are passed on to the health-care system and absorbed by the government and its taxpayers. While also burdening the system, out-of-pocket payers could lose everything; in 2007, medical payments caused a stunning 62 % of all personal bankruptcies in the United States [17].

Free Care

Many Americans do not purchase health insurance and cannot afford health care at the point and time of service. If patients are over 65, they are enrolled in Medicare. Citizens can pursue either private insurance or Medicaid coverage when they are younger than 65. For those without any type of coverage, the most common recourse is going to the emergency room (ER) when they are very sick. ER care is more expensive and is intended for emergencies, not for untreated sickness. However, uncovered patients even go to the ER for routine outpatient care.

When people wait until their illness warrants ER service, the total amount of ER care increases and overall health-care costs rise. Very often hospitals pay for this care, with assistance from state or federal "uncompensated care pools." These pools have to be very large to cover all ER care, so all Americans bear the cost to support uncompensated ER care.

Free clinics are another important place for people to seek health care. Many of these clinics provide a full range of primary care services, but not for complicated conditions that require more capital-intensive care. Funding for free clinics comes from elective, private sources. Importantly, these clinics provide for poor citizens and draw away costly traffic from hospital ERs, but cannot replace hospital-based care or even more complex outpatient evaluation and management.

Where Does the Money Flow?

In this chapter, we want to focus on where health-care money comes from, but we must also have a feel for where the money goes:

- *The money flows from*: America's total national health expenditure in 2010 was $2.6 trillion. 32 % of this was from private health insurance—the largest source of funding. However, combined public funding for health care comprised half of national health expenditure: the bulk of this is from Medicare at 21 % and Medicaid/CHIP at 16 % [2]. Other private, public, and out-of-pocket spending made up the remaining spending.

- *The money flows to*: in 2009, 30.5 % of the total American health expenditure went to hospital care [18]. The second largest slice of spending was paid for physician or clinical services: 20.3 %. Spending also went to prescription drugs (10.1 %), other personal health care (14.9 %), nursing home care (5.5 %), home health care (2.7 %), and other health spending (15.9 %). The specific flow of cash from consumer (or contributor) to provider is extremely complicated and beyond the scope of this chapter. Helpful details about reimbursement can be found in Chap. 15.

Quick Recap

In the early twentieth century, groundbreaking advances in medical technology led to the formalization of the health-care industry. Part of this formalization was the creation of third-party insurance, which was a way to spread financial risk and adverse effects of a unique health-care economy. Health insurance allows Americans to hedge against the uncertainties and information asymmetries in the market for medical services. In a private fee-for-service (FFS) system, payments for health care come from a number of sources. By examining each source, we can track the origins of significant health cost increases in the latter half of the twentieth century. In the next section, we will zoom out to understand key problems and possible solutions related to health-care affordability in the United States.

Problems Leading to Rising Costs in the Market for Health Care

The United States has a historically "fee-for-service" health-care system, which means that physicians charge fees commensurate with the type and amount of services they provide to patients. This system was tweaked with the emergence of basic managed care and is being markedly altered by different versions of "capitation," a type of payment system we will address in this chapter. However, it is critical to note that although we have many ways to pay for health services, in the end it is always the patient/consumer that pays. However the final bill is rerouted, consumers tend to bear the brunt of cost increases as America heads into the twenty-first century.

What is remarkable is that, because our insurance system is both employer and government based, very few individuals know how substantially they are affected by increasing health-care and insurance costs. Whereas the financial hurt is obvious when you write a larger check to your insurance company, it is hard to notice the raise you did *not* get because your employer's health-care costs were rising, eating away profits that would have gone to you in an increased salary. Below we demonstrate how costs have risen, and then we investigate how risks have been managed and distributed in response to increased costs.

Profit-Maximizing Behavior and the Rising Costs of Health Care

"The failure of the market to insure against uncertainties has created many social institutions in which the usual assumptions of the market are to some extent contradicted." This quote by Kenneth Arrow, one of the most influential health-care economists in history, effectively illustrates that the creation of health insurance to solve one problem—the unaffordability of unexpected care—created a new set of problems. Rising health-care costs are the main sequelae, and we explain them here.

The Adverse Effects of Technology (on Costs)

The cost of health care depends predominantly on medical costs. In the chapter breaking down health insurance, it was evidenced how rapidly advancing medical technology leads to rapidly rising health-care costs. Although imaging is often cited as a cause of the increasing costs, the problem is more system-wide. In 2012, routine MRIs cost $1,080 in the United States, somewhat more than the cost of an MRI in other developed countries (in Switzerland the cost is $903; in Germany the cost is $599). However, the cost of a hospital visit is $15,734 in America, *three times* the going rate in Germany [19]. With more hospital care than ever before in the United States (30 % of expenditures) and more life-threatening illnesses that require those services, our health-care system is very much based on treatment and not prevention. America is richer, sicker, and more medically advanced today than ever. This is why procedures like coronary artery bypasses cost an average of $68,000 in the USA today [19].

The Adverse Effects of Providers (on Costs)

In a fee-for-service (FFS) health-care system without government price controls, joint provider-insurer price agreements, or substantial free-market regulation, it is well documented that the quantity and cost of medical services will increase progressively [20]. FFS health-care payments, aggressive pharmaceutical and medical device marketing campaigns, and ever-rising medical costs create incentives for doctors to provide more treatments. Whether or not providers are aware of their practices, an FFS system will encourage the following financial conflicts of interest: to avoid integrated care, practice self-referral, and put a premium on quantity over quality. Predictable cost increases ensue from such practices.

Cost increases and overutilization of health care reinforce each other, so at the turn of the century, doctors find themselves practicing "hamster health care": decreasing patient care time and increasing patient turnover just to keep their practices afloat [21]. This practice might raise $1 of professional income for doctors, but the final medical bill could increase $5—the multiplier effect in health care. This system is exacerbated by the still-common practice of price-discrimination, where doctors charge more to those who can pay more. They negotiate a higher price with the private market in order to balance out discounts for low-income and nonpaying customers. Private *and* public insurance costs rise as a result of price discrimination.

One last point related to providers: the system for training and becoming a licensed medical doctor restricts the number of qualified doctors. When fewer doctors are available, they will more readily be able to discriminate between patients who can afford their services and those who cannot; restricted supply perpetuates the out-of-control hamster wheel that is health care, and thus, the costs will continue to rise.

The Adverse Effects Due to Consumers (on Costs)

Overutilization of health care is due to many factors other than physicians. If a hospital increases the bed count, those beds will most likely be filled in the short term. In this case, "supply begets demand" of health services, even if people are not getting more ill in the short term [22]. Observing human nature in America, there is little a family will not do to keep loved ones alive. If there is an elderly high-income patient requiring a coronary heart bypass with little chance of survival, few patients (or their family) will choose against measures to stay alive, regardless of the chances. Americans are living longer, and health becomes more expensive after age 65. Consequently, short- and especially long-term care of senior citizens makes up an inordinate share of health-care expenditure [23]. Last-year-of-life expenses constituted 22 % of all medical spending in the United States [23]. And, overall, the highest-spending 5 % of patients (many of whom are the very sick and/or senior citizens) accounted for over half of total health-care expenditures in the United States in 2012 [24].

Those with a high ability to pay, or extreme readiness to seek paid or unpaid services, utilize most medical care; this is a type of reverse price/service discrimination. However, insurance coverage allows more people to pursue these costly services. Having purchased insurance premiums to spread risk, patients feel shielded from paying for health services [25]. In the short term, they could opt for emergency health procedures that cost twice as much. In a medical version of the prisoner's dilemma [26], patients will usually opt for more care if they do not have to pay for it in the short term, even if the services will have minimal health benefits. However, in the long run, everyone will pay higher premiums, including the patient who "benefited" from costly care.

Applying his economic lens to health care, Kenneth Arrow labels overconsumption of health care due to insurance a "moral hazard." In an "inefficient moral hazard," many patients make the same choices (to seek unnecessary medical care because "they can") that make everybody worse in the long term—a net welfare loss. Some scholars will make the case for an "efficient moral hazard," where increased consumption allows individuals to attain better health outcomes in the long term—a net welfare gain [27]. Regardless, the moral hazard undoubtedly inflates the cost of health care.

The Adverse Effects of Insurance (on Cost)

Because of these collective incentives for doctors and consumer/patients to overutilize health care, insurance companies charge higher premiums to offset the resulting increased costs. Eventually, there is a significant group of patients that can no longer afford to insure against health risks. Through new insurance policies denying coverage to people with preexisting conditions and refusing to cover certain services, more patients have been added to this group. The newly uninsured either seek uncompensated care through the ER or forego necessary care while their conditions continue to worsen. Both options hurt not only the individual but also systemic health-care costs and quality.

Insurance companies make a profit by minimizing the "medical loss ratio" (MLR), which means that they cover less in insurance claims than they earn by collecting premiums [28]. If an insurer is not making a profit, they will exit the health-care market. So when medical services and costs rise, insurance corporations will automatically pass on these costs to the consumer in the form of premiums, coinsurance, or deductibles.

The Adverse Effects of Government (on Cost)

As will be demonstrated later in this section, the government can do a lot to decrease costs. However, there are a few current policies that tend to exacerbate the rising cost of medical care. First of all, the government grants tax exclusions for most employer contributions to employees' health insurance plans. This exemption has helped to keep the American system predominantly employer based and does in fact lead to more total coverage. However, employers end up over-purchasing insurance, which increases cost [12]. Secondly, publicly provided insurance can increase coverage but will also systemically underpay for these hospital and professional services; this forces providers to negotiate higher fees for those covered under private insurance.

Possible Departures from Profit-Maximizing Behavior

Health insurance economist Mark Pauly suggests this situation:

Consider two companies A and B: company A offers health insurance on top of a relatively low salary. Company B does *not* offer health insurance, but workers are paid a higher salary. Company A might prefer to offer discounted insurance instead of extra direct pay, especially since employees put a premium on jobs that supply insurance. However, those employees *could* otherwise be given that same money in hand, were it not that individual private insurance was more risky for the third party and more expensive for the patient.

Health-care insurance is so ingrained into American employment that we rarely stop to think about its cost to the employee/patient/consumer. While workers for Company A see insurance as an important benefit, they do not usually perceive how expensive that benefit really is. For example, if a worker *did* transfer to a viable Company B—one that had the same amount of resources for worker compensation—he or she would earn a much higher salary. While the average American family treats their premium contributions and co-pays as their health-care expenditure, their hidden cost could be 20 % of their salary. An $80,000 annual salary could otherwise be $100,000, but the American public does not always perceive it this way. Only after they underutilize preventive care and overutilize curative treatment do they see health-care costs severely reduce their paychecks.

To make a very long story short, in most cases consumer/patients will bear the brunt of increased medical costs in a fee-for-service (FFS) health-care system. The fact that consumers feel the shock in the long term is largely the problem. There have been many efforts to contain health-care costs in the United States, many of which included dramatic structural changes to how medical care is offered and paid for. These new methods have had varying degrees of success. Here we will briefly survey the most important attempts to reform health-care payment structures.

Managed Care

As described in the previous chapters, managed care was the first concerted system-wide effort to reign in American health-care costs. Managed care organizations (MCOs), the first of which were HMOs, put constraints on medical service usage through utilization review and "gatekeeping" to more effective, integrated care [29]. Managed care augmented the delivery of traditional insurance and effectively slowed cost growth in the 1980s. Even public programs adopted managed care structures, and it was popular opinion that health care was more efficient alongside the emerging practice of evidence-based medicine (as opposed to multiple-approach medicine) [30].

However, total health expenditures rose again in the late 1980s, alongside a transformation in managed care itself. There were many reasons for the decline of managed care as it was originally built to be. As managed care became more widely used, providers were progressively more resistant to let insurance plans determine which practitioners and hospitals were covered. At the same time, consumers were dissatisfied when they were denied services or received insufficient claims from their plans. Very often both doctors and patients would file for damages against what they thought were faulty business practices [31].

In the late 1990s, dissent grew enough that insurance companies relaxed many of their regulations. Plans now allowed greater access to specialists and referrals for certain hospital procedures. Because utilization review and PCP gatekeepers were the key cost-containment mechanisms for MCOs, something had to take their place. MCOs in turn shifted the responsibility for health-care decision making to consumers/patients. Plans encouraged subscribers to increase preventative care and modify health-related behaviors, with the help of newly created websites. Instead of using time and resources to advocate for their subscribers, MCOs offered wellness programs and disease management.

This was the beginning of what is termed "consumer-driven" health care. Managed care plans started to deny high-risk patients access to their pools, sometimes withdrawing from Medicare and Medicaid entirely [32]. For the consumers that could be covered, a product called the "high-deductible health plan" (HDHP) was created, with fewer premiums in order to control costs. These plans were supposed to insure against catastrophic conditions, and having an HDHP was the only way to qualify for health savings accounts (HSAs) and health reimbursement accounts (HRAs). These accounts were tax deductible and only to be used on health expenses, leaving patient/consumers to make their own spending decisions. In essence, this new type of managed care was becoming increasingly similar to insurance systems before managed care, just adorned with new institutions.

Two examples of these new institutions would be coinsurance and deductibles. In order to limit health cost growth, managed care organizations would keep premiums slightly lower for patients, but they would have to contribute a co-pay for pharmaceuticals, tests, and doctors' appointments.

Additionally, patients would now have to pay out-of-pocket for a minimum of health services annually, a limit called a deductible. Basically, today MCOs still are very liable for insurance claims, but they've transferred some of the initial bill to consumers. Patients continue to be asked to contribute more: from 2006 to 2012, the percentage of workers paying deductibles over $1000 rose from 10 % to 34 % [10].

FFS patients today are increasingly responsible for their out-of-pocket expenses, but they are also less shielded from cost increases due to provider or third-party behavior. Insurance companies, after intense provider and consumer pressure, have shifted cost risks to consumers once again.

Capitation

The most obvious problem with fee-for-service (FFS) with regards to increased costs is the adverse incentive to treat more and therefore charge more. With this structural pressure, insurance companies avoid covering high-risk patients, and doctors treat the sickest patients with the most medical "firepower" possible. In the 1980s, providers and HMOs started to create radically new models for physician reimbursement. The new thinking was that 3rd parties should pay in the aggregate in order to discourage overtreatment and moderate the medical costs incurred. Fully extrapolated, this idea would end in full capitation, which means "pay by the head" [33].

DRGs

A precursor and more widely accepted payment methodology to full capitation was the system of diagnosis-related groups (DRGs), originally 467 classifications by Medicare for inpatient hospital diagnoses. Beginning in 1983, Medicare would assign a treatment cost for each DRG, which would be paid regardless of how long a patient was hospitalized [34]. Comorbidities and confounding health-related variables are accounted for in assigning DRGs. As expected, it took decades to refine these groups to represent contingencies and new diagnoses. Medicare used this practice to slow down skyrocketing prices in the 1980s, and DRGs have been moderately successful since.

There are two possible glitches with implementing DRGs. First of all, when patients are sicker than expected and require more hospitalization, doctors might assign a new DRG code with a higher charge. If this reassignment is easy enough, the incentive to limit treatment (to what is necessary) disappears, and the DRG system becomes a de facto fee-for-service payment method. On the contrary, if the hospital does not allow the updating of DRG codes, physicians have the adverse incentive to discharge patients early. This latter incentive is disappearing as Medicare is now penalizing hospitals for readmissions [35].

Full Capitation

In a fee-for-service payment structure, doctors get paid for every piece of work they do. Under capitation, HMOs pay provider groups monthly payments for everyone they insure. After this payment, the provider must (within limits) give care to enrolled people, regardless of whether they accrue tremendous treatment costs or they never fall ill. This payment structure limits health-care cost increases in the short term because providers have incentive to limit unnecessary care. If they do not, doctors cannot make money, and the only recourse is to raise total capitation rates in the long term.

Capitation and FFS programs face *opposite* problems. In an FFS system, doctors' salaries depend on how much care they provide. Under capitation, doctors receive identical revenue whether they provide 2 days or 10 days of inpatient care. However, they will profit much more off of a 2-day hospital stay. Insurers are passing off to providers their responsibility to manage risk. Provider networks now must figure out how to divvy up a monthly set of payments among PCPs and specialists, how to reconcile the desire to increase quality with the incentive to decrease quantity of care, and how to calculate the risks of their patients falling ill, which used to be the insurer's job, using the insurance company's data and techniques.

By nature, provider networks have less actuarial experience in analyzing health risks compared to professional insurance companies. They are also much smaller than HMOs and therefore have fewer patients per insurance pool over which to spread risk. In essence, insurance companies have transferred their financial risk onto providers, who are less-qualified financial managers. The worry with full capitation is that providers will need to sacrifice the quantity of health care, to the detriment of quality. By extension, instead of bearing the financial risks of health services, consumer/patients will now bear more health risks.

Bundled Payments

A bundled payment system represents the "middle ground" between fee-for-service and full capitation systems [36]. In a bundle system, physicians are paid a negotiated lump sum for each hospital visit, rather than a sum for each service provided (FFS), or a sum per month for each patient, irrespective of services provided (full capitation).

In response to issues with diagnosis-related groups, experiments in the late 1980s created "case rates for episodes of illness," basically paying hospitals for a defined period of treatment. This fee would cover any necessary health-related costs, possibly including follow-up clinic visits. The first trial of bundled payments by the Texas Heart Institute in 1984 maintained that this approach lowered costs while maintaining a high quality of care [37]. Trials much later by the Geisinger Health System in Pennsylvania (2006–2007) would show that patients utilizing "ProvenCare"—their bundled payment system—had shorter total lengths of stay, lower readmission rates, and a greater likelihood of being discharged to home [38].

Although bundles have worked in certain situations, they have not been tested outside of these very careful controls. Without sufficient evidence for bundled payments so far, the effect of widespread bundling on health outcomes is "uncertain" [36]. Some concerns with bundles: physicians might still undertreat patients—as is the problem in DRGs. In capitation, repeat visits to the hospital are still covered by the monthly fee, but with bundling if patients are discharged and return for care after the "global payment period ends," a new bundle starts. While it is possible to regulate against this tendency, doctors will still be incentivized to hospitalize patients unnecessarily [39] and to favorably input patients that can pay more. At risk populations could be left further behind.

A series of other problems are possible, depending on the type of bundling: the hospital might have disagreements with specialists over how to divide payments [33]; academic medical centers will be at a financial disadvantage by using resources for research, teaching, and technology; and it might be excessively difficult to specify what constitutes certain "episodes" and their corresponding "fair compensation rates" [40].

Not a Perfect Solution

With all three approaches—DRGs, capitation, and bundled payments—providers have a reason to reign in care, which can also achieve the goal of reigning in costs. However, providers may be incentivized to do "too little for more money." In 2009, health economists Stuart Altman and Robert Mechanic said: "Considering the advantages and disadvantages of fee-for-service, pay for performance, bundled payment for episodes of care, and global payment such as capitation... 'episode payments' are the most immediately viable approach" [41].

There are many proposed ways to protect against the disadvantages of bundles. One possible way is to give providers a penalty for allowing the cost of a bundle to be upgraded after initial diagnosis or for adverse health outcomes due to insufficient treatment at the point of service. The problem with these solutions is differentiating adverse outcomes that could have been prevented from those that occur due to random variation. Preventing upgrading a bundle or charging for treatment in the latter circumstance is unfair to the treating community.

Alternatively, physicians could receive bonuses for voluntarily cutting down on unnecessary services, leading to a reduced health-care bill. There is the natural response though that it is perverse to incentivize a physician to earn more by doing less. The goal must be to do better. For the first time in history, Medicare is attempting to employ many of these techniques while rolling out a national pilot for bundled payments, specifically for acute and post-acute care [42].

The Problem

After understanding two major approaches to sharing risk—fee-for-service and capitation—there are seemingly intractable trade-offs in the attempts to reform health care in the United States [43]. These trade-offs have the potential to adversely affect the costs, quantity, and quality of health services.

Costs

In seeking quality health for Americans, low costs are not the inherent goal, but high costs are the predominating obstacle. In trying to decrease the cost of medical care, we are faced with what seems like a Catch-22: we must either give out less medical care or pass the cost of more care onto patient/consumers. It does not help that 5 % of Americans require 50 % of our national health expenditures. These high-risk patients are expensive to insure, but if no one insures them, those expenses are borne by "the system" after the patients grow even more sick. Consumers (and sometimes doctors) want to take advantage of services they perceive as free—from either uncompensated pools or insurance claims—but all patients see their premiums rise in the process.

Quantity

The tremendous costs of health care distort the health-care provision in the United States. In a FFS payment system, more services are offered to those who can pay for them; as a result, basic services become unavailable to certain income brackets. There are extensive arguments about whether more is better, and there are clear examples of where it is not. That said, the population continues to demand more care, and setting up and spreading systems to provide better care rather than more care has thus far proven elusive [44]. To exacerbate the decline in American health care, there is a massive shortfall in the provision of preventative medicine. Part of the problem here is that people frequently change insurers, and thus, a given insurance company does not have the incentive to invest in an individual's health and subsequently sends that investment to a competitor. Even as preventative care increases, the consumer/patient uptake of these services is far from ideal.

Quality

The quality of the top medical care in the United States is unparalleled, but many citizens do not have access to this care. Costs are an important reason why quality suffers. Very few insurance plans cover the full expense of emergent or chronic care, and those plans are unaffordable for most Americans. Many of the worst conditions could be attacked early on through preventive care, but the American health-care system historically shies away from cautionary treatment or wellness programs, as these do not prove lucrative for medical professionals. Insurance companies and consumer/patients alike must deal with the financial risks of catastrophic health in the long term, risks that could be reduced through comprehensive preventative measures. Unfortunately, consumers pay with poor health and extreme expenses, much more so than risk-averse insurance giants.

The Solution

As described previously, two "inevitabilities" of health care have resulted, despite concerted policy efforts to avoid them. Firstly, we have an "iron triangle" encompassing the three essential aspects of health-care systems: quality, cost, and access. Traditionally, health scholars maintain that you cannot affect one aspect without adversely affecting one or both of the others. Secondly, the consumer/patient always tends to "lose," either by paying too much for health care, not receiving ideal quality health care, or by not getting care at all.

However, opponents of the "iron triangle" contend that there is no consistent, direct correlation between the cost of care and its quality, especially since there is a substantial "cost of poor quality" due to overuse, misuse, and waste in American health care. This waste could comprise up to 30 % of health-care spending [45].

A case in point: in 2009 physician-journalist Atul Gawande studied McAllen, Texas, the town with the most expensive health-care costs in America, costs greater than the town's average income. McAllen has the same demographics and comparable technology to El Paso, Texas, but double the per capita health-care spending. Interestingly, despite comprehensive malpractice reform in both cities, McAllen orders 50 % more specialist visits, and its patients are two-thirds more likely to see ten or more specialists in a 6-month period.

On a greater scale in America, there is a negative correlation between the states' levels of Medicare expenditure and their health-care quality rankings [46]. Furthermore, the four states with the highest levels of health-care spending rank at the bottom nationally for quality of patient care [44]. On a much more encouraging note, Mayo Clinic in Rochester, Minnesota, features the highest level of technological capability and quality indicators, while also offering this care at costs in the country's lowest fifteenth percentile [44]. Further studies in Grand Junction, Colorado, and with the Geisinger Health System in Pennsylvania, suggest that Mayo is not an aberration [44]. Solutions exist to overhaul health-care quality alongside health-care costs.

The solution seems to be one with many facets, as there has not really been one cure-all for health-care cost increases. Because of the key problems in American health-care economics—many of which were explained in this chapter—the solution lies in making health care sustainable. The rate of health-care cost increases is unsustainable, even to the United States as a whole. At 17 % of GDP and growing, these costs are the primary driver of American debt [47]. In order to bring down costs and ensure effective medical provision in the future, we must make sure everyone feels cost increases and quality decreases.

In order to do this, many assert that we need to align incentives—for providers, patients, and 3rd parties—to decrease cost and increase quality/access. Early models and techniques for doing so, some included in the Patient Protection and Affordable Care Act (PPACA), emphasize sharing of financial risks as well as incentivizing quality provision of health care for all players. Chapter 15 features in-depth explanations on new payment methods, but it is critical to first understand the significance of these methods to health-care economics.

When considering this, it is also worth noting our hypothesis that physicians in general want lower-risk jobs. They do not seek high variability in their income and prefer a reliable solid income rather than the chance at a very high income in exchange for the risk of a low income (a risk tolerance more common to Wall Street). As such, these models that transfer risk to doctors transfer it to a group of people not only ill-equipped mathematically to deal with the risk but also ill-equipped in preference to do so.

The Obamacare/PPACA

PPACA, known by supporters and detractors as "Obamacare," features many initiatives for risk sharing and incentivizing quality. The effectiveness of these strategies has yet to be proven one way or the other, but the law is an instructive lens through which to study options for the future. One of the main vehicles through which the US government can set new health-care precedents is through Medicare; its significant purchasing role is "policymakers' most powerful lever to alter negative trends" [48]. Most of PPACA's new ideas will first be trialed through Medicare.

Integrated Care

Health-care policymakers consistently agree that medical care needs to be more seamless and integrated. Streamlining care usually involves improvement in information-sharing technologies and both vertical (primary, secondary, and tertiary care) and horizontal integration (multidisciplinary specialist teams). Most reforms in PPACA contribute to integrating care, and each has potential benefits and drawbacks.

Pay for Performance

Pay for performance (P4P), or "value-based purchasing," is a central strategy in aligning incentives in American health care today. This model is the newest version of managed care, first trialed in California (2001) [49]; in short, providers are rewarded for achieving quality and efficiency

standards. One example would be receiving a percentage of all savings underneath the index value for a set of procedures (or patients). P4P oftentimes stipulates disincentives for providers that incur unnecessary costs—due to mistakes and ordering of superfluous tests. At one extreme, payers may refuse to pay for specified "never events" such as avoidable inpatient infections.

One difficulty with implementing P4P is drawing up performance metrics that cover every contingency and yet do not present negative externalities. If certain outcomes are incentivized, providers might select cases they can easily manage and select against the sickest patients with the most uncertain outcomes. If certain procedures are stipulated as "proper care," physicians might overutilize radiographs or lengthen hospital stays. In both cases, defensive medicine is oftentimes an adverse solution that actually yields suboptimal physician performance. Finally, if decreased costs are incentivized, doctors might do the opposite; they would provide "too little for more money"— as is a problem with capitation—but they would also be given a reward for doing so.

P4P has produced a mixed bag of outcomes. Initial studies suggest that P4P implementation shows small gains in quality for the money spent [50]. Start-up administration costs for P4P systems are extremely high, so these studies call into question the P4P models as they stand today. Supporters of P4P stress the unmeasurable performance improvements that result from the model; they also argue that as performance metrics become more nuanced (to reflect particular social and economic circumstances), medical services will improve more significantly.

Accountable Care Organizations (ACOs)

PPACA provides for trials of Accountable Care Organizations (ACOs), a much newer entity that employs some P4P and other capitation ideals. ACOs are doctors' organizations, which means that consumer/patients can see any ACO physician without being restricted to a preselected group of providers. The providers, however, are at risk for the expenses of the patient and thus are incentivized to keep the patient within their own system.

The PPACA enacted regulations in October 2011, outlining requirements for ACOs. Basically, hospitals or groups of physicians can unite under an ACO, receiving a stamp of approval for quality, cost, and patient-interaction measures. The US Department of Health and Human Services (DHHS) allows physicians to participate in their ACO program through the Medicare Shared Savings Program (MSSP) for a minimum of 3 years, with requirements for patient assessment and engagement. As described thoroughly in Chap. 15, there are two models for new ACOs through Medicare, one featuring shared savings (between payers and providers) without shared risks (for providers) and the other featuring greater shared savings for providers but with some shared risks if the cost of care exceeds CMS benchmarks [51].

There are distinguishing traits of ACOs. Firstly, providers are incentivized to integrate care to improve quality and decrease costs simultaneously, without the risks of losing money. Secondly, physicians have a lot of freedom to lead in the structuring of new ACOs. Potential disadvantages can arise with this lack of a specific structure for ACOs. Start-up costs can be high, coordination with patients and payer risks being disorganized, and overorganization could violate antitrust laws and drive up health-care costs.

Government Regulation

PPACA will be more thoroughly covered in Chap. 19 but deserves brief coverage in the context of payments. While it does give government a more active role in organizing health care, it does not constitute a government take-over. It is important to note that, before PPACA, the Federal Government did indeed run Medicare/Medicaid, just as it does Social Security, but not all transfer payments qualified as a rich-to-poor redistribution. Today, Bill Gates and "Joe Sixpack" both receive Medicare and Social Security payments, and very often Medicaid covers sicker patients and not just poorer patients.

PPACA creates a new "triangle" of policies—those of guaranteed issue, community rating, and an individual mandate—which are the lynchpin to the expansion of coverage in the private market. Guaranteed issue requires health insurance plans to offer insurance to every American regardless of preexisting conditions. These plans must be community rated such that an individual cannot be charged a higher premium for uncontrollable factors like a family history of cancer, a diagnosis of heart disease, or even gender. The mandate is well known and requires that every citizen must have insurance. In order to quell concerns with these three requirements, the government will subsidize many plans in order to facilitate universal coverage, and it will also allow grandfathering of individuals' insurance plans.

The government will build an exchange, which can be thought of as an "Amazon.com" for insurance, letting private (and not public) insurers to place their products on the exchange. They demand a minimum level of coverage for a plan to be listed but otherwise leave it as a wide-open competitive market. The government will then subsidize poor individuals, enabling them to purchase on the open market. The overall theme here is to maximize choice and, as much as possible, to keep the government out of health insurance decisions while ensuring that everyone is insured.

It is important to note that arguments against the individual mandate have many misperceptions. If the mandate is struck down, as was unsuccessfully attempted in 2012 [52], the remaining two tenants of Obamacare would destroy the private insurance market as we know it. If people can always get affordable health care (through guaranteed issue and community rating), but do not have to buy it today, they will just choose to buy it tomorrow if and when they get sick. Eventually, private insurance companies will exit the market because there is no incentive to cover the sickest people without seeing commensurate compensation. The result would be single-payer health care. The health economist's takeaway from studying the PPACA: If you want to ensure that anyone with preexisting conditions can be affordably insured (and guaranteed issue and community rating) in the private market, the individual mandate must exist. The three were meant to work in synchrony.

Conclusion

Over the last 100 years, the health-care system has gone through remarkable changes. Hand in hand, the explosion of medical capabilities, augmented by the distribution of risk and insulation from the cost consequence of care provided by third-party insurance, has led to a system that is increasingly taking over the economy. Most agree that the current trends are untenable and that some change must be made in the marketplace to ensure that insurance and the provision of health care do not bankrupt the federal government and state governments, and that these changes do not make business uncompetitive in the international marketplace. There is little agreement on what changes need to be made, but most all agree that the current incentives in the system, both for patients and providers, have perverse consequences and need to be modified in some way. The question for the next decade and for the policymakers of today and tomorrow is how to do this while protecting patients.

Looking towards the future, health care is taking up a larger percentage of persons' total income and could reach 30 % in the not too distant future. The problem with this is that in addition to its obvious costs mentioned in this chapter, growth in health care can crowd out other jobs in the American economy. Throughout both the Bush and Obama administrations, the health-care industry is one of few growing industries alongside otherwise stagnant growth. To make medical care more efficient, we need to figure out how to bend the cost curve. Especially considering efforts with managed care, it seems that many strategies to reduce costs cause a one-time shock, followed by a subsequent rise in prices. New models, including some we have mentioned directly previously in this chapter, could cause similar shocks.

However, health economist Robert Shapiro maintains that, despite our attempts to reform the way medical care is provided, the real problem is in demand for health care [53]. The dearth of preventive care in America, coupled with a growing willingness to seek and provide curative care, makes prices soar. In these situations, providing access to health services is not necessarily the solution in bending the cost curve. If health-care utilization gets more excessive, we could even be looking at health-care cost controls in our country's future. Therefore, we should all examine the root of the problem—patient health—and see what we can do to help quell demand for health care in the future.

References

1. Anderson GF, Reinhardt UE, Hussey PS, et al. It's the prices, stupid: why the United States is so different from other countries. Health Aff. 2003;22(3):89–105.
2. Centers for Medicare and Medicaid Services, Office of the Actuary. Updated National Health expenditure projections 2009–2019. 2011 Jan. https://www.cms.gov/Research-Statistics-Data-and-Systems/Statistics-Trends-and-Reports/NationalHealthExpendData/downloads/proj2009.pdf
3. Healthcare payment and delivery reform: is it capitation 2.0?Accenture; 2011. http://www.accenture.com/SiteCollectionDocuments/PDF/Accenture_Health_Healthcare_Payment_Reform_Final_Electonic.pdf
4. The Kaiser Family Foundation. Health care spending in the United States and selected OECD countries. 2011 Apr. http://www.kff.org/insurance/snapshot/oecd042111.cfm
5. The Kaiser Family Foundation. Health care costs: a primer. The Kaiser Family Foundation. 2012 May;1. http://www.kff.org/insurance/7670.cfm
6. The joint Commission. Health care at the crossroads: guiding principles for the development of the hospital of the future. 2008;11. http://www.jointcommission.org/assets/1/18/Hosptal_Future.pdf
7. Kenworthy L. America's inefficient health-care system: another look. Consider the evidence (blog). 2011 July 10. http://lanekenworthy.net/2011/07/10/americas-inefficient-health-care-system-another-look/
8. Jefferson Thomas, editor. Scanned image of the Jefferson's "original rough draught" of the declaration of independence, written in June 1776, including all the changes made later by John Adams, Benjamin Franklin and other members of the committee, and by Congress. Declaration of independence: Jefferson's draft as amended and accepted by Congress. http://www.loc.gov/exhibits/declara/images/draft1.jpg. The United States of America: Library of Congress.
9. Sullivan A, Sheffrin SM. Economics: principles in action. Upper Saddle River: Pearson Prentice Hall; 2003. p. 524.
10. Kaiser Family Foundation. Calculations and slides using NHE data from Centers for Medicare and Medicaid Services. Office of the Actuary. National Health Statistics Group. http://www.cms.hhs.gov/NationalHealthExpendData/

11. Young DA, Wildsmith TF. Perspective: individual versus employer insurance markets: digging deeper into the difference. Health Aff (Millwood) 2002 Jul–Dec; Suppl Web Exclusives:W391-4. http://content.healthaffairs.org/content/suppl/2003/12/03/hlthaff.w2.182v1.DC1

12. Lyke B. Congressional research service. The tax exclusion for employer-provided health insurance: policy issues regarding the repeal debate. CRS report; 2008 Nov 21.

13. Medicare Chartbook. Sources of payment for medicare fee-for-service beneficiaries' health care spending, 2006. 4th ed. 2010. http://facts.kff.org/chart.aspx?cb=58&sctn=168&ch=1785

14. Centers for Medicare and Medicaid Services. Medicaid program information. CMS website. http://medicaid.gov/Medicaid-CHIP-Program-Information/Medicaid-and-CHIP-Program-Information.html

15. Wilensky GR. Reforming medicare's physician payment system. N Engl J Med. 2009;360:653–5.

16. Hospital & physician cost shift: payment level comparison of medicare, medicaid, and commercial payers. Milliman; 2008 Dec. http://publications.milliman.com/research/health-rr/pdfs/hospital-physician-cost-shift-RR12-01-08.pdf

17. Himmelstein DU, Thorne D, Warren E, et al. Medical bankruptcy in the United States, 2007: results of a National study. Am J Med. 2009;122(8):741–6.

18. Rublee DA, Schneider M. International health spending: comparisons with the OECD. Health Aff. 1991; 10(3):187–98.

19. Andrews A. The high cost of medical procedures in the U.S. Graphic, International Federation of Health Plans. Article, Washington Post; 2012 Mar 2. http://www.washingtonpost.com/wp-srv/special/business/high-cost-of-medical-procedures-in-the-us/

20. Emanuel EJ, Fuchs VR. The perfect storm of overutilization. JAMA. 2008;299(23):2789–91.

21. Morrison I. Hamster health care: time to stop running faster and redesign health care. Br Med J. 2000;321:1541–2.

22. Roemer MI. Bed supply and hospital utilization: a natural experiment. Hospitals. 1961;1:35, 36–42.

23. Hoover DR, Crystal S, Kumar R. Medical expenditures during the last year of life: findings from the 1992–1996 medicare current beneficiary survey. Health Services Research; 2002 Dec. http://www.ncbi.nlm.nih.gov/pmc/articles/PMC1464043/

24. Cohen SB, Yu W. The concentration and persistence in the level of health expenditures over time: estimates for the U.S. Population, 2008–2009. Medical Expenditure Panel Survey, Agency for Healthcare Research and Quality. http://meps.ahrq.gov/mepsweb/data_files/publications/st354/stat354.pdf

25. Pauly MV. Taxation, health insurance, and market failure in the medical economy. J Econ Lit. 1986; 24(2):629–75.

26. Poundstone W. Prisoner's dilemma. New York: Anchor Books/Doubleday; 1992.

27. Frick KD, Chernew ME. Beneficial moral hazard and the theory of the second best. Excellus Health Plan; 2009 June. http://www.rwjf.org/content/rwjf/en/research-publications/find-rwjf-research/2009/06/beneficial-moral-hazard-and-the-theory-of-the-second-best.html

28. Robinson JC. Use and abuse of the medical loss ratio to measure health plan performance. Health Aff (Millwood). 1997;16(4):176–87.

29. Health Insurance Association of America. Managed care: integrating the delivery and financing of health care – Part A. 1995;9. http://www.amazon.com/dp/1879143267

30. Sackett DL et al. Evidence based medicine: what it is and what it isn't. PubMed Central, Free Articles. BMJ. 1996;312(7023):71–72.

31. Havighurst CC. Consumers versus managed care: the new class actions. Health Aff. 2001;20(4):8–14.

32. Lagoe R, Aspling DL, Westert GP. Current and future developments in managed care in the United States and implications for Europe. Health Res Policy Syst. 2005;3(4):6.

33. Bodenheimer, TS, Grumbach K. Capitation or decapitation: keeping your head in changing times. Health care policy: a clinical approach; 1996 Oct. http://jama.jamanetwork.com/article.aspx?articleid=408553

34. Jain SH, Besancon E. Reimbursement: understanding how we pay for healthcare. In: Sethi MK, editor. Health policy for physicians. New York: Springer; (2013).

35. Rau J. Medicare to Penalize 2,217 hospitals for excess readmissions. Kaiser Health News; 2012 Aug. http://www.kaiserhealthnews.org/Stories/2012/August/13/medicare-hospitals-readmissions-penalties.aspx

36. RAND Corporation. Overview of bundled payment. Comprehensive Assessment of Reform Efforts (COMPARE). 2011. http://www.rand.org/health/projects/compare.html

37. Edmonds C, Hallman GL. Cardiovascular care providers. A pioneer in bundled services, shared risk, and single payment. Tex Heart Inst J. 1995;22(1):72–6.

38. Asale AS, Paulus RA, Selna MJ, et al. ProvenCareSM: a provider-driven pay-for-performance program for acute episodic cardiac surgical care. Ann Surg. 2007;246(4):613–21. discussion 621–3.

39. Medicare Payment Advisory Commission. A path to bundled payment around a hospitalization. Chapter 4. Report to the Congress: reforming the delivery system. Washington, DC: Medicare Payment Advisory Commission; 2008. pp. 80–103.

40. Robinow A. The potential of global payment: insights from the field. Washington, DC: The Commonwealth Fund; 2010.

41. Mechanic RE, Altman SH. Payment reform options: episode payment is a good place to start. Health Aff (Millwood). 2009;28(2):262–71.

42. Sood N, Huckfeldt PJ, Escarce JJ. Medicare's bundled payment pilot for acute and postacute care: analysis and recommendations on where to begin. Health Aff (Millwood). 2011;30(9):1708–17.

43. Berenson RA, Rich EC. US approaches to physician payment: the deconstruction of primary care. J Gen Intern Med. 2010;25(6):613–8.

44. Gawande A. The cost conundrum. The New Yorker; 2009 June 1. http://www.newyorker.com/reporting/2009/06/01/090601fa_fact_gawande

45. The factors fueling rising health care costs, 2008. America's Health Insurance Plans; 2008 Dec. http://www.ahip.org/uploadedFiles/Content/News/Press_Room/2008/Resources/TheFactorsFuelingRisingHealthcareCosts2008.pdf

46. Baicker K, Chandra A. Medicare spending, the physician workforce, and beneficiaries' quality of care. Health Aff (Millwood). 2004 Jan–Jun; Suppl Web Exclusives:W4-184-97. http://content.healthaffairs.org/content/early/2004/04/07/hlthaff.w4.184.short

47. Quast T. Is there a relationship between HMO quality of care and financial performance? Evidence from Texas HMOs. Sam Houston State University. http://www.shsu.edu/~tcq001/paper_files/wp10-07_paper.pdf

48. Pham HH, Ginsburg PB. Unhealthy trends: the future of physician services: medicare could lead the way to integrated care by moving away from fee-for-service payment policies. Health Aff (Millwood). 2007;26(6):1586–98.

49. Advancing quality through collaboration: the California pay for performance program. Integrated Healthcare Association; 2006 Feb. http://www.iha.org/pdfs_documents/p4p_california/P4PWhitePaper1_February2009.pdf

50. Rosenthal MB, Frank RQ, Li Z, Epstein AM. Early experience with pay-for-performance: from concept to practice. JAMA. 2005;294(14):1788–93.

51. Health Policy Brief. Accountable care organizations. Health Aff. 2010 July 27. http://www.healthaffairs.org/healthpolicybriefs/brief.php?brief_id=20

52. O'Connor MC, Jackson WO. Analysis: U.S. Supreme court upholds the affordable care act: Roberts rules? The National Law Review; 2012 June 29. http://www.natlawreview.com/article/analysis-us-supreme-court-upholds-affordable-care-act-roberts-rules

53. Litow M, Shapiro B. Consistently framing the design and analysis of health care proposals. Visions for the future of the U.S. Health Care System. Society of Actuaries. http://www.amcp.org/WorkArea/DownloadAsset.aspx?id=13476

Part III

Understanding Systems of Health Care

The American Health-Care System: Understanding How the Pieces Come Together

12

Roshan P. Shah and Samir Mehta

Learning Objectives

After completing this chapter, the reader should be able to answer the following questions:
- Understand the complexity of the US health-care system.
- Identify the major players involved in the US health-care system.
- Identify the relevant factors that have influenced the classical physician-patient relationship.
- Characterize the benefits and flaws of the design of the US health-care system.

Introduction

The American health-care system is a complex, fragmented collection of competing interests and a multitude of central and peripheral characters that are loosely coordinated but indelibly intertwined. Unlike those of other developed nations, the health-care system in the USA is not centrally controlled. Instead, it comprises an amalgam of public and private financing, a collection of regulatory authorities, and a patchwork system of providing access to care. A sophisticated understanding of the US health-care system accepts that it is a massive, multifaceted, organizational

behemoth that does not neatly fit into a coherent set of interests, goals, and values. It is a uniquely American enterprise that, in many ways, defines its predominance in innovation and technological advancement by the individual incentives and capitalistic rewards that exist in direct conflict with other components of the system. The recipients of health care are not the same as those paying for it; providers complicate their fiduciary duties to patients by alliances with industry, payers, and hospitals; a variety of administrators and insurance businesspeople exert an invisible hand on the practice of medicine; and the same government concerned with managing the costs and delivery of health care condones toxic industries like tobacco, alcohol, and firearms. In spite of, and perhaps because of, the complexities, contradictions, and capitalistic incentives, the US health-care system remains preeminent among industrialized nations for the actual delivery of care. Foreign dignitaries and the international elite consistently choose US institutions for their

R.P. Shah, M.D., JD • S. Mehta, M.D. (✉)
Department of Orthopedic Surgery, Hospital of the
University of Pennsylvania, Philadelphia,
PA 19104, USA
e-mail: roshan.shah@uphs.upenn.edu;
samir.mehta@uphs.upenn.edu

Fig. 12.1 This figure depicts the integration of the many different facets of the US health-care system. It is viewed as a sphere, with a single interest occupying the core—that of the patient—and surrounding layers comprised of the other elements of the system

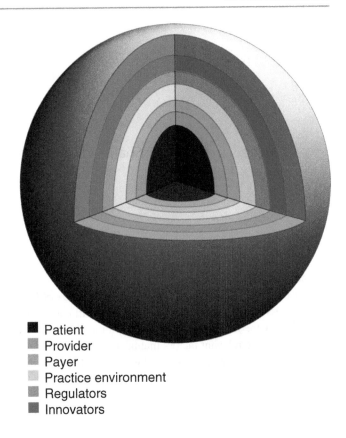

■ Patient
■ Provider
■ Payer
■ Practice environment
■ Regulators
■ Innovators

personal health care. US-trained physicians are highly regarded throughout the world, and the best and brightest physician hopefuls from across the globe strive to train in the USA.

As discussed throughout this book, the poor control over cost and access mars an otherwise successful health-care system. The difficulty in finding solutions to our problems lies in part with the complexity of the system. This chapter attempts to encapsulate the different elements of US health care to give the reader an understanding of how they come together to form a system. The integration of the many different facets is viewed as a sphere, with a single interest occupying the core—that of the patient—and surrounding layers comprised of the other elements of the system (Fig. 12.1).

The Central Figure: The Patient

Viewing the complex and nuanced landscape of the American health-care system, one can easily lose sight of the central figure of importance–the patient. This is excusable to an extent, given that the functional health-care system we have is anything but patient centric. As discussed throughout this book, layers and layers of generalists, specialists, administrators, and single-service participants cloud the central integral relationship within any health-care system: patient and provider.

According to the Census Bureau, the population of US residents in 2011 was 311,591,917 [1]. The Department of Homeland Security has estimated an illegal population of 11.5 million in 2011 [2]. There were 62.7 million visitors to the United States in 2011 [3]. All in all, the number of actual and potential patients in the United States is staggering, and the system in place is capable of providing at least emergency care, and usually more, for all who seek it. The CDC estimates that 82.2 % of adults and 92.1 % of children had some contact with a health-care professional in 2010, amounting to 1.2 billion visits during the year to physician offices, hospital outpatient, and emergency departments [4]. In 2009, there were 48 million inpatient surgical procedures performed [5].

Access to medical care has been positioned as a cornerstone of contemporary health-care reform. According to the CDC, 6.9 % of Americans failed to obtain medical care due to cost in 2009 [6]. In 2010, 48.6 million people under 65 were uninsured, with 35.7 million people uninsured for more than 1 year. The overall uninsured rate represents an increase of over 10 million people since 2000 [7]. It is interesting to note that the lack of insurance does not necessarily mean a lack of access to health care. Effectively, however, access to care through self-pay is too burdensome for most Americans. All patients can have emergency care through any emergency department. Thus, this scenario has given rise to the problem of the uninsured accessing emergency room care as a substitute for primary medical care, rather than acute emergencies. Indeed, the CDC estimates that 14.6 % of Americans do not have a "usual place to go for medical care" [6].

To an extent, the patient remains at the forefront of discussions of our health-care system and of reforms and alternate visions. It is important to keep the patient central to any consideration of the system, as they are the true common denominator by which all systems are judged. As the following sections will show, the outer layers of our health-care sphere all exert some effect on the patient and their experiences navigating medical care.

A New Development: The Health Advocate

Just as lawyers train to be legal advocates for their clients, a new breed of advocates has arisen as a cottage industry to help shepherd patients through an increasingly complex and frustrating health-care system. Health advocates have gained in popularity since 1980 when the first Masters training program started at Sarah Lawrence College. In 2008, more than 3,000 corporate employers included independent health advocates on their list of perquisites. Today, even more are finding that access to an advocate can improve the patient experience and even reduce costs.

Independent health advocates, who are often former nurses or other health-care professionals, can help patients navigate health care- and insurance-related issues. They can help explain diagnoses or treatment plans, help find the right specialists, battle insurance companies and claim denials, and help organize eldercare for loved ones. They can attend medical appointments and help patients ask the right questions of providers. Interestingly, this service is usually offered for free by employers, who ultimately save money and improve workforce efficiency by redirecting their employee's attention away from medical complexities [8]. For many, they are navigators in an otherwise indiscernible maze. It remains to be seen whether this class of advocates can justify their cost and remain in the system.

The Provider

In the early days of American medicine, providers of health care were easy to identify. Physicians and surgeons provided medical knowledge and guided medical decision-making, with nurses as care intermediaries and few other authority figures in the arena. This simplistic character scheme has evolved into a web of providers with a variety of educational training, certifications, and accreditations.

There are nearly 17 million people employed in health care and social services, according to the Bureau of Labor Statistics [9]. Of these, nearly six million fill rolls ranging from physicians and nurses to dentists, optometrists, pharmacists, physician assistants, physical and occupational therapists, respiratory therapists, speech pathologists, midwives, laboratory technicians, paramedics, dieticians, athletic trainers, and more. There are alternative care providers, like chiropractors, podiatrists, and a variety of culturally based philosophies, like shamanism, ayurveda, acupuncturists, and other healers. Each of these different types of providers undertakes a broad range of educational milestones, apprenticeship training paths, board testing, and sacrifices to achieve their expertise. Just over 540,000 providers have been traditionally trained in allopathic or osteopathic medical school. Where formerly a hierarchical system existed in caring for patients, today those relationships are increasingly dissolving due to work-hour restrictions and the increased specialization and fragmentation of medicine. The hospital health-care team is comprised of physicians, nurses, pharmacists, physical therapists, nutritionists, respiratory therapists, social workers, and case managers. It is increasingly common to see congregations of these providers rounding and collectively determining health-care plans.

Providers do not prescribe treatments and health-care plans with impunity. That is, the autonomy enjoyed in the early days of American health care no longer characterizes the modern practice of medicine. Foremost are the desires and influences of the patient and patient's family. The art of modern day medicine lies in part with crafting therapies around a patient's social, personal, cultural, or religious framework of beliefs. With easily accessible information on the Internet, both accurate and skewed, health literacy has deepened and changed the physician-patient relationship tremendously. When the self-education is accurate, the encounter becomes more efficient, and the system is benefited by the informed patient. When the information is inaccurate or unrelated, health-care delivery is impeded. Occasionally, physicians will even acquiesce to clinically inappropriate treatments when faced with misinformed patients [10].

The payer is another factor that influences diagnostic and treatment choices. As discussed in the preceding chapters, an early attempt at bending the cost curve aimed to reign in providers' free autonomy by instituting the oversight of a managed care organization. When the Nixon administration announced the adoption of health maintenance organizations (HMOs) in the early 1970s, there were only 30 such organizations in the country. By 1996, that number grew to over 600, enrolling about 65 million people, or close to one-fourth of the US population [11]. Through mechanisms like requiring prior approval, managed care can obstruct and deter physicians away from costly treatment decisions [12]. The provider's practice also influences the range of diagnostic and treatment options available for patient care. Programs like utilization review committees, formularies, and therapeutic interchange

have been instituted to restrict access to more expensive options and to review whether less expensive options exist. Programs to increase cost awareness among physicians have been successful in reducing costs, underscoring the relevance and importance of these factors that influence diagnostic and treatment choices [13].

The provider, as a segment of the US health-care system, is an evolving role, with each generation entering the part with different expectations and antecedent beliefs. The core fiduciary relationship with patients will remain unchanged and must be preserved in any future iteration of the health-care system.

The Payer

The third-party payer in the US health-care system has had a growing influence on the physician-patient relationship over time. Being backed by a payer is a prerequisite of almost all non-emergent health-care delivery. Furthermore, both primary and subspecialty physician practices can differentiate access to their care based on the type of insurance held.

In 2010, 256.2 million people had health insurance, with 64.0 % coming from private health insurance. The proportion of people getting insurance benefits through work is 55.3 %. About 31.0 % of coverage comes from government health insurance; Medicare enrollees number about 47.2 million, while Medicaid enrollees number about 50 million [14–16]. Chapters 2, 3, and 4 cover these insurance programs.

When viewing the health-care crisis, cost pressures, and central position of the patient, many consider the private health insurance industry to be least essential and most interchangeable. A payer is, after all, a payer. It is remarkable, and somewhat startling, to view the financial statements of the biggest health insurance companies (Table 12.1). The largest ten companies banked a whopping $13.3 billion in profits on revenues of over $300 billion in 2012 [17].

With such staggering revenues and profits, it is no wonder that many frustrated patients and physicians inquire about the rationality of their

Table 12.1 Revenues, profits, and margins for the 10 largest health insurance companies

Insurance companies	Revenues ($, million)	Income ($, million)	Profit margin (%)
United Health Group	110,620.00	5,530.00	5.00
WellPoint	61,710.00	2,660.00	4.31
Humana	39,130.00	1,220.00	3.12
Aetna	36,600.00	1,660.00	4.54
Cigna	27,070.00	1,560.00	5.76
Coventry Health Care	14,110.00	487.06	3.45
Health Net	11,280.00	24.81	0.22
Centene	8,700.00	1.86	0.02
WellCare Health Plans	7,410.00	184.73	2.49
Molina Healthcare	587.00	9.79	1.67
Total	317,217.00	13,338.25	

Revenues and income are reported for the trailing 12 months
Source: Data from Ref. [17]

rejected claims and preauthorization denials. The proportion of health insurance premiums spent on real health-care claims (and not administration, marketing, or profits) is termed the *medical loss ratio (MLR)*. The MLR varies tremendously by geographic region, occurrence of natural calamities, and chance. Between 1994 and 1995, the MLR for a selected group of large insurance companies ranged from 58 % to 110 % [18]. The Patient Protection and Affordable Care Act (see Chap. 19 for further discussion) mandated that health insurance companies maintain a MLR of at least 80 % or 85 % depending on their size or else issue rebates to their enrollees. For 2011, the first year of implementation of the MLR requirement, a Kaiser Family Foundation report, estimated that $1.3 billion in excess profits were realized and would be issued to consumers as rebates [19]. Thus, even the level of 15 % of revenues from premiums was a difficult target for administrative costs for these companies.

The payer is the key variable that distinguishes the US health-care system from that of peer nations. It exerts a significant influence over the state of affairs of the system; however, it is far enough away from the system's core—the patient—that it becomes vulnerable to substantial changes in health-care reform proposals.

The Practice Environment: The Hospital, Emergency Room, and Ambulatory Clinic

The patient-physician encounter can occur in a wide variety of physical locations, including a hospital, emergency room, ambulatory clinic, nursing home, rehabilitation center, community health center, workplace, or even a sporting stadium. In 2009, there were 1.3 billion visits to physician offices, hospital outpatient departments, and hospital emergency rooms. Of these, one billion were to physician offices, 96 million were to hospital outpatient departments, and 136 million were to hospital emergency departments [20].

In 2010, there were 5,754 hospitals registered in the United States [21]. The makeup of these hospitals is given in Table 12.2. There are about 941,995 hospital beds in total in the United States, and, in 2010, there were nearly 37 million admissions. The CDC estimates that the average length of stay is about 4.9 days [22]. This generated expenses of $750 billion in 2010 [21].

The practice location can predict the number of care providers and complexity of care given. In 2009, an average of 49.1 % percent of office-based physicians reported the use of nurse

Table 12.2 Hospital types in US system

Nongovernmental nonprofit hospitals	2,904
For-profit hospitals	1,013
State/local government hospitals	1,068
Federal hospitals	213
Number of rural hospitals	1,987
Number of urban hospitals	2,998

Source: Data from Ref. [3]

practitioners, certified nurse midwives, or physician assistants [23]. Health care provided in the hospital rarely exists as care between so few providers and a patient. Usually, in addition to the primary provider, many other physician services are enlisted. These can include anesthesiology, radiology, pathology, laboratory medicine, and innumerable specialists as warranted by the admission diagnosis. In addition, countless other ancillary care providers are enlisted in the care of hospital inpatients. These include the floor nursing staff, specialty nurses like wound care and specialty IV placement nurses, nutritionists, physical and occupational therapists, respiratory therapists, phlebotomists, radiology technicians, chaplains, and more. The web of interrelated services within a hospital can be large and explains the thickness of bedside charts and the massive charges generated to the health-care system.

Regulators and Government Agencies

The practice of medicine is not regulated by the Food and Drug Administration (FDA), Centers for Medicare and Medicaid Services (CMS), Department of Health and Human Services (HHS), or Centers for Disease Control and Prevention (CDC) (for further discussion, please see Chaps. 16 and 17). Generally, where there is oversight of the practice of medicine, the source of the authority is state police powers. Thus, in controlling licensing, state medical boards exert their influence on the practice of medicine. Individual medical decision-making, however, rarely conjures state police powers.

The most obvious examples involve euthanasia, mandatory state reporting of communicable diseases, and mandatory notification laws related to child, spousal, and elder abuse.

The FDA regulates the entry of pharmaceuticals and medical devices into the marketplace and the ability of companies to market those products. That a product does not have FDA approval for a given indication, in and of itself, has no bearing on whether a physician can prescribe that product for the unapproved condition. Where it does become relevant is when the physician asks to be reimbursed by a third-party payer. In many circumstances, unapproved indications will not be covered by insurance companies. As will be discussed in later chapters of this book, the HHS is an arm of the executive branch of the federal government, charged with "protecting the health of all Americans and providing essential human services, especially for those who are least able to help themselves." The CDC's mission is "collaborating to create the expertise, information, and tools that people and communities need to protect their health—through health promotion, prevention of disease, injury and disability, and preparedness for new health threats."

Technology and Innovation

The American ideals of innovation and entrepreneurship extend to and thrive in the health-care system. The promise that a new drug, device, or therapy will reap bountiful pecuniary rewards motivates a massive national research and development program. The US government and countless private sector philanthropies fund biomedical research programs. Nearly every major disease has a supportive organization that coordinates and distributes research funding.

Whereas the technological innovation characterized by the US health-care system helps to define its excellence in the delivery of medical care, it can exacerbate problems of cost and access. When discoveries translate into therapeutic advances, frequently they are incremental improvements rather than paradigm-shifting breakthroughs. These small advances compel premium pricing and can inflate the expenses associated with the health-care system. Patients, physicians, hospitals, and industry marketing will tout the latest technological offerings which compound the impact of these costly discoveries on the system. Nonetheless, innovation and rapidly evolving standards of care are integral characteristics of the US health-care system and influence nearly all aspects of health-care delivery.

The Influence of Medical Malpractice

As will be discussed in detail in Chap. 17, the specter of malpractice varies by geographic region and can have an influence on the patient-physician relationship ranging from significant defensive medicine to nothing more than a fleeting thought. The US health-care system exists alongside a cultural embracement of litigation and the prospect of climbing the economic ladder. The threat of suit is not just the unfortunate reality of physicians but also for insurance companies, hospitals, pharmaceutical and device companies, and all other levels of providers. The practice of defensive medicine consists of excess documentation, otherwise unnecessary imaging and laboratory testing, and superfluous subspecialty consultation. The influence of litigation avoidance constrains the practice of medicine. Instead of relying on physician autonomy and expertise, the standard of care forces conforming to cookie-cutter consensus statements and decision trees.

Conclusion

The different facets of US health care come together to form an immense, complex, and decentralized system. There are layers of competing interests, aligned and misaligned players, and a variety of social and cultural factors that surround the central-core patient. It is helpful to have an understanding of how the different topics of this textbook fit together and interrelate in practice.

References

1. United States Census Bureau. Population, 2011 estimate. 2012. census.gov, 8/16/2012 2012 [cited 2012 Aug 31]. http://quickfacts.census.gov/qfd/states/00000.html
2. Hoefer M, Rytina N, Baker B. Estimates of the unauthorized immigrant population residing in the United States: January 2011. Edited by Department of Homeland Security. Washington, DC: DHS Office of Immigration Statistics; 2012.
3. Fast facts: United States travel and tourism industry, 2011. Edited by Office of Travel and Tourism Industries. Washington, DC; 2012.
4. US National Center for Health Statistics. Ambulatory care use and physician visits. Office of Health Statistics. 2012 Aug 20 [cited 2012 Aug 31]. http://www.cdc.gov/nchs/fastats/docvisit.htm
5. US National Center for Health Statistics. Inpatient surgery. National Center for Health Statistics. 2012 May 16 [cited 2012 Aug 31]. http://www.cdc.gov/nchs/fastats/insurg.htm
6. US National Center for Health Statistics. Access to health care. National Center for Health Statistics. 2012 Aug 20 [cited 2012 Aug 31]. http://www.cdc.gov/nchs/fastats/access_to_health_care.htm
7. DeNavas-Walt C, Proctor BD, Smith JC. Income, poverty, and health insurance coverage in the United States: 2010. Washington, DC: U.S. Government Printing Office; 2011.
8. Young L. Advocates who help you negotiate health care. Businessweek Magazine, 2007 Oct 21.
9. May 2011 National Industry-Specific Occupational Employment and Wage Estimates, Sector 62 – Health Care and Social Assistance (including private, state, and local government hospitals). U.S. Bureau of Labor Statistics, 2012 Mar 27 [cited 2012 Aug 31]. http://www.bls.gov/oes/current/naics2_62.htm
10. Murray E, Lo B, Pollack L, Donelan K, Catania J, Lee K, Zapert K, Turner R. The impact of health information on the Internet on health care and the physician-patient relationship: national U.S. survey among 1.050 U.S. physicians. J Med Internet Res. 2003; 5(3):e17.
11. A brief history of managed care. Tufts Managed Care Institute; 1998.
12. Carroll NV. How effectively do managed care organizations influence prescribing and dispensing decisions? Am J Manag Care. 2002;8(12):1041–54.
13. Johnson CC, Martin M. Effectiveness of a physician education program in reducing consumption of hospital resources in elective total hip replacement. South Med J. 1996;89(3):282–9.
14. The Hi-SMI trend table shows the unduplicated count of persons enrolled in either or both parts of the program (HI and/or SMI). Edited by Centers for Medicare and Medicaid Services. Washington, DC: CMS.gov; 2012.

15. Synder L, Rudowitz R, Ellis E, Roberts D. Medicaid enrollment: June 2011 data snapshot, Kaiser commission on medicaid facts. Washington, DC: The Henry J. Kaiser Family Foundation; 2012.

16. Income, poverty and health insurance coverage in the United States: 2010 (Press Release). Washington, DC: U.S. Census Bureau; 2011.

17. http://finance.yahoo.com on 2/26/2013. Accessed 26 Feb 2013.

18. Robinson JC. Use and abuse of the medical loss ratio to measure health plan performance. Health Aff. 1997;16(4):176–87.

19. Keller M, Palosky C. Kaiser analysis: estimated health insurance rebates under the health reform law total $1.3 billion dollars in 2012. News Release. Menlo Park: The Henry J. Kaiser Family Foundation; 2012.

20. US National Center for Health Statistics. Health, United States, 2011: with special feature on socioeconomic status and health. Hyattsville: Department of Health and Human Services, Centers for Disease Control and Prevention; 2012.

21. Fast facts on US Hospitals. 2012. Jan 3 [cited 2012 Aug 19]. http://www.aha.org/research/rc/stat-studies/fast-facts.shtml

22. US National Center for Health Statistics. Hospital utilization (in non-Federal short-stay hospitals). National Center for Health Statistics, 2012 Aug 20 [cited 2012 Aug 31]. http://www.cdc.gov/nchs/fastats/hospital.htm

23. Park M, Cherry D, Decker SL. Nurse practitioners, certified nurse midwives, and physician assistants in physician offices. NCHS data brief. Hyattsville: National Center for Health Statistics; 2011.

Alternative Systems of Care and Consumer-Driven Health Care

13

Daniel Guss

Learning Objectives

After completing this chapter, the reader should be able to answer the following questions:

- How one defines value in health care.
- The implication of moral hazards for both patients and providers.
- The overarching aim of consumer-driven health care.
- The fundamental importance of financial risk in health care as well as who bears it.
- The potential role for accountable care organizations especially as it pertains to provide incentives and opportunities for innovation in the delivery of care.

Abbreviations

ACO   Accountable Care Organization
CDHC Consumer-Driven Health Care
HDHP High-Deductible Health Plan

D. Guss, M.D., M.B.A. (✉)
Department of Orthopedic Surgery,
Massachusetts General Hospital, Boston,
MA 02114, USA
e-mail: dguss@partners.org

Introduction

The fundamental aspiration of any health-care system is to maximize the value it provides to patients. Historically, clinical advancement has been at the epicenter of this aim, but skyrocketing costs and inconsistent correlation of increased spending with improved outcomes have precipitated the search for system-wide alternatives. Any successful health-care system must ultimately integrate patients, providers, and payers in a manner that promotes quality while containing costs. Doing so requires defining value in health care as well as understanding the implications of moral hazards.

Defining Terms

As alluded to in the introduction, understanding the health-care system requires first defining terms, specifically value and moral hazard.

Value

One proposed definition of value in health care relates the quality of patient outcomes to the cost of attaining those outcomes [1, 2]. It is the ratio of health quality attained per dollar spent and therefore intrinsically represents efficiency in health care. Thus, promoting value must encompass both quality and cost, and health-care systems cannot maximize value by focusing solely on one aspect of the equation such as cutting costs without attention to the resultant effect on outcomes. Quality and cost are not invariably in conflict, however, and may in fact be inversely correlated from a system-wide perspective. Improving the quality of care can potentially reduce overall costs by virtue of preventing events like medical complications and hospital readmissions.

Moral Hazard

Moral hazard refers to the human tendency to alter behavior once benefiting from, but no longer bearing, the full cost of a given action. For example, a bank may pursue riskier investments with higher potential payoffs if it knows the federal government will intervene to prevent bankruptcy. Along this line, humans are prone to an "all-you-can-eat buffet phenomenon," wherein one tends to overconsume when paying a predetermined fee to enter the buffet without an incremental charge for additional portions. Health care similarly risks overconsumption by patients and over-prescription by providers, both of whom potentially benefit from increased utilization without necessarily bearing the incremental costs associated with additional resource use.

The Patient (A.K.A. the Consumer)

Consumer Economics

At the heart of economics is the need to reconcile limited resources against limitless human desires [3]. In the majority of realms, people reconcile this tension by how they use their purchasing dollars as shaped by personal preferences and budget constraints. In health care, insurance companies or other payment intermediaries stand between the patient and the provider and collectively pool resources, so that patients generally spend money that is not immediately their own. Accordingly, while out-of-pocket health-care expenses for patients have risen in absolute terms over recent decades, they have shrunk in relative terms as a percentage of overall health-care spending. National health-care expenditures totaled $2.6 trillion in 2010, representing 17.6 % of United States Gross Domestic Product (GDP) and are up from 12.0 % of GDP in 1990 and 5.1 % in 1960 [4–6]. In contrast, out-of-pocket expenditures as a percent of overall health-care spending were 12 % in 2010, down from 20 % in 1990, and 48 % in 1960. Therein lies one side of the moral hazard in health care. Patients do pay increasing amounts for health care, be it in the form of higher premiums, lower real wages due to employer-sponsored insurance, or higher taxes, but the removed nature of such spending insulates behavior from the influence of costs [7].

Furthermore, in most industries, altered spending patterns represent the primary lever by which value is maximized for consumers. Specifically, when there is a competitive marketplace with sellers vying for buyers, goods tend to improve in quality and decrease in cost over time, as exemplified by industries ranging from automobiles to personal computers [8]. Adam Smith in his "The Wealth of Nations" described the so-called invisible hand inherent to such marketplaces, which "direct[s] that industry in such a manner as its produce may be of the greatest value" [9]. In health care, the dissociation of patients from their spending dollars mitigates the effect of the invisible hand. Competition on quality and cost, and therefore value as defined in this chapter, is less prominent.

Consumer-Driven Health Care

Consumer-driven health care (CDHC), as it was originally conceived, aimed to empower individuals to make their own health-care decisions while minimizing the collective influence of third-party payers. The overarching idea was that patients, when equipped with appropriate information and incentives, can manage their own care better than even a well-intentioned third party [3]. To some degree a backlash against managed care, it envisioned a health-care system in which insurance covered unpredictable, catastrophic events, but individuals otherwise paid directly for predictable, low-cost provider services under high-deductible health plans (HDHPs). By virtue of putting patients in a position to manage their own care not only medically but also financially, CDHC espoused countermeasures to the moral hazard issue while attempting to harness the value-creating potential of the marketplace. Cheaper HDHPs empowered patients to choose among an array of providers and treatment plans, but also forced patients who benefited from utilization to directly incur the cost of their decision-making. These expenses could be subsidized through vehicles such as health-saving accounts, which allow tax-exempt saving towards health-care expenses, as well as other government supports for lower income brackets. CDHC also envisioned that providers would be free to set their own prices, and independent rating agencies would provide a clear assessment of quality and cost. Armed with this information, patients could then vote with their dollars as they do in other industries, thereby sparking competition among providers to improve quality while lowering costs, ultimately maximizing the value for patients.

While there has been limited implementation of some aspects of CDHC, HDHPs as part of its vision have become increasingly common [10].

In 2011, an estimated 17 % of workers covered by employer-sponsored plans were enrolled in an HDHP with a tax-preferred saving option (i.e., a health care–specific saving account set aside pretax), double the rate of 8 % in 2009 [11]. Such plans have a minimum deductible of $1,200 for individual coverage or $2,400 for family coverage [12]. Some supporters have touted the ability of such plans to rein in health-care spending [13]. Critics, however, have in turn raised concerns about the potential health implications of passing financial risk onto the patient [14]. While HDHPs do appear to decrease utilization such as emergency room visits, it is unclear the degree to which patients also forgo appropriate care [15–17]. Hybrid models have therefore emerged that exempt necessary preventative care from the full value of the deductible, and some have recommended "smarter" cost sharing that varies out-of-pocket expenses based on the implication of a given service towards future health and costs [18]. Another critical issue is that empowering patients to make value-driven decisions requires access to sufficient information on quality, efficacy, and cost, which is frequently unavailable [19]. Patients participating in self-pay markets for procedures such as laser-assisted in situ keratomileusis (LASIK) eye surgery and in vitro fertilization (IVF) have historically relied on word of mouth and physician recommendations for this reason [20]. When information about quality and cost is made available in a well-designed format, however, studies have found that patients do gravitate towards high-value providers, underscoring the need to effectively measure and disseminate such information [21]. Critics have also expressed other general concerns about CDHC, including the challenges of care coordination in a marketplace environment, the potential migration of healthier individuals to HDHPs leaving traditional health insurance plans with predominantly sicker patients, and the associated risk of insolvency (i.e., adverse selection), as well as the potential erosion of medical professionalism that could result from introducing commercial competition to the physician-patient relationship [3, 22].

Ultimately, the final version of CDHC is likely to evolve as it adapts its original vision to real-world conditions. Its overarching attempt to empower patients through choice, while counteracting their proclivity to utilize more when spending other's money, may need to be complemented by institutional support structures that offset some of CDHC's shortfalls as well as help patients successfully navigate the complexities of health care [23].

The Provider (A.K.A. the Supplier)

Cost-sharing instruments such as HDHPs focus on modulating the demand side of the health-care equation by altering patient-driven utilization. A supply side also exists, however, and coherent restructuring of the health-care system must also encompass providers. Indeed, some have argued that the provider side of the equation provides a more apt target because, while both patients and providers decrease utilization with cost-sharing initiatives, increased out-of-pocket expenses for patients may result in decreased use of appropriate care, while no similar predilection has been demonstrated in the provision of care [24]. The latter may be due to the information advantage among health-care providers further buttressed by professional ethics. Perhaps more importantly, however, providers at the forefront of delivering care arguably represent one of the most fruitful sources of system-wide innovation.

Supplier Economics and Risk

In its simplest form, total health-care spending equals the quantity of goods and services provided multiplied by their price. Accordingly, efforts to curb the growth in health-care spending have historically focused on one of these two factors [25]. Private insurance, for example, utilized deductibles and copayments for patients as well as service utilization reviews for providers to curb the volume of services. Meanwhile, public payers such as Medicare and Medicaid tended to focus on the price of services, set administratively at the federal and state level. What is frequently lacking from a discussion focused solely on quantity and price is the concept of risk and who bears it.

Insurance by definition exists to mitigate risk, be it the risk of fire offset by home insurance or the risk of poor health offset by health insurance. The unpredictability of events at the individual level, but the actuarial ability to pool risk at the population level, makes this possible. Individuals are unable to accurately determine whether or not they will personally fall ill nor, once requiring care, the ultimate outcome of treatment. Third-party payers mitigate this risk by pooling it across large swaths of the population, but can potentially vary the degree of risk they assume. At one end of the spectrum, in an environment where providers are paid exclusively on a fee-for-service basis and patients have no out-of-pocket expenses, the entirety of risk is borne by third-party payers. Neither patients nor providers assume the increased costs associated with higher utilization. Furthermore, while providers generally espouse a professional and ethical obligation to maximize quality, there is no incentive to do so in a cost-effective manner. Value, defined as quality divided by costs, is not necessarily maximized. At the other end of the spectrum, where patients pay entirely out of pocket or physicians are capitated to provide all care at a predetermined price irrespective of costs, the risk has been transferred in its entirety onto the patients and providers, respectively.

Historically, both private and public payers had backstops for risk. Specifically, private insurance could simply increase premiums, and public programs such as Medicare could simply receive additional government funding. Health-care costs have risen faster than US GDP, however, and unchecked growth now infringes on other public spending ranging from education to infrastructure [26, 27]. A newfound urgency has therefore reinvigorated the focus on the provider's role in the health-care system, including the possibility of stimulating quality and cost improvements by transferring some of the risk onto providers.

Accountable Care Organizations

One proposed mechanism for restructuring health-care systems is the accountable care organization (ACO). Broadly speaking, ACOs aim to reorganize health-care delivery into groups or networks of providers whose financial reimbursement is, at least to some degree, tied to measurably improving the quality of care for a defined patient population while cutting the rate of cost increases [28, 29]. Thus, providers assume some financial responsibility for patient outcomes, as well as the cost of achieving those outcomes, and are therefore incentivized to find innovative ways to improve overall value in health care. ACOs can form at multiple levels of care, ranging from large primary care groups to hospital systems [30]. In turn, they can range from a low-risk model, wherein providers are reimbursed within a fee-for-service framework but may share in the money saved from reaching quality and cost-reduction targets, to one where providers assume more risk by committing to care for a defined patient population at a predetermined per-episode or time-based fee, but with a higher potential share in any accrued savings [31]. Financial rewards may also be offset by financial penalties should providers fail to reach predetermined benchmarks. The idea is to find a balance between the fee-for-service reimbursement model, where reimbursement increases lockstep with the volume of services provided and which therefore risks overutilization, and a capitated model, under which providers are paid a fixed amount for each patient regardless of expenses and which thereby risks underutilization [32]. The ACO concept recognizes that there are inherent barriers to achieving high-value care, including fragmentation of care that makes care coordination challenging, volume-based reimbursement that is independent of quality or cost-effectiveness measures, and a general belief that more care equates with better care (and by extension that any reduction in care is tantamount to rationing) [33]. By virtue of passing some financial risk onto the providers, however, ACOs recognize not only that the current health-care system is fraught with opportunities for quality improvement and cost cutting, but also that providers rather than third parties are best equipped to recognize and capitalize on such opportunities. In addition to incentivizing care coordination as a means to achieving higher quality care, ACOs also aim to inject a degree of provider "accountability" through a

commitment to public transparency of quality measures, which aids patients and payers in selecting among providers [34]. Undoubtedly, transforming the concept of ACOs from theory into reality will be an ongoing and iterative process. Even at the most basic level, ACOs face the challenges of delineating what defines quality and elucidating how to risk adjust for sicker patient populations. Nonetheless, the concept of incentivizing and empowering providers by ceding to them a degree of risk remains.

Ultimately, the recent focus on providers seeks to spark system-wide pursuits of value in health care. A strong ethical and professional code imbues the practice of medicine, and no orthopedic surgeon, for example, realistically desires that a total hip replacement become infected in order to economically benefit from additional procedures nor does an internist hope that an elderly patient with pneumonia get readmitted shortly after discharge in order to increase hospital bed utilization. But some argue that professionalism can only go so far in mitigating the inherent moral hazard of a fee-for-service system that rewards volume above all else [31]. Such a system does little to force reevaluation of health interventions from the perspective of efficacy and cost, nor does it explicitly spark innovation in the coordination of care, which has become increasingly necessary given the complexity of modern health-care systems. Skyrocketing health-care costs now infringe not only on government funding of other critical public goods, such as education, but also erode a vast majority of real income gains for US families and make US workers less competitive on a global scale due to the rising corporate expense of employer-sponsored health insurance [5, 7]. Questions remain about the implications of placing increased risks on the shoulders of providers. For example, insurance companies generally harbor cash and liquid asset reserves to offset potential losses. Should some of this cash now be transferred to providers alongside the newfound risk? Regardless, the ultimate idea is that providers themselves, when appropriately incentivized, are well positioned to provide the "disruptive innovations" that have revolutionized other industries [35].

Summary

Rising health-care costs have broadened the requisite scope of health-care innovation from one that focuses primarily on clinical advancement to one that also encompasses the concept of value. The ultimate question is how to maximize quality while minimizing costs, and any solution must successfully integrate patients, providers, and payers. Key questions include who benefits from and who bears the costs of decision-making in the context of moral hazards, and how does a potential system-wide solution effectively distribute risk to incentivize innovations that maximize value?

References

1. Porter ME. A strategy for health care reform–toward a value-based system. N Engl J Med. 2009;361(2): 109–12.
2. Porter ME. What is value in health care? N Engl J Med. 2010;363(26):2477–81.
3. Robinson JC, Ginsburg PB. Consumer-driven health care: promise and performance. Health Aff (Millwood). 2009;28(2):w272–81.
4. Chernew ME, Hirth RA, Cutler DM. Increased spending on health care: how much can the United States afford? Health Aff (Millwood). 2003;22(4):15–25.
5. Iglehart JK. Changing health insurance trends. N Engl J Med. 2002;347(12):956–62.
6. Keehan SP, Sisko AM, Truffer CJ, Poisal JA, Cuckler GA, Madison AJ, Lizonitz JM, Smith SD. National health spending projections through 2020: economic recovery and reform drive faster spending growth. Health Aff (Millwood). 2011;30(8):1594–605.
7. Auerbach DI, Kellermann AL. A decade of health care cost growth has wiped out real income gains for an average US family. Health Aff (Millwood). 2011;30(9):1630–6.
8. Herzlinger R. Who killed health care? America's $2 trillion medical problem – and the consumer-driven cure. New York: McGraw-Hill; 2007.
9. Smith A. An inquiry into the nature and causes of the wealth of nations. In: Bullock JC, editor. New York: PF Collier & Son; 1909. p. 351.
10. Reed M, Fung V, Price M, Brand R, Benedetti N, Derose SF, Newhouse JP, Hsu J. High-deductible health insurance plans: efforts to sharpen a blunt instrument. Health Aff (Millwood). 2009;28(4):1145–54.
11. Claxton G, Rae M, Panchal N, Lundy J, Damico A, Osei-Anto A, Kenward K, Whitmore H, Pickreign J. Employer health benefits, 2011 annual survey. Menlo Park/Chicago: The Kaiser Family Foundation and Health Research & Educational Trust; 2011.
12. Publication 969, Health Savings Accounts and Other Tax-Favored Health Plans. Department of the Treasury, Internal Revenue Service. 2011. http://www.irs.gov/pub/irs-pdf/p969.pdf. Accessed 1 June 2012.
13. Haviland AM, Marquis MS, McDevitt RD, Sood N. Growth of consumer-directed health plans to one-half of all employer-sponsored insurance could save $57 billion annually. Health Aff (Millwood). 2012;31(5):1009–15.
14. Lee TH, Zapert K. Do high-deductible health plans threaten quality of care? N Engl J Med. 2005;353(12):1202–4.
15. Dixon A, Greene J, Hibbard J. Do consumer-directed health plans drive change in enrollees' health care behavior? Health Aff (Millwood). 2008;27(4):1120–31.
16. Greene J, Hibbard J, Murray JF, Teutsch SM, Berger ML. The impact of consumer-directed health plans on prescription drug use. Health Aff (Millwood). 2008;27(4):1111–19.
17. Reed M, Graetz I, Wang H, Fung V, Newhouse JP, Hsu J. Consumer-directed health plans with health savings accounts: whose skin is in the game and how do costs affect care seeking? Med Care. 2012 Jul;50(7):585–90.
18. Rowe JW, Brown-Stevenson T, Downey RL, Newhouse JP. The effect of consumer-directed health plans on the use of preventive and chronic illness services. Health Aff (Millwood). 2008;27(1):113–20.
19. Bloche MG. Consumer-directed health care. N Engl J Med. 2006;355(17):1756–9.
20. Tu HT, May JH. Self-pay markets in health care: consumer Nirvana or caveat emptor? Health Aff (Millwood). 2007;26(2):w217–26. Epub 2007 Feb 6.
21. Hibbard JH, Greene J, Sofaer S, Firminger K, Hirsh J. An experiment shows that a well-designed report on costs and quality can help consumers choose high-value health care. Health Aff (Millwood). 2012;31(3): 560–8.
22. Berenson RA, Cassel CK. Consumer-driven health care may not be what patients need–caveat emptor. JAMA. 2009;301(3):321–3.
23. Robinson JC. Managed consumerism in health care. Health Aff (Millwood). 2005;24(6):1478–89.
24. Rosenthal MB. What works in market-oriented health policy? N Engl J Med. 2009;360(21):2157–60.
25. Ginsburg PB. Reforming provider payment–the price side of the equation. N Engl J Med. 2011;365(14): 1268–70.
26. Fuchs VR. Major trends in the U.S. health economy since 1950. N Engl J Med. 2012;366(11):973–7.
27. Song Z, Landon BE. Controlling health care spending–the Massachusetts experiment. N Engl J Med. 2012;366(17):1560–1.
28. Berwick DM. Making good on ACOs' promise–the final rule for the medicare shared savings program. N Engl J Med. 2011;365(19):1753–6.
29. McClellan M, McKethan AN, Lewis JL, Roski J, Fisher ES. A national strategy to put accountable care

into practice. Health Aff (Millwood). 2010;29(5): 982–90.

30. Shortell SM, Casalino LP. Health care reform requires accountable care systems. JAMA. 2008; 300(1):95–7.

31. Health Affairs. Health policy brief: accountable care organizations. 2010 July 27. http://www.healthaffairs.org/healthpolicybriefs/brief.php?brief_id=20

32. Goldsmith J. Analyzing shifts in economic risks to providers in proposed payment and delivery system reforms. Health Aff (Millwood). 2010;29(7): 1299–304.

33. Fisher ES, McClellan MB, Bertko J, Lieberman SM, Lee JJ, Lewis JL, Skinner JS. Fostering accountable health care: moving forward in medicare. Health Aff (Millwood). 2009;28(2):w219–31.

34. Crosson FJ. Analysis & commentary: the accountable care organization: whatever its growing pains, the concept is too vitally important to fail. Health Aff (Millwood). 2011;30(7):1250–5.

35. Hwang J, Christensen CM. Disruptive innovation in health care delivery: a framework for business-model innovation. Health Aff (Millwood). 2008;27(5): 1329–35.

National Healthcare Systems: A Worldview

14

Benjamin S. Hooe, Perrin T. Considine,
and Manish K. Sethi

Learning Objectives

After completing this chapter, the reader should be able to answer the following questions:
- What are basic tenants of other healthcare systems across the world, including the United Kingdom, France, Republic of Korea, Switzerland, and Canada?
- What similarities tie these healthcare systems together, and what sets them apart?
- What principals can one take from international systems to improve health care in the United States?
- How have other countries dealt with the rising costs of health care?

Introduction

To gain further insight into American health care, it is important to examine healthcare systems in other countries, so that one can assess and compare various plans and paths of reform.

B.S. Hooe, BS, B.A. • P.T. Considine, BS
Vanderbilt University School of Medicine,
Nashville, TN 37232, USA
e-mail: benjamin.s.hooe@vanderbilt.edu;
perrin.t.considine@vanderbilt.edu

M.K. Sethi, M.D. (✉)
Director of the Vanderbilt Orthopaedic Institute Center for Health Policy, Assistant Professor of Orthopaedic Trauma Surgery, Department of Orthopaedic Surgery and Rehabilitation, Vanderbilt University School of Medicine, Nashville, TN 37232, USA
e-mail: manish.sethi@vanderbilt.edu

Health systems in the United Kingdom, France, South Korea, Canada, and Switzerland provide a broad international sampling that includes another massive North American country (Canada), three European powers (France, Switzerland, and the UK), and a rising Asian superpower (South Korea). In examining these nations' healthcare structures, we must understand that their efficacy and outcomes are influenced by several modulating factors besides the system's inherent design: politics, history, and economics must all be considered when assessing a foreign system and translating successful strategies appropriately to the landscape of American health care.

For example, though the UK's National Health Service has retained its basic structure since its formation in 1948, it was not until 2001–2003—when political action established financial incentives for high-performing doctors and hospitals—that the British quality of care rose to what it is today. The Republic of Korea faces the logistical problem of supporting a rapidly growing and aging populace with the funds of a yet-developing economy. Switzerland's both famous and infamous healthcare system reflects its government's commitment to allowing individual choice within a mandatory coverage.

This examination explores not just what alternative healthcare systems are possible but *why* they are possible, given the different political and historical landscapes of individual countries. How might these various international systems affect our understanding of American health care?

United Kingdom

The United Kingdom—comprised by England, Scotland, Wales, and Northern Ireland—organizes its health care through four separate national systems that arose from dividing the common UK National Health Service (NHS) in 1999. While each of the four new national systems has taken slightly divergent paths since "devolution," the British NHS can be described as a fair representative of the essential system: that is, a single-payer system with publically provided care [1]. Worldwide, the British health system is known for its economy: the UK only spent $3,503 per capita on health care in 2010 [2] (compared to $8,233 per capita in the USA) [3]. Because the NHS is directly responsible for regulating both payment, as managed through the taxpayer-funded NHS, and reimbursement, by employing the majority of physicians, and funding most hospital operations costs, the British government has tight control over how much it spends on health care and what services it will pay for [4].

The NHS was originally formed in 1948 to provide health care to citizens who could not afford to pay at the time of service. This original iteration established a universal single-payer system funded by general taxes, allowing any UK citizen to receive health care free at the point of delivery. Individuals could—and still can—purchase private insurance to receive additional perks (such as shorter waiting lists for appointments and procedures), but this did not preclude them from paying their income-dependent NHS taxes. As of 2000, only 11.5 % of UK citizens chose private insurers, with the vast majority of the country receiving health care through either the NHS or employer-based private insurance [5].

After the NHS receives taxpayer money, it channels it directly to doctors and hospitals, both of which are reimbursed depending on performance, specialty, and volume of patients. Most doctors are employed directly by the NHS and hence have their income tightly regulated in many ways by the NHS. For example, in regulating the income of general practitioners (GPs), the NHS (1) mandates that all of its subscribers have a GP, (2) controls the total number of GPs trained and employed, and (3) determines the level of capitation, along with other reimbursements, that these physicians receive. Recent developments to this model include a 2004 "pay-for-performance" scheme that incentivizes general practitioners with up to $77,000 for providing thorough preventative care; successfully managing chronic conditions; keeping thorough, easy-to-access health records; and satisfying patients [5]. Specialist physicians receive salaries for their public work—though some also receive fee-for-service from private insurance companies.

Because the NHS determines both the money received from taxpayers and money paid for services, the British government is in a uniquely strong position to choose what will or will not be standard practice, by choosing which practices it will pay for. Strict budgets can actually be adhered to, resulting in low spending. The NHS extended its "pay-for-performance" model to hospitals [4] to increase quality and timeliness of care. Healthcare recipients themselves—because they choose their own GPs—can also influence quality of care through their role in free market competition between GPs.

The process of health care follows a hierarchy that starts with a local general practitioner and continues regionally. GPs are truly the "gate-keepers" to care, such that—excepting emergencies—one can only access specialist services through a GP referral. Patients with difficult problems must go first to their GP, get a referral (usually) to a local hospital, and if their problems warrant more treatment, progress to a regional teaching hospital. Hospitals are responsible for the entire population within their geographic vicinity. This allows cheaper care to be provided with fewer specialists.

However, a side effect of having fewer specialists is long wait lines: the 1995 UK "charter standard" for the waiting period between a referral and a specialist appointment was 6 months for an outpatient visit and 18 months for an inpatient visit [5]. Recent efforts to improve quality have lowered the 2009 target waiting period to 3–6 months for an inpatient visit. Yet, perhaps the most notable benefit of private insurance in the UK remains the ability to jump in queue or bypass long waiting lines.

2003 studies showed that the British are generally satisfied with the cost of their health care, with only 6 % of Brits (compared to 48 % of Americans) citing cost as a major problem with health care. However, 39 % of British patients (and 3 % of Americans) cited long waiting times as one of the most important problems of their national health system [4].

The British NHS's current success can be understood as the result of two major, targeted political pushes in 2001 and 2002 to incentivize quality improvement. As recently as the 1990s, the UK had "the highest mortality from major diseases" compared to other European countries in addition to its then-infamous waiting times.[1] In an attempt to move past a phase where "hospitals with long waiting lists and times [were] rewarded with extra money to bail them out," Prime Minister Tony Blair introduced a "target-driven culture" in which receiving NHS funding for hospitals became contingent on meeting Treasury targets for basic measures of healthcare success such as "reducing mortality rates from major killers, narrowing health inequalities, treating patients at a time that suits their medical need, reducing waiting times, and increasing patient satisfaction" [6].

This culture shift was enacted in order to reduce the gap in quality between private and public health care, because this gap necessarily reflects the income-based inequity of health care. Specifically, the NHS hoped to move past the dichotomy of "a privately financed high-quality service for those who can afford to pay for it and a publicly funded service of low quality for the rest." Part of this era of accountability included publishing the names of all NHS organizations along with "star ratings" of their performances to encourage good practices while simultaneously "naming and shaming" subpar hospitals.

Yet, the target-driven system, though effective, also allowed people to attempt to "game" the system. As noted by Bevan, narrow targets can successfully be used to achieve wide health goals, but often not without some idiosyncrasies:

> It is often said, and it is true, that government targets can lead to perverse consequences. Ambulances wait outside hospitals because there is a target that no patient should wait more than four hours in A & E[2]... Ninety-eight per cent of patients do, indeed, now get seen in A & E in less than four hours. [7]

In 2002 and 2003, the flavor of British healthcare reform began emphasizing provider competition over "targets." By allowing patients to attend whichever hospital they chose, and reimbursing hospitals and physicians with a blend of capitation[3] and salary, the British government ensured that "money follow[ed] the patient." As a cumulative result of these reforms, British health care is now a success story in terms of manufacturing its own competition to increase the quality

---

[1] Despite these criticisms, the UK gained a 1997 "Overall health system attainment" score of 91.6/100 and a 9th best ranking out of all WHO Member States. That year Switzerland placed 2nd, France placed 6th, Canada 7th, the USA 15th, and the Republic of Korea 35th.

---

[2] Accident and Emergency.

[3] Pay determined by the number of patients seen rather than quality of care.

of state-provided health care [8]. The percentage of the population reporting being "quite satisfied" or "very satisfied" with the general running of the English NHS increased from 35 % in 1996 to over 50 % in 2006 [5].

France

In 2000, the French healthcare system was ranked No. 1 by the World Health Organization. Although some have criticized the methods of assessment used in this report, overall satisfaction ratings and health status indicate that the French system is worthy of attention. The French healthcare system combines universal health insurance coverage with a mixed public-private system of hospital and ambulatory care. In addition, it provides higher levels of resources and greater volumes of care than the American system while maintaining significantly lower costs [9].

It is important to note that the French healthcare system, the National Health Insurance (NHI) system, was implemented in stages in response to a national call for greater coverage. The original program, passed in 1928, covered low-income, salaried industry, and commerce workers. It was not until 2000 — following several expansions of program coverage throughout the century — that France achieved true universal health insurance coverage [10]. Public health insurance benefits are available to all citizens, regardless of employment status.

NHI in France revolves around a system of reimbursement for medical care; patients pay their physicians directly and are reimbursed[4] by specific health insurance funds [9]. All workers in France are required to pay a portion of their income into a specific health insurance fund,[5] the sum of which is then used to reimburse medical expenses at predetermined rates. This process helps to mutualize health risks between individuals. Although workers are grouped into different health insurance funds based on their employment, the funds all share a common legal framework, and competition between funds is prohibited.[6] Retirees and the unemployed receive automatic coverage by the fund that corresponds to their previous occupational category [11].

The government shapes this process by determining which health services are considered reimbursable[7] and the rate at which those services will be reimbursed.[8] Physicians are permitted to set and collect their own fees, but services will only be reimbursed at the predetermined government rate [10]. In this way, fees remain fairly competitive, as patients are likely to choose the service with the smallest difference between the physician and reimbursement rates.

The French NHI is relatively generous in terms of benefits, covering a broad range of services such as hospital care, outpatient services, prescription drugs, and nursing home care; dental and vision care are covered to a lesser extent, and small differences in coverage exist between different NHI funds. Competitive private insurance is available to cover gaps in NHI and expand benefits. Private insurance is often employer subsidized or is government provided for low-income citizens [12].

The French NHI was founded on the principle of solidarity: the notion that "health insurance is a right for all — sick and well, high and low income, active and inactive — and that premiums ought therefore to be calculated on the basis of ability to pay, not anticipated risk" [13]. Essentially, the sicker a person becomes, the less they are expected to pay. For example, patients are exempted from co-pay requirements and receive complete reimbursement of healthcare costs if they are diagnosed with one of thirty

---

[4] Presentation of Sécurité Sociale card, enhanced with a microchip, at a physician's office allows for an electronic transfer of funds to the patient's bank account. This transaction takes place almost immediately.

[5] Workers are automatically enrolled in a group based on employment. Three major health insurance funds exist: [1] commerce and industry workers, [2] agriculture workers, [3] nonagriculture workers and the self-employed.

---

[6] Examples of competition would include the lowering of health premiums and the micromanagement of health care.

[7] Most medical services are considered reimbursable.

[8] Reimbursement typically ranges from 70 % for procedures such as x-rays to 95 % for minor surgeries or childbirth.

specified chronic conditions or if their hospital stay exceeds 30 days. This is in direct contrast to the American healthcare system, where chronic illness and long-term recovery are associated with increased costs for the afflicted individual.

South Korea

Over the past 50 years, South Korea's economy has grown rapidly, earning it a place among the G-20 major economies. As the nation's economy developed, so did its standard of living expectations and thus its need for a quality, affordable healthcare system. In an attempt to maintain continued economic growth and political stability, the South Korean government developed a health insurance program intended to improve the social welfare of its citizens [14]. In just 12 years, South Korea was able to implement a system of universal health insurance, bringing coverage to over 96 % of its population.

South Korea's first compulsory health insurance act was signed into law in 1977.[9] In addition to establishing several health insurance societies, this act required all companies with more than 500 employees to provide health insurance to their workers. By 1989, through a series of government-directed program expansions, South Korea had achieved universal health insurance coverage, requiring health insurance of both public and private sector employees, as well as the self-employed.

Eleven years later, in 2000, the nation's multiple health insurance societies were merged into a solitary government-run, single-payer system, the National Health Insurance (NHI) program. Until this point, health insurance had been provided primarily by private insurance societies, with the government offering direct coverage to those who were unable to obtain private insurance[10] [15]. All people are eligible for coverage

under the NHI program, and, as of 2006, 96.3 % of South Koreans were insured under its umbrella.[11] The remaining 3.7 % were covered by the nation's Medical Aid Program (MAP), which is similar to the American Medicaid program [16].

The National Health Insurance program uses a combination of public and private financing derived from government subsidies, tobacco surcharges, and individual contributions (premiums). While a uniform contribution amount[12] is set for those who are employer-insured, expected contributions for the self-employed are determined based on income.[13] Co-payments for medical services are also collected, with costs being dependent upon the services provided [14].

The South Korean healthcare plan, while providing comprehensive care, does little to address the root of the nation's health issues, choosing to focus on the treatment of disease rather than its prevention. In addition, an increase in expenditures for chronic degenerative diseases has followed an increase in South Korean life expectancy, placing a financial and social burden on younger populations [16]. As the American healthcare system continues to progress and develop, it should take into account the need for both an emphasis on preventative services and a strategy for the management of age-related costs.

Canada

The Canadian province of Saskatchewan founded the first publicly-financed universal hospital insurance program in North America in 1947, and the other provinces soon followed suit. In 1957, the Canadian government passed the Hospital Insurance Act, creating a national universal hospital insurance program to replace the

---

[9] Prior to this time, health insurance enrollment was voluntary.

[10] According to the Center for Health Market Innovations, 90 % of South Koreans were covered through private insurers prior to 1997; direct coverage through the government was provided to the remaining 10 %.

[11] 57.7 % were employer insured and 38.6 % were self-employed.

[12] Employer-insured premium rates are levied as a percentage of the employee's gross income; the employer and employee each pay 50 % of the premium amount. The premium rate was 5.08 % in 2008.

[13] Income calculations include factors such as property value, age, and gender.

Table 14.1 Healthcare expenditures: USA versus Canada

	Total healthcare expenditure	Total current expenditure (individual and collective health care)				
		Services of curative and rehabilitative care	Services of long-term nursing care	Medical goods	Prevention and public health services	Health administration and health insurance
United States	$8,232.9	$5,486.0	$463.0	$1,105.2	$286.1	$569.8
Canada	$4,444.9	$1,990.4	$624.7	$853.5	$291.7	$143.9

Note: Values expressed are per capita costs, in US$ purchasing power parity

fragmented provincial one. Although the creation of this program was a large step toward universal health insurance coverage, the program covered only hospital services, not physician services. A true universal health insurance plan was passed in 1966, and the program was fully implemented in 1971 [4].

The Canadian universal health insurance program, named Medicare, is a public, single-payer[14] system that is financed through taxation. As of 2010, the federal government financed 33 % of the cost of provincial health services[15] [4]. The provinces themselves use a variety of taxes to finance their health budgets, including compulsory premiums,[16] and payroll, income, and sales taxes [17].

In contrast to many other systems, the Canadian Medicare system has completely separated health insurance from employment; every Canadian receives the same benefits, regardless of occupation or employment status. Benefits under the program are broad, covering physician, hospital, and ancillary services[17] [4]. Canadian patients are free to choose their own primary care physicians (PCP) and are able to see specialists without referrals from their PCP.[18] Physicians are typically prohibited from billing above the provincially-mandated service fees [18].

The Canadian system is also unique in that it prohibits citizens from purchasing private health insurance that duplicates the basic benefits covered under the national plan. This policy is designed to prevent physicians from offering preferential treatment to patients with private insurance. Private insurance may be purchased, but only to cover gaps in coverage[19] or for special amenities such as private hospital rooms [18].

Compared to costs for care in the United States, Canadian healthcare expenditures are relatively low [19]. Several key differences between the USA and Canadian systems account for the variance in cost of health services between the two nations. In the USA, administrative costs are more than 300 % greater than in Canada. American physicians also utilize expensive, high-tech services (such as MRI scans) at a much higher rate than their Canadian counterparts. Finally, hospital stays in general are more expensive in the USA, as are physician fees and pharmaceutical prices (Table 14.1) [20].

Although the cost for care is significantly lower in Canada than in the United States, health-related expenditures in Canada have risen in recent years, and, in 2010, Canada was reported as having the fifth highest per capita healthcare costs among developed nations.[20] Since that time, Canada has taken steps to curb health costs and increase federal funding to provinces. Tax expansions have increased the federal payout to provinces, while a planned reorganization of the

[14] Within each Canadian province, the provincial government is the single payer.

[15] The Canadian federal government originally financed 50 % of health services costs in the 1970s.

[16] British Columbia and Alberta provinces.

[17] Ancillary services include diagnostic, therapeutic, and custodial services.

[18] Specialists receive a specialist fee, but only if the patient is referred by a PCP. For this reason, many specialists refuse to see patients without a referral.

[19] Dental care, physical therapy, prescription drug coverage, etc.

[20] According to a report published by the Organisation for Economic Co-operation and Development (OECD).

Medicare system aims to simultaneously decrease administrative costs and improve efficiency [4].

Overall, the Canadian universal insurance program has been successful in providing a means for the fair distribution of healthcare services. Critics of the system target long wait times for elective procedures and decreased access to primary care physicians compared to insured Americans [12]. In addition, payments to Canadian physicians on a fee-for-service basis have been said to emphasize volume of patient visits over quality of patient care [18].

Switzerland

Switzerland provides the classic model of universal coverage achieved through highly regulated private insurance companies. An individual mandate requires all Swiss to purchase at minimum a "basic plan," with a minimum, predetermined amount of coverage. These basic plans are heavily regulated by the government to ensure quality and affordability, though private plans are available to those who can afford them. As a whole, Switzerland's health system is known for retaining a great plurality of consumer options and promoting consumer autonomy around the standard for minimum individual coverage—though critics often dispute its cost-effectiveness [21].

Swiss health care, though possibly successful through its own design, must nevertheless be considered in the context of the Swiss history of government, with its limited federalism and emphasis on individual autonomy. For the latter half of the twentieth century, Switzerland had already established for itself "universal social insurances" in case of widowhood, orphanage, unemployment, or disability [22]. From this history of social support came the federal 1996 Law on Health Insurance, which set forth an individual mandate for health insurance, along with measures to maintain the individual's options for coverage and providers.

These protective measures allow the Swiss complete freedom to define their own health coverage, as long as they meet the individual

mandate.[21] In fact, insurance companies are prohibited by federal law from penalizing citizens who switch healthcare plans. Individuals are thus encouraged to take an active role in choosing from the 90 or so private insurers in Switzerland, thus shaping the free market and perhaps leading to better coverage and service [23]. To increase transparency in selecting from the multitude of insurance choices, the Swiss government publishes an annual list of insurance companies along with their rates for "basic" plans, which are identical in form and provide essential coverage as defined by federal law. Besides monthly premiums, healthcare recipients must also pay for their own co-pays; this is to encourage patients to participate in the process of keeping healthcare costs low—for example, by declining unnecessary lab tests their doctor might otherwise have ordered.

"Basic insurance," by Swiss law, provides the same services and benefits (including sick treatment, preventative care, and approved prescriptions) to all insured under it, for premiums legally determinable only by age and geographic location. While the Swiss government does not fix specific prices for these basic plans, it directly prohibits insurance companies from profiting from them. Theoretically, since the numerous basic plans are identical in content, insurers will compete for customers via secondary services, such as customer service and administrative support.

Insurance companies may also offer "private plans" that offer greater amenities (such as private hospital rooms) or more advanced treatments (such as those that are infeasible to provide to the entire population) [18], and it is legally permissible to profit from these private plans. While companies are prohibited from using most personalized information to determine basic premiums, they may—in determining private premiums—consider gender, risk factors,

---

[21] Swiss government revolves around the individual; as a direct democracy, *any* of its laws or decisions can be delayed, or decided by public referendum, if enough signatures are obtained. This is in contrast to indirect democracy, which is used in the USA.

and preexisting conditions. Insurers may even reject applicants for private insurance, while they are required to insure anyone who seeks a basic plan from them.

A Swiss citizen has increased freedom in choosing not only insurance plans but providers as well. Furthermore, there is no requirement that a general practitioner "keep the gates" and make referrals in Switzerland, so an individual may choose and seek specialist treatment directly. The only limitation, outside times of emergency, is that one must seek treatment within the confines of one's geographic subdivision or "canton."

Cantons are responsible for running local hospitals, determining insurance subsidies for low-income families, and determining reimbursement amounts for services. Though hospitals are primarily funded by insurance companies based on diagnoses and/or lengths of hospital stays, cantons provide additional funds to cover any deficits [18]. However, because cantons operate independently from each other, the health care experience of a Swiss resident can depend greatly on where they live within Switzerland. As an extreme example, a Swiss family of four living on $42,000 PPP[22] in 2007 might have spent anywhere between 4.4 % and 16.4 % of their income on health care depending on their local canton's health premium subsidies for low-income families [22].

Theoretically, segmentation might allow competition between cantons, that is, if people were to relocate according to their preferences for canton-provided health care.[23] However, due to the actual reality of relocation, as well as differences in language and culture between the cantons, this seems unlikely to be a great determinant of Swiss health care. Further criticisms of the canton system include that it "encourages the creation of regional monopolies and segmentation of hospital supply" and lacks the benefits of a centralized federal system, such as economies of scale and coordination of effort.

In summary, health care provided by cantons must still conform to federal standards that require that: (1) all individuals purchase insurance; (2) identical, "basic insurance" plans covering the minimum amount of health coverage for an individual are available from each of the 90 or so private insurance companies; (3) private insurance companies offer these basic plans not for profit (companies may profit off supplementary plans that provide increased comfort and/or service); and (4) individuals have great freedom in choosing providers and hospitals.

Conclusion

The United Kingdom, France, Switzerland, Republic of Korea, and Canada have evolved different healthcare solutions to differing sets of circumstances; yet, each system aims to save money and maximize human potential by redistributing the flow of time, money, and attention through different venues under differing sets of restriction.

In this international analysis, all of the examined countries achieved universal health care, and the majority of the healthcare models (UK, France, Republic of Korea, and Canada) offered public insurance. Switzerland alone differs in this respect, as it lacks government-provided coverage, relying instead on a great multiplicity of private insurers. Yet, Swiss insurers are so heavily regulated that their basic coverage plans may be considered as essentially similar to public plans, but without direct government administration.

The USA, in contrast, is far from universal coverage and does not yet have universally available public insurance. Health costs per capita are greatest in the USA and Switzerland ($8,233 and $7,812, respectively) and least in the UK and the yet-developing Republic of Korea ($3,503 and $1,439). France is in between with $4,691 per capita spending. When these costs are viewed relative to their country's economic strength, however, we see that each of the international systems spent approximately 10–12 % of the GDP on health care, while the USA spent closer to 18 %. See Table 14.2 for a comparison of healthcare systems between the United Kingdom,

---

[22] PPP = product purchasing power, a quantified representation of the buying power of a currency in its home nation, translated roughly into USD.

[23] As Crivelli and Bolgiani put it, "voting with their feet."

Table 14.2 Comparison of healthcare systems between the United Kingdom, France, Republic of Korea, Switzerland, Canada, and the United States

	Insurance type	Single payer?	Payment singularities	Amount of GDP spent on health care (%)	Gross national income per capita (US dollars)	$ USD spent on health care per capita
United Kingdom (*National Health Services*)	Public, universal	Yes	Free at the point of delivery; state money follows the patient	9.6	$30,600	$3,503
France (*National Health Insurance*)	Public, universal	No	Patients pay physicians and are reimbursed by the state	11.9	$29,700	$4,691
Republic of Korea (*National Health Insurance*)	Public, universal	Yes	Institutions provide care to patients and are later reimbursed by the state	12.4	$24,900	$1,439
Switzerland	Private (heavily regulated), universal	No		11.5	$42,700	$7,812
Canada (*Medicare*)	Public, universal	Yes		11.3	$32,800	$5,222
United States	Mixed public + private, not universal	No		17.6	$38,900	$8,233

France, Republic of Korea, Switzerland, Canada, and the United States.

It is clear that there are multiple functional models for funding and delivering health care, and, within those models, there are many modes of variation. Even grossly similar systems, such as those in Canada and the UK, may achieve different results depending on the timing, implementation, and politics involved. It is important to keep in mind both the strengths and weaknesses of each of the systems described as our American healthcare system continues to progress.

References

1. Greer Scott L. Four way bet: how devolution has led to four different models for the NHS. UCL: the constitution unit. 2004 Feb. http://www.ucl.ac.uk/spp/publications/unit-publications/106.pdf. Accessed 13 Oct 2012.
2. United Kingdom, Country statistics. Global health observatory data repository. World Health Organization. http://apps.who.int/ghodata/?theme=country, Accessed 13 Oct 2012.
3. Haden A, Campanini B (eds). The world health report 2000: improving performance. World Health Organisation. http://www.who.int/whr/2000/en/whr00_en.pdf. Accessed 11 Oct 2012.
4. Bodenheimer T, Grumbach K. Understanding health policy: a clinical approach. 6th ed. New York: McGraw-Hill Medical; 2012.
5. Connolly S, Bevan G, Mays N. Funding and performance of healthcare systems in the four countries of the UK before and after devolution. London: The Nuffield Trust; 2011. http://www.nuffieldtrust.org.uk/sites/files/nuffield/funding_and_performance_of_healthcare_systems_in_the_four_countries_report_full.pdf. Accessed 12 Oct 2012.
6. The NHS Plan: A plan for investment; A plan for reform. Presented to parliament by the secretary of state for health by command of Her Majesty. 2000 July. http://www.dh.gov.uk/prod_consum_dh/groups/dh_digitalassets/@dh/@en/@ps/documents/digital-asset/dh_118522.pdf. Accessed 12 Oct 2012.
7. Bevan G, Hamblin R. Hitting and missing targets by ambulance services for emergency calls: impacts of different systems of performance measurement within the UK. J R Stat Soc. 2009;172(1):1–30.
8. Bevan G. Have targets done more harm than good in the English NHS? No. BMJ. 2009;338:a3129.
9. Dutton PV. Differential diagnoses: a comparative history of health care problems and solutions in the United States and France. Ithaca: ILR Press; 2007.

10. Rodwin V. The health care system under French National Health Insurance: lessons for health reform in the United States. Am J Public Health. 2003;93(1):31–7.

11. Sandier S, Paris V, Polton D. Health care systems in transition: France. Copenhagen: WHO Regional Office for Europe on behalf of the European Observatory on Health Systems and Policies; 2004.

12. Schoen C, Osborn R, Squires D, Doty MM, Pierson R, Applebaum S. How health insurance design affects access to care and costs, by income, in eleven countries. Health Aff. 2010;29(12):2323–34.

13. Rodwin V. The marriage of national health insurance and La Medecine Liberale in France: a costly union. Milbank Mem Fund Q Health Soc. 1981;59(1):16–43.

14. Chun C-B, Kim S-Y, Lee J-Y, Lee S-Y. Republic of Korea: health system review. Health Syst Transit. 2009;11(7):1–184.

15. Lee J-C. Health care reform in South Korea: success or failure? Am J Public Health. 2003;93(1):48–51.

16. Song Y. The South Korean health care system. Jpn Med Assoc J. 2009;52(3):206–9.

17. Health Care Funding: Canadian health care. http://www.canadian-healthcare.org/. Accessed 13 Oct 2012.

18. Commonwealth Fund: International profiles of health care systems: Australia, Canada, Denmark, England, France, Germany, Italy, the Netherlands, New Zealand, Norway, Sweden, Switzerland, and the United States. New York: The Commonwealth Fund. http://www.commonwealthfund.org/~/media/Files/Publications/Fund%20Report/2010/Jun/1417_Squires_Intl_Profiles_622.pdf (2010). Accessed 15 Oct 2012.

19. Organisation for Economic Co-operation and Development: OECD Health data 2012: How Does Canada Compare. http://www.oecd.org/health/health-policiesanddata/BriefingNoteCANADA2012.pdf (2012). Accessed 12 Oct 2012.

20. Organisation for Economic Co-Operation and Development: Health expenditure and spending. OECD.StatExtracts: http://stats.oecd.org/Index.aspx?DataSetCode=SHA (2012). Accessed 13 Oct 2012.

21. Roy A. Why Switzerland Has the World's Best Healthcare System. Forbes. 29 Apr 2011. http://www.forbes.com/sites/aroy/2011/04/29/why-switzerland-has-the-worlds-best-health-care-system/. Accessed 12 Oct 2012.

22. Crivelli L, Bolgiani I. Consumer-Driven Versus Regulated Health Insurance in Switzerland. Ed. Okma, Kieke G. H.. Six countries, six reform models: the healthcare reform experience of Israel, the Netherlands, New Zealand, Singapore, Switzerland and Taiwan: healthcare reforms "under the radar screen". Hackensack: World Scientific, 2010. Electronic reproduction. Palo Alto, Calif.: Febrary, 2010. Available via World Wide Web. Accessed 13 Oct 2012.

23. Federal Office of Public Health. Your questions, our answers: The compulsory health insurance in Switzerland. Federal Department of Home Affairs, Swiss Confederation. Swiss Federal Office of Public Health. 1 Jan 2012. http://www.bag.admin.ch/shop/00013/00548/index.html?lang=en&print_style=yes. Accessed 14 Oct 2012.

Reimbursement: Understanding How We Pay for Health Care

15

Sachin H. Jain and Elaine Besancon

Learning Objectives

After completing this chapter, the reader should be able to answer the following questions:
- Understand the history and shortcomings of fee-for-service payment models
- Introduce and describe past approaches to payment reform
- Outline several proposed models for reform
- Discuss the effect of payment reform on physician practice

Introduction

American health-care costs have risen steadily over the past several decades, and interventions to curtail them have met with minimal success. Increasing attention is being paid to payment reform—changing the ways in which we structure and organize payments for health-care services—as potential sources for saving as well as a potential driver for quality improvement. As health-care expenditure nears 20 % of GDP—a proportion more than double that of most other industrialized nations—the need for solutions has never been greater [1].

S.H. Jain, M.D., M.B.A. (✉)
Boston VA Medical Center, Harvard Medical School,
and Merck and Company, Boston, MA 02115, USA
e-mail: shjain@gmail.com

E. Besancon, M.D.
Department of Internal Medicine, Brigham
and Women's Hospital, Boston, MA 02115, USA
e-mail: ebesancon@partners.org

Reforming our health-care payment systems will have a dramatic impact on how health care is delivered—and hospital-based care, in particular. In this chapter, we (1) address the history and shortcomings of fee-for-service payment models, (2) introduce and describe past approaches to payment reform, and (3) outline several proposed models for reform.

The chapter concludes with a discussion of payment reform's effects on physician practice.

The History and Shortcomings of Fee-for-Service Payment in Health Care

Payment for both inpatient and outpatient health-care services has historically been grounded in fee-for-service approaches to payment. In a fee-for-service model, third-party payers contract with doctors and hospitals to compensate them in proportion to the volume of services delivered to patients. Therefore, each office visit, test, or procedure is assigned a level of coverage by the third-party payer and is reimbursed individually according to this schedule, regardless of any other services being provided.

Fee-for-service approaches to payment have held several distinct advantages. They have been relatively easy to administer; they reward physicians and hospitals for the full complement of services delivered; and because payment is not tied to a particular network or provider group, they typically allow patients to choose their own physicians and hospitals [2, 3].

Yet, fee-for-service has been subject to significant criticisms that have fueled calls for major reform.

For its detractors, fee-for-service payment models encourage waste and overutilization of health-care services in the form of unneeded services that bolster revenues but have an uncertain link to outcomes [4]. This consideration has become particularly relevant as costly new technologies and therapies have become available that offer questionable benefit.

Fee-for-service models of payment also treat all physicians and hospitals as essentially equivalent, regardless of *quality* or *appropriateness* of the care delivered [4]. Under most contracts with third-party payers, a physician with outstanding outcomes and experience is paid similarly to a new practitioner with uncertain performance. Many physicians bristle at the ways in which fee-for-service models treat health-care services as a priced commodity.

Finally, fee-for-service models typically pay physicians for managing sickness—not promoting and maintaining patient health. Physicians have little financial incentive to promote patient wellness in a system that rewards them highly for intervening to manage care of sick patients but compensates them minimally for efforts to prevent morbidity [5]. Some observers have noted that fee for service is the basis for a "sick care" system instead of a "health-care" system [6].

Previous Models of Reform

The shortcomings of fee-for-service medicine have been long evident, and efforts to reform fee-for-service systems have a deep history. The most significant reform efforts have been managed care, the introduction of diagnosis-related group payment (DRG), pay for performance (P4P), and, most recently, the introduction of nonpayment for preventable complications of care. Each of these will be discussed in the following sections. Table 15.1 compares these reimbursement models using diabetes as an example.

Table 15.1 Comparison of reimbursement models: diabetes as an example

Payment type	Metric by which payment is determined	Example
Fee for service	Individual procedures and services	Compensation is given for checking labs and prescribing medication to a diabetic in clinic
Pay for performance	Bonuses for meeting quality metrics	Bonus is given for good blood sugar control in a diabetic patient
Capitation	Paid set amount to cover all patients in a population	An organization is paid a set amount to take care of all of it's patients for a year, adjusted based on how much this particular population usually costs
Diagnosis related groups	Paid set amount per hospitalization for a given diagnosis	A hospital is paid a set amount for any admission related to complications of diabetes, regardless of actual cost
Payment bundling	Paid set amount for all care for a given diagnosis	An organization is paid a set amount to take care of a patient who was admitted with complications of diabetes for the duration of the hospitalization and the next 30 days, regardless of actual cost

Managed Care

Managed care is a broad term that encompasses two primary models of health-care payment and delivery: staff- and contract-model health maintenance organizations (HMOs).

Staff-model HMOs and prepaid group practice—the most prominent example of which is Kaiser Permanente—are delivery systems that insure patients and provide health-care delivery within a closed network to physicians and hospitals. Physicians and hospitals that are part of staff-model HMOs work to conservatively manage resources and maintain patient health because they are at risk for any costs above and beyond the insurance premiums they collect from patients. Staff-model HMOs have gained recognition for their lower costs of care delivery and superior outcomes in patients with chronic illnesses [7, 8].

In contrast, contract-model HMOs are payment models in which third-party payers push the risk for managing care of patients onto physicians. In exchange for a per-patient-per-month fee (capitation) paid by an insurance company, physicians assume full risk for the patient's health [9]. If the patient remains healthy and does not use any health-care services, the physician or his/her group keep their capitation payment as profit. If the patient uses health-care services (i.e., lab tests, radiologic studies, hospitalization), the costs for these services are counted against the capitation payments received by the physicians. In theory, physicians in contract-model HMOs have strong incentives to promote the health and well-being of the patients for whom they assume responsibility.

While staff- and contract-model HMOs have their respective strengths—and were, for a time, popular models of paying for health care—they, too, have suffered critical backlash.

While outcomes in HMOs were typically similar to outcomes in fee-for-service models of care delivery, staff-model HMOs became unpopular among many patients who wished to preserve their choice of doctor or hospitals [10]. The efficiencies that were sometimes gained by creating a closed network of physicians were ill-recognized

by patients who felt that they were trapped in a closed system.

Both staff- and contract-model HMOs suffered from the perception that doctors were withholding needed treatments because of a profit motive. Whether real or imagined, managed care's emphasis on more appropriate resource utilization was received by patients as the delivery of inferior or substandard care, a lasting perception that persists today [10].

Finally, both types of HMOs were criticized for selecting favorable risk by seeking to attract young and healthier patients to plans whose health-care needs and expenditures would be minimal. If providers were at risk for the health-care expenditures of their patients, it only made sense to try to attract members with low resource utilization needs [11].

And doctors, too, found critical failures with managed care that challenged its sustainability. In both staff and contract models, managed care altered the nature of a physician's job to incorporate resource utilization and management, an uncomfortable shift for which few were adequately prepared [12].

Physicians in staff- and contract-model HMOs alike often complained of an excessive focus on productivity and profit; doctors used to practicing in "unmanaged" environments complained about the overly prescriptive nature in which they are expected to deliver care [1].

Finally, in contract-model HMOs, physicians often suffered because of their inability to manage risk and closely manage patient utilization. Many physicians and physician groups that were ill-equipped to manage risk incurred significant financial losses.

Diagnosis-Related Group (DRG) Models

While managed care has had an ebb and flow, the diagnosis-related group model of payment (DRG) has had a sustained impact on how we pay for and deliver care.

Prior to the implementation of DRGs, the Medicare program saw an average increase of

17.1 % per year in expenditures associated with inpatient hospitalization [13]. At the time, hospitals were largely paid on a fee-for-service basis that reflected their "allowable charges." Healthcare costs grew rapidly and with little restraint.

In 1983, Medicare introduced the use of diagnosis-related groups (DRGs) to reform payment for inpatient hospital care (Medicare Part A) [14]. DRGs are a collection of more than 500 types of hospitalizations that, in principle, should have standardized resource utilization and payment [13].

Whether a patient stayed 10 days in the hospital or two, DRGs standardized payment for the hospitalization of a patient with a particular illness [15]; illnesses were further stratified by up to eight comorbidities and up to six procedures performed during the patient's inpatient hospitalization. DRGs covered nursing services, room and board, and diagnostic and ancillary services [16]. Outpatient and physician services were covered separately by Medicare Part B.

In addition to the primary diagnoses and intervention, payments were based on the location and designations of the hospital, the prevailing wages in a particular community, and the indirect medical education costs for teaching hospitals [15, 16]. Special allowances were made for higher payments for patients who qualified as cost outliers and had much higher than average costs for the full length of their stay [17].

While the prospective payment system for inpatient hospitalizations has been adjusted somewhat since it was first introduced, it has remained largely intact as a model for paying for inpatient hospital care. The survival of the program is rooted in its early success.

In the first years after it was introduced, growth in hospital expenditure declined significantly. In the first 6 years after DRGs were introduced, the rate of increase in Medicare inpatient hospital spending slowed from 17.1 % to 5.7 % per year [13]. Many commercial payers subsequently adopted DRGs model for reimbursing care costs.

Despite initial success, hospital costs have again continued to rise and overall spending along

with it. Some have argued that while diagnosis-related group models of payment move away from fee-for-service payment, it does not do so completely. To the contrary, a hospitalization made more costly by an error, infection, or complication allows a hospital to code a higher DRG than it otherwise might and, in this way, at least partially resembles a fee-for-service approach [18].

Pay for Performance

With increasing recognition of gaps in quality of care, a movement emerged to try to provide specific incentives for physicians and hospitals to fill those gaps. *Pay-for-performance* models of payment provide additional payments to providers and hospitals if they demonstrate compliance with particular process guidelines or, in rare instances, demonstrate achievement of specific clinical outcomes.

Pay-for-performance programs became widely in vogue in both the public health plans (Medicare and Medicaid) and in private, commercial health plans, but have met with mixed success and reception.

Advocates of pay for performance note that the program is an important mechanism for aligning incentives for quality with patient care.

While in some cases pay-for-performance programs have led to higher rates of compliance with evidence-based guidelines for care delivery [19–21], critics argue that clinical performance is not appropriately boiled down into a few metrics, that the improvements achieved are not worth the extra costs incurred, and that focus on isolated metrics could potentially cause hospitals and doctors to focus on certain elements of the care delivery experience to the exclusion of others [22]. Studies of outcomes achieved by pay-for-performance programs have had mixed results [20, 23–25].

Furthermore, because of the difficulty of adequately risk-adjusting payment models, pay-for-performance programs focus excessively on process metrics that have an uncertain impact on outcomes [26–28].

Nonpayment for Preventable Complications of Care

Over the past several years, a movement has emerged to eliminate payment for adverse events that are entirely preventable and inexcusable in the course of health-care delivery. Under traditional models of payment, such complications have led to higher payment because additional services are consumed [29]. Under reformed models of payments, so-called "never events" are not reimbursed. In 2008, Medicare moved to eliminate payment for 11 such events: air embolism, blood incompatibility, catheter-associated urinary tract infection, certain manifestations of poor control of blood sugar levels, DVT or PE after total knee and hip replacements, falls/trauma, retained foreign bodies in surgery, pressure ulcers, certain surgical site infections, and vascular catheter-associated infections [29, 30].

While the results of this and similar initiatives are uncertain at this point, they have certainly led to an increasing focus on avoidance of preventable complications in the inpatient setting [31]. Increasing managerial and clinical attention is being applied to implementing protocols to ensure that preventable complications are avoided.

Emerging Models of Payment Reform

The future of health-care payment will clearly be informed by its past. Lessons learned around the implementation of managed care, DRG models, pay-for-performance programs, and nonpayment for preventable complications will help shape payment policies going forward. The ultimate goals of reformers remain the same: (1) lowering health-care costs, (2) increasing alignment between payment and the provision of quality care, and (3) improving incentives to deliver high-quality care. This section addresses several concepts relevant to payment reform that have gained considerable recent attention in discourse around health-care delivery reform including (1) accountable care organizations, (2) bundled payments, and (3) other approaches.

Accountable Care Organizations

While defined in other chapters in this book, these terms are crucial to understanding the future of payment, and as such we will review them here. The Patient Protection and Accountable Care Act (PPACA) established authority for the Center for Medicare and Medicaid Services (CMS) to establish accountable care organizations (ACOs). Payers will make per capita payments to these organizations—made up of hospitals and groups of providers—to manage the health care delivered to a defined population of patients. The hospitals and providers would share whatever savings they achieve in delivering care to that population as profit. Any cost overruns about the per capita payments would be absorbed by the payer [32]. The accountable care organization (ACO) model has many potential benefits. By creating organizations—virtual or real—that have an incentive for spurring lower overall health-care utilization for a defined population, health-care providers are incentivized to consider ways to improve the overall health of the patient populations they manage [33]. ACOs would correct many of the problems with fee-for-service payment models by rewarding providers for services *not* rendered and for proactive management of population health. In this regard, ACOs are in some ways like managed care.

An important distinction in contrast with managed care, however, is that patients are not locked into receiving care at a particular ACO. While patients' costs will be attributed to a particular ACO, patients will continue to have the option of receiving care from any provider or hospital that they choose [34]. In this way, there is a decoupling of payment and an individual patient's selection of a provider. Furthermore, the ACO, while incentivized to manage costs and improve health, is not at risk if overall costs exceed the per capita payment they receive for managing a patient's care.

As with all payment reform models, the effectiveness of the ACO approach to managing health-care finance will be based on the skill with which it is executed and how effectively organizations and policy-makers manage unintended consequences.

The administrative complexity of attributing health-care costs to individual patients and to ACOs will be significant; decisions about how to distribute payment within an ACO can be equally challenging. So too will be the challenge of measuring quality within an accountable care organization.

Various aspects of the execution of the ACO model will be dependent on local area variation; attribution of patients to an ACO will be far simpler in noncompetitive rural health-care markets than in competitive urban environments, where several hospitals and provider groups aspire to serve the same set of patients.

CMS has launched several programs based on these concepts in the last decade. From 2005 to 2010, CMS conducted the Physician Group Practice Demonstration, which enrolled 10 large medical care organizations with the dual goals of shared savings and improved quality. Participants were assigned spending goals based on historical spending data for each organization [35]. These organizations were eligible to share up to 80 % of any savings they achieved if they also met certain quality metrics [36]. They did not share in any risk should their spending exceed target rates. While the demonstration did result in overall cost savings and the majority of quality metrics were met by most organizations, several criticisms also surfaced. For example, although in aggregate the spending numbers looked impressive, the average cost saved per Medicare beneficiary was only $121 over 5 years, prompting some to suggest that offering shared savings without any shared risk was not a sufficiently powerful motivator [37]. Additionally, most of the cost savings occurred in the outpatient rather than inpatient setting. In fact, none of the participating groups that were affiliated with a nonacademic hospital achieved cost savings, leading to speculation that the conflicting interests of hospital ownership discouraged meaningful reduction in practices like unnecessary admissions [36].

With the passage of the Health Reform Law, CMS announced two new ACO programs in 2011 informed by the experience of the PGP demonstration: the Medicare Shared Savings (MSS) Program and the Pioneer ACO Program.

Like the PGP demonstration, the goals for these two programs were shared savings and improved quality. The MSS Program offers two enrollment options: one similar to the PGP structure with shared savings but no shared risk and another with shared risk but a higher proportion of shared savings (50 % vs. 60 %) [37]. Based on a projection that 270 ACOs will be formed, CMS estimates that savings in the first four years will total $940 million [37]. The Pioneer ACO Program is designed for more experienced groups who desire to share both a greater proportion of savings and risk. If groups enrolled in this program meet savings goals for 2 years, they have the option of switching over to a partial capitation-based payment method [38]. CMS has stated that they hope that the Pioneer ACO Program will result in 1.1 billion dollars saved over 5 years [37]. Additionally, the capitation method may allow Pioneer ACOs to focus on providing services that have not been well compensated by current fee-for-service models. However, this program has been criticized for many of the same issues as the PGP demonstration and the MSS, namely, that it may be difficult for groups to actually achieve significant spending reductions. Additionally, the Pioneer ACOs will face significantly more potential risk when they switch over to capitation, risk which has previously been borne by insurance companies, and may be challenging for many health organizations to absorb. Regardless, as the members of the Pioneer ACO Program are all experienced organizations, they are likely the best initial group to test the theory that ACOs and capitation-based payments are a sustainable model for the future.

Table 15.2 shows a comparison of recent CMS reform programs.

Bundling for Episodes of Care

Another approach that has been proposed and increasingly implemented to manage health-care costs is the use of bundled payments or episode-based case rates. Payment bundling gives a provider a fixed case rate for managing all of the inpatient and outpatient costs associated with a

Table 15.2 Comparison of recent CMS reform programs

	PGP demonstration	MSS	Pioneer ACO
Reimbursement method	Fee for service	Fee for service	Initially fee for service with option of switching to partial capitation
Maximum proportion of savings shared	80 %	50 % if no risk, 60 % if risk assumed	70 %
Assumption of risk?	No	Depends	Yes

particular condition, procedure, or illness. Paying for services as a bundle—as opposed to a discrete set of services—aims to incentivize the provider to deliver care that has fewer associated complications and extraneous costs because any overruns in expenditure are attributed to the provider.

As an example, a provider or provider group might be given a single risk-adjusted payment for inpatient management and subsequent follow-up care for an inpatient admitted with pneumonia. Under a current fee-for-service model of payment, the provider has no monetary incentive to promote close follow-up of the patient to avoid rehospitalization. If, as part of a bundle, the provider group were given responsibility for managing the inpatient care for the patient and 30 days of follow-up care, the provider group might work to ensure that the patient has adequately coordinated follow-up, close monitoring of medication adherence, and any other services that would contribute to the overall well-being of the patient. Providers would profit if and when patients remained healthy and would assume risk for losses if patients required high-service utilization.

Bundled payment models have been tested on a small scale in a variety of settings with mixed success [4, 39, 40]. The model that has gained the most attention in recent discourse has been the Prometheus Model of Payment that focuses on acute myocardial infarction, hip replacement, congestive heart failure, diabetes, and asthma [39, 41]. In the Prometheus Payment Model, all services related to a single condition or illness are covered; "covered services are determined by commonly accepted clinical guidelines or expert opinion that lay out the tested, medically accepted method for best treating the condition from beginning to end" [42]. The Prometheus model—as well as other approaches to bundling

payments—is being considered and tested by public and private payer organizations.

A key challenge with any bundled payment approach is determining the appropriate criteria by which the services and patients to be included in a given bundle are chosen [5, 43]. While a bundled approach may lead to an efficient form of service delivery for a particular condition or intervention, any system of bundled payment must take into account whether or not the intervention is indicated or if the patient was appropriately classified. Absent such tests and measures of appropriateness, bundled payment systems may lead to untoward distortions in the delivery of services.

Other Approaches

While accountable care models and bundled payments are two of the most often discussed approaches to reforming payment and delivery, they are by no means the only solutions. Other models of reforming payment and delivery have focused on targeting the care of patients with specific diseases, i.e., end-stage renal disease, or utilization patterns, i.e., patients with multiple repeated hospitalizations in a 1-year period. Other models still focus on modifying or enhancing pay-for-performance programs, maximizing compliance with evidence-based standards through comparative effectiveness research, improving management of complex patients through disease management, and the use of health information technology to coordinate care. Indeed, there is no shortage of ideas of how to improve care delivery. While many of these ideas will be tested and applied in isolation of each other, much broader payment reform models such as accountable care organizations may provide a broader framework in which to test and measure interventions that improve health and health-care delivery and, importantly, reduce health-care costs.

Impact on Physician Practice

Given that all payment reform efforts have, as an intention, improved coordination of care and reduced utilization of inpatient services, the impact of payment reform efforts on physicians will be profound.

While there is already a growing orientation in the field towards managing and ensuring close follow-up, the emphasis on post-acute care will only redouble in the face of efforts to manage health-care costs and utilization. Physicians of all stripes will likely be called upon to ensure appropriate coordination of post-acute care plans and may be charged with measuring and assessing adherence to these plans.

In inpatient settings, physicians will be increasingly seen as marshals of how resources are deployed. With both accountable care and bundled payment models, there will be increasing trends towards conservatism in use of laboratory tests, diagnostic imaging, and other interventions.

Physicians will be critical in helping build the infrastructure to actually execute upon payment reform models. Because interventions such as bundled payments will require broad agreement upon standards of care, physicians and their associated societies can take a leadership role in helping to establish these standards.

The history of health-care payment reform suggests that there will be no single solution to managing the ongoing crisis in health-care costs and that every solution will bring a set of unintended consequences that must be managed. The physician community would be wise to participate in reform as engaged actors, as they will have to practice and take leadership in the new world of health-care delivery that is being created.

References

1. Fuchs V. Major trends in the US health economy since 1950. N Engl J Med. 2012;366:973–7.
2. Jegers M, Kesteloot K, De Graeve D, Gilles W. A typology for provider payment systems in health care. Health Policy. 2002;60(3):255–73.
3. Davis K, Collins K, Schoen C, Morris C. Choice matters: enrollees' views of their health plans. Health Aff. 1995;14(2):99–112.
4. Mechanic RE, Altman SH. Payment reform options: episode payment is a good place to start. Health Aff(Project Hope). 2009;28(2):w262–71.
5. Miller H. From volume to value: better ways to pay for health care. Health Aff. 2009;28(5):1418–28.
6. Harkin S. Health care, not sick care. Am J Health Promot. 2004;19(1):1–2.
7. Luft H, Greenlick M. The contribution of group-and staff-model HMOs to American medicine. Milbank Q. 1996;74(4):445–67.
8. Iglehart J. The American health care system: managed care. N Engl J Med. 1992;327:742–7.
9. Wagner E. Types of managed care organizations. In: Kongstvedt PR, editor. The managed health care handbook. 4th ed. Gaithersburg: Aspen Publishers; 2001.
10. Bodenheimer T. The HMO, backlash—righteous or reactionary? N Engl J Med. 1996;335(21):1601–4.
11. Morgan R, Virnig B. The Medicare-HMO revolving door—the healthy go in and the sick go out. N Engl J Med. 1997;337(3):169–75.
12. Simon S, Pan R. Views of managed care—a survey of students, residents, faculty, and deans at medical schools in the United States. N Engl J Med. 1999;340:928–36.
13. Davis M, Burner S. Three decades of Medicare: what the numbers tell us. Health Aff. 1995;14(4):231–43.
14. Wennberg J. Will payment based on diagnosis-related groups control hospital costs? N Engl J Med. 1984;311(5):295–300.
15. Altman SH. The lessons of Medicare's prospective payment system show that the bundled payment program faces challenges. Health Aff (Project Hope). 2012;31(9):1923–30.
16. Mayes R, Berenson R. Medicare prospective payment and the shaping of US health care. Baltimore: The Johns Hopkins University Press; 2008.
17. Mistichelli J. Diagnosis related groups (DRGs) and the prospective payment system: forecasting social implications. georgetown.edu [Internet]. [cited 2012 Dec 14]. http://www11.georgetown.edu/research/nrcbl/publications/scopenotes/sn4.pdf
18. Wald HL, Kramer AM. Nonpayment for harms resulting from medical care: catheter-associated urinary tract infections. JAMA. 2007;298(23):2782–4.
19. Calikoglu S, Murray R, Feeney D. Hospital pay-for-performance programs in Maryland produced strong results, including reduced hospital-acquired conditions. Health Aff. 2012;31(12):2649–58.

20. Lindenauer P, Remus D. Public reporting and pay for performance in hospital quality improvement. N Engl J Med. 2007;356(5):486–96.
21. Sutton M, Nikolova S, Boaden R. Reduced mortality with hospital pay for performance in England. N Engl J Med. 2012;367(19):1821–8.
22. Tanenbaum SJ. Pay for performance in Medicare: evidentiary irony and the politics of value. J Health Polit Policy Law. 2009;34(5):717–46.
23. Ryan AM. Effects of the premier hospital quality incentive demonstration on medicare patient mortality and cost. Health Serv Res. 2009;44(3):821–42.
24. Epstein AM. Will pay for performance improve quality of care? The answer is in the details. N Engl J Med. 2012;367(19):1852–3.
25. Werner R, Kolstad J, Stuart E, Polsky D. The effect of pay-for-performance in hospitals: lessons for quality improvement. Health Aff. 2011;30:690–8.
26. Shahian D, Meyer G, Mort E. Association of National Hospital Quality Measure adherence with long-term mortality and readmissions. BMJ Qual Saf. 2012;21(4):325–36.
27. Morse RB, Hall M, Fieldston ES, McGwire G, Anspacher M, Sills MR, et al. Hospital-level compliance with asthma care quality measures at children's hospitals and subsequent asthma-related outcomes. JAMA. 2011;306(13):1454–60.
28. Patterson ME, Hernandez AF, Hammill BG, Fonarow GC, Peterson ED, Schulman KA, et al. Process of care performance measures and long-term outcomes in patients hospitalized with heart failure. Med Care. 2010;48(3):210–16.
29. Rosenthal M. Nonpayment for performance? Medicare's new reimbursement rule. N Engl J Med. 2007;357(16):1573–5.
30. Mattie A, Webster B. Centers for Medicare and Medicaid Services'" Never Events": an analysis and recommendations to hospitals. Health Care Manag. 2008;27(4):338–49.
31. Lee GM, Kleinman K, Soumerai SB, Tse A, Cole D, Fridkin SK, et al. Effect of nonpayment for preventable infections in U.S. hospitals. N Engl J Med. 2012;367(15):1428–37.
32. Addicott R. What accountable care organizations will mean for physicians. BMJ. 2012;345:e6461.
33. Berwick D. Launching accountable care organizations—the proposed rule for the Medicare shared savings program. N Engl J Med. 2011;364:e32.
34. Ginsburg P. Spending to save—ACOs and the Medicare shared savings program. N Engl J Med. 2011;364:2085–6.
35. Trisolini M, Aggarwal J, Leung M, et al. The Medicare physician group practice demonstration: lessons learned on improving quality and efficiency in health care. [Internet]. The Commonwealth Fund. [cited 2012 Aug 27]. http://www.commonwealthfund.org/Publications/Fund-Reports/2008/Feb/The-Medicare-Physician-Group-Practice-Demonstration--Lessons-Learned-on-Improving-Quality-and-Effici.aspx#citation
36. Iglehart JK. Assessing an ACO prototype–Medicare's physician group practice demonstration. N Engl J Med. 2011;364(3):198–200.
37. Berenson R. Health policy brief: next steps for ACOs. 2012 [cited 2012 Dec 12]. http://www.urban.org/url.cfm?ID=1001587
38. Alternative Payment Arrangements for the Pioneer ACO Model. [Internet]. Centers for Medicare & Medicaid Services. [cited 2012 Aug 27]. http://innovations.cms.gov/Files/x/Pioneer-ACO-Model-Alternative-Payment-Arrangements-document.pdf
39. Hussey P, Ridgely M, Rosenthal M. The PROMETHEUS bundled payment experiment: slow start shows problems in implementing new payment models. Health Aff. 2011;30(11):2116–24.
40. Struijs J, Baan C. Integrating care through bundled payments—lessons from the Netherlands. N Engl J Med. 2011;364:990–1.
41. De Brantes F, Camillus J, Fund C. Evidence-informed case rates: a new health care payment model. Pharm Ther. 2009;34(3):119–23.
42. McKesson and HCI3 Form Partnership to Support Large-Scale Bundled Payment Programs [Internet]. [cited 2012 Dec 14]. http://www.mckesson.com/en_us/McKesson.com/About%2BUs/Newsroom/Press%2BReleases%2BArchives/2012/McKesson%2Band%2BHCI3%2BForm%2BPartnership%2Bto%2BSupport%2BLarge%2526%252345%253BScale%2BBundled%2BPayment%2BPrograms.html
43. Mechanic R. Opportunities and challenges for episode-based payment. N Engl J Med. 2011;365(9):777–9.

Part IV

Understanding the Politics in Health Policy

How Health-Care Policy Is Made in Washington: Understanding the Players and the Game

16

Eleby R. Washington IV , Ilisa Halpern Paul, Amy L. Walker, and A. Alex Jahangir

> **Learning Objectives**
>
> *After completing this chapter, the reader should be able to answer the following questions:*
> - An introduction to the United States Congress and how laws are passed.
> - A discussion on Congressional committees responsible for health-care issues.
> - A discussion about physicians in Congress.
> - A discussion on how to get involved in advocacy and why it is important to do so.

Introduction

Most physicians enter medicine for the purpose of wanting to improve the life of their fellow man while practicing a profession that is challenging and rewarding. Fulfilling this basic desire is what drives many to fight through the rigors of medical school and residency and keeps them motivated enough to wake up every day and face the unique and always evolving challenges presented by the US health-care delivery system. However, the ability of physicians to provide quality patient care is impacted directly – and indirectly – by the influence of government on the health-care system.

For most physicians, understandably, the majority of their time is spent practicing medicine rather than paying close attention to the politics of health care and the consequences of health-care policy – both legislative and regulatory – on the practice of medicine. However, it is imperative that all physicians – current and future – recognize and appreciate the powerful impact and role that government and policy have on the practice of medicine. From the resources available to support graduate medical

E.R. Washington IV, B.A.
Meharry Medical College, Nashville,
TN 37208, USA
e-mail: elebywash@gmail.com

I.H. Paul, MPP • A.L. Walker, B.A.
Government and Regulatory Affairs
Practice Group, Drinker Biddle & Reath LLP,
Washington, DC 20005, USA
e-mail: ilisa.paul@dbr.com; amy.walker@dbr.com

A.A. Jahangir, M.D. (✉)
Department of Orthopedic Surgery,
Vanderbilt University Medical Center,
Nashville, TN 37232, USA
e-mail: alex.jahangir@vanderbilt.edu

M.K. Sethi and W.H. Frist (eds.), *An Introduction to Health Policy: A Primer for Physicians and Medical Students*,
DOI 10.1007/978-1-4614-7735-8_16, © Springer Science+Business Media New York 2013

education (GME), to the implementation and enforcement of HIPAA (the Health Insurance Portability and Accountability Act), to the amount of money and number of grants offered for biomedical and clinical research, to the number of residency slots for a given medical specialty, and to the relationship that physicians can and cannot have with pharmaceutical companies, the federal government's authority and influence reign supreme. As such, physicians who understand the basics of the federal policymaking process and occasionally take the time to weigh in with policymakers on issues of importance often will find that they can influence the outcome of policy deliberations to the benefit of their specialty, profession, and patients.

This chapter is focused on providing a better understanding of how federal health-care policy is made by taking a closer look at the power players involved in the political landscape, specifically those who affect the health-care system on the macro level. The first part of this chapter reviews the process by which laws are made in the United States, discusses the roles of Congressional committees, and provides an overview of the physicians currently serving in Congress. The second half of the chapter provides information on how medical students and physicians can play an active role in creating and influencing health policy.

The US Congress and How Bills Become Law

The legislative branch of the US government is responsible for developing and passing the laws that govern this country. The legislative branch, known as the Congress, is comprised of the US House of Representatives and the US Senate. While most Americans learn some American civics in elementary school, before digging into the details of health-care policymaking, it is worth reviewing the basics, as without a solid understanding of the institution of Congress and its operations, it is very difficult

to influence it.[1] See Table 16.1 for an overview of Congress.

The primary responsibilities of the US Congress are crafting new policy; conducting oversight and evaluation of existing policies, programs, and agencies; investigating problems and developing remedies; and allocating funding each year to the federal government's operations. There are numerous other constitutionally enumerated responsibilities for the Congress (e.g., advising and consenting on nominations, ratifying treaties), which will not be discussed here. Principally, this chapter will focus on the development of health-care policy and the funding of health-care programs and agencies.

The legislative process establishes new laws and is the medium through which new public policy is born. A bill can start in either of the two chambers of Congress: the House of Representatives or the Senate. New policy comes in a number of forms; the most significant of which include authorization bills that create and/or continue federal programs and agencies and annual appropriations bills that provide funding for all the departments, agencies, and programs of the federal government. Ideas and original drafts for laws can come from virtually anyone or anywhere: individuals; loosely organized groups of citizens (e.g., neighbors who share a common concern); national, state, or local organizations (e.g., American Public Health Association, American Medical Association); trade associations (e.g., National Association of Manufacturers,

---

[1] The focus of this chapter is on influencing the legislative branch. However, it is important to note that physicians have an important role to play in impacting federal laws once they are enacted; the implementation process, undertaken by federal agencies, such as the Centers for Medicare and Medicaid Services (CMS), often affords the opportunity for public comment, expert testimony, and input from individuals with expertise and/or who will be impacted by new programs, regulations, rules, etc. As such, physicians also should take time to understand the regulatory and rule-making process and weigh in when appropriate. For the basics of the federal regulation/rule-making process, see Federal Regulations: The Laws Behind the Acts of Congress at usgovinfo.about.com/od/uscongress/a/fedregulations.htm.

Table 16.1 Congress at a glance

US Congress	House	Senate
Number of elected officials	435	100
Duration of term (*No term limits*)	Two years (Entire House – all 435 Member seats up for election every 2 years – 2012, 2014, 2016, etc.)	Six years (1/3 of the entire Senate up for election every 2 years – 33 Senate seats up for election in 2014)
Jurisdiction of representation	A single Congressional District – on average, approximately 700,000 people	An entire state
Chamber control	Majority rules – the House is generally a winner takes all environment; the minority party has very little power	A simple majority (51) gives one party control over committees, budgets, and the floor schedule; however, Senate rules generally require a supermajority (60 votes) to bring most legislation to the floor
Americans' (except those in the District of Columbia) three-member delegation	One representative	Two senators
A session of Congress	Two years – commencing in odd years and ending in even years. For example, the 112th Congress commenced in January 2011 – its first session was in 2011 and its second session was 2012. The first session of the 113th Congress will commence in January 2013, and the second session of the 113th Congress will begin in January 2014	

US Chamber of Commerce); lobbyists[2] who represent a specific interest or entity, the executive branch, or Members of Congress [1]. Although anyone can generate an idea for legislation and draft a bill, proposed law only can be introduced in the Congress by a Member of Congress [1]; this Member is referred to as the primary sponsor. Other Members of Congress can show support for a bill by officially adding their names to the roster of supporters of the legislation, known as cosponsors. Lists of cosponsors of legislation are made public and available at the official website of the US Congress – the Library of Congress THOMAS site (thomas.loc.gov).

Once the sponsor introduces the bill, it is assigned a number (starting with H.R. in the House and starting with an S. in the Senate: e.g.,

H.R. 123 and S. 456) and then referred to one or several standing committees based on the rules of jurisdiction in that particular chamber [1]. In the Senate, the committees do not share or split jurisdiction over issues, so legislation is referred to a single committee. Senate bill referral is made by the Presiding Officer, with guidance from the Parliamentarian [1]. In the House of Representatives, the Speaker of the House decides to which committee(s) – or subcommittee(s) – a bill is referred [1, 2]. House committees can share or split jurisdiction over issues, and it is not uncommon for a single bill to be referred to two or more committees (known as joint referral). Thousands of bills are introduced in each session of Congress and in each respective chamber, with more measures usually being introduced in the House than the Senate. The vast majority of bills do not see legislative action, and if they are not acted on before the end of a Congress, which lasts 2 years, they "die." However, the role of advocates is the difference between a bill moving forward or dying in committee.

For those proposals that see legislative action, they undergo a thorough review process that may

---

[2] The term "lobbyist" generally refers to an individual who is employed by an organization or company to engage in outreach to elected officials and/or agency officials to influence policy deliberations. The term "lobby" is used to refer to the activities in which individuals or organizations engage to impact policymakers' views and the subsequent outcome of public policy. In this chapter we use "lobbying" and "advocacy" interchangeably.

involve obtaining reports from government departments and agencies, seeking advice from the Government Accountability Office (GAO), and holding hearings and hearing public witness testimony regarding the bill [1]. Often, the committee chairperson assigns a subcommittee the task of evaluating – and making recommendations on – a piece of legislation before the full committee reviews the legislation and makes a final determination on the proposal. A subcommittee may hold hearings and markup (which involves reviewing the bill text line by line and considering amendments) and then vote on the measure. If the subcommittee votes on the proposal favorably, it is then passed forward to the full committee for similar action and consideration. The full committee makes its revisions to the legislation and reports the bill as either favorable or unfavorable. The committee also can decide not to report a bill, effectively tabling the legislation [1]. In the House, if the bill has been referred to more than one committee, the other committees with jurisdiction also need to take action on the measure – or waive jurisdiction – before it can go to the full House chamber for a vote.

Once the committee reports a bill, the legislation typically is placed onto a calendar and then brought before the full chamber for debate, amendment, and vote for final passage [2]. At this stage the bill can be passed, denied, referred back to the committee, or tabled. In the House of Representatives, a simple majority is required for passage. However, in the Senate, depending on the type of legislation and due to the complexities of Senate procedure, favorable floor consideration involves either a simple majority or a 60-vote "supermajority." If the bill is passed in one chamber, it is then sent to the other chamber for consideration. If a measure is passed by both chambers but the House and Senate bills differ, the legislation will be referred to a conference committee that is comprised of Members from both parties and both chambers. Conference committees are charged with resolving discrepancies between the versions of the legislation and are instructed to create a single, uniform measure. Once the conference committee has reached a resolution, a final bill (known as a conference report) is produced and sent back to both the House and Senate for a final vote; a conference report cannot be amended on the floor and must be passed – or disapproved – as is.

After both chambers pass the exact same version of a bill, it is then sent to the President, who has 10 days to approve and sign the bill. The President holds the power to veto the bill, which can only be overturned by a 2/3 majority vote from both chambers of Congress. If the President does not sign the bill in 10 days, the bill automatically becomes law if Congress is in session. If Congress is not in session and the President does not sign the bill, it is "pocket vetoed" – it does not become law [2].

Congressional Committees and Health Policy

As noted earlier, there are two main types of legislation – authorizing and appropriating. Authorizing legislation typically creates, continues, or amends programs, policies, regulations, and/or agencies. Appropriations legislation is, in essence, a legislative check that draws money out of the US Treasury to support the policies, programs, agencies, and departments of the federal government. Congressional committees play a vital role in this process of developing and enacting both authorizing and appropriations legislation.[3] Each chamber of Congress operates standing committees, select committees, and joint committees. Standing committees are per-

---

[3] Authorizing legislation provides the authority for the federal government to undertake a particular endeavor and may include a specific dollar amount permitted to be allocated to such an undertaking. However, an authorizing bill does not actually draw money out of the US Treasury for the activity. A separate appropriations authorization is necessary to provide the actual funds from the US Treasury to the particular program, agency, department, etc., for the authorized activity. It is not uncommon for Congress to enact authorizing legislation and then subsequently choose not to provide funding to the authorized program, effectively making it as the program did not exist. This is referred to as being authorized but not appropriated. Similarly, initiatives can receive funding in an appropriations bill but not have underlying statutory authorization; this is referred to as being appropriated but not authorized.

manent committees with legislative duties and oversight responsibilities over various federal agencies and government programs. Select committees are temporary committees created to conduct special investigations or make decisions on unique measures where there may be overlapping or complex jurisdictional issues. Joint committees are committees made up of Members of both chambers of Congress [3]. The Senate and House of Representatives have 16 and 20 standing committees, respectively [2, 3]. At the beginning of each session of Congress, individuals are selected to serve on these standing committees. Each party uses a selection committee and a variety of factors (e.g., tenure/seniority, expertise) to choose which of its Members will serve on which committees; committee assignments must be approved by both the full party and the entire chamber of Congress. The majority party has more seats on each committee than the minority party [3]. The chairperson for each committee comes from the majority party. The highest ranking Member of the minority party on each committee is referred to as the "Ranking Member."

As mentioned previously, committees analyze, review, amend, and make recommendations on legislation referred to the committee before it is presented to the respective chamber for further consideration. The outlook of a proposed bill is tied directly to and influenced by the actions of the committee(s) to which it is assigned and the priorities, interests, and dynamics of the committee leadership and Membership. As a result, the process by which a committee is assigned jurisdiction over a bill is very important. While the committee referral process generally is determined by established guidelines, there can be some degree of variability in this process because of overlap with respect to committee jurisdiction over a variety of legislative issues. This has contributed to internal Congressional chamber politicking to both protect existing legislative responsibilities and secure new jurisdiction [4]. The nature of the committee referral process places a lot of the power in the hands of the referees, the Speaker of the House in the House of Representatives, and the Parliamentarian and Presiding Officer in the Senate.

Nowhere is the complexity of the legislative referral process more apparent than in the health-care arena. Legislation impacting health care is wide-ranging – from child nutrition to medical malpractice to hazardous wastes – to name a few issues. In fact, if all legislation related to health were assigned to a single committee, almost all domestic health policy items would be given to the panel, overwhelming a single committee and undermining the Congressional division of labor [4]. To account for the wide variety of issues and concerns that make up health policy, both the House of Representatives and the Senate have a number of different committees and subcommittees with the responsibility of reviewing health-related legislation. This has created a complex policy environment in which there are many players in the US Congress who are in a position to influence health policy. Tables 16.2 and 16.3 summarize the different House and Senate committees that hold jurisdiction over some portion of the health sector and, thus, play a significant role in health policy [5].[4]

Physicians in Congress

Physicians have been community leaders since the beginning of the United States and were critical in the foundation of American government. In fact, the Continental Congress included 31 physicians (8.5 % of the total Members), and 6 (10.6 %) of the signers and 2 (5.1 %) of the writers of the constitution were physicians [6]. However, over time, physician representation in government has markedly declined. If one compares the first 100 years of Congress to roughly the last 40 (1960–2004), physician representation in Congress has fallen significantly, from 4.6 % in early years to 1.1 % more recently [7].

In the 113th Congress (2013–2014), there are 18 Members of the House of Representative and three Senators who are physicians (Tables 16.4 and 16.5). Of those 21 physician-legislators, 17 are Republican and represent many different

---

[4] To learn which Members of Congress serve on which committees, visit www.house.gov and www.senate.gov.

Table 16.2 Senate committees

Senate Appropriations Committee	Responsible for allocating federal funding each year to all the functions of the federal government. The Labor, Health and Human Service (HHS), Education and Related agencies (LHHS) Subcommittee holds the primary responsibility for health-related program funding. While mainly centered on HHS (e.g., National Institutes of Health, Medicare, Medicaid, Centers for Disease Control and Prevention), funding for federal health programs also is provided by other Subcommittees, including Defense (military health research) and State and Foreign Operations (global health), among others
Senate Budget Committee	Develops and recommends an annual federal budget blueprint, which includes proposed spending targets for health-care-related agencies and programs in the form of a budget resolution. The budget resolution does not have the force of law
Senate Environment and Public Works Committee	Has jurisdiction over health issues as they relate to the environment; maintains two health-related subcommittees: the Children's Health and Environmental Responsibility and the Superfund, Toxics, and Environmental Health Subcommittees
Senate Finance Committee	Maintains responsibility over tax-related measures. The Senate Finance Committee and its Health Subcommittee have a significant impact on the health policy landscape through jurisdictional control over the Social Security Act and its components related to health care, which include Medicaid, Medicare, and the Children's Health Insurance Program (CHIP). The Senate Finance Committee played a leadership role in the health reform debate and the shaping of the Affordable Care Act (ACA)
Senate Health, Education, Labor and Pensions (HELP) Committee	Holds legislative jurisdiction over a number of areas within the health sector, including biomedical research, public health, and occupational health. The committee also has oversight and legislative control over numerous issues, such as those relating to the Food and Drug Administration, children's health, immunization, and elder abuse.[a] Subcommittees with health-related responsibilities include the Children and Families Subcommittee, the Employment and Workplace Safety Subcommittee, and the Primary Health and Aging Subcommittee
Senate Homeland Security and Governmental Affairs Committee	Contains two relevant health-related subcommittees: the Permanent Subcommittee on Investigation that studies and investigates crimes that have implications of national health and the Subcommittee on Disaster Recovery and Intergovernmental Affairs which oversees the activities of the Department of Homeland Security as related to emergency preparedness and recovery in the wake of national disaster
Senate Judiciary Committee	Responsible for providing oversight to the Department of Justice, reviewing executive nominations for various government agencies as well as judicial nominations, and reviewing proposed legislation from a number of different areas.[b] With respect to health, the Senate Judiciary Committee holds jurisdiction over legislation related to medical malpractice, tort reform, and product liability

Source: Data from[5]

[a]About the Committee. Senate Budget Committee. http://budget.senate.gov/democratic/index.cfm/aboutcommittee. Accessed May 11, 2012; Jurisdiction. The United States Senate Committee on Finance. http://www.finance.senate.gov/about/jurisdiction/ Accessed May 11, 2012; About the HELP Committee. The United States Committee on Health Education Labor and Pensions. http://www.help.senate.gov/about/ Accessed May 11, 2012

[b]Subcommittees. The United States Committee on Health Education Labor and Pensions. http://www.help.senate.gov/about/ Accessed May 11, 2012; Subcommittees. U.S. Senate Committee on Homeland Security and Governmental Affairs. http://www.hsgac.senate.gov/subcommittees Accessed May 11, 2012; Committee Jurisdiction. United States Senate Committee on the Judiciary. http://www.judiciary.senate.gov/about/jurisdiction.cfm Accessed May 11, 2012

specialties including anesthesiology, family practice, emergency medicine, several surgical subspecialties, and obstetrics and gynecology [8]. Interestingly, some physicians serve on committees vital to the enactment of health policy legislation, such as the House Ways and Means Committee, while others serve on committees that are less involved with health-care matters.

During the health-care reform debate in 2009, only seven of the physicians then in Congress were Members of committees directly involved in the crafting of the health-care reform bill [9].

Regardless of whether physicians in Congress serve on committees with jurisdiction over health-related legislation, physician-legislators do impact the health policy discussion on Capitol Hill in

Table 16.3 House of representatives csommittees

House Appropriations Committee	As in the Senate, the Appropriations Committee is responsible for allocating federal funding each year to all the operations and programs of the federal government. Like the Senate, the House LHHS Subcommittee holds the primary responsibility for health-related program funding. While mainly centered on HHS (e.g., National Institutes of Health, Medicare, Medicaid, Centers for Disease Control and Prevention), funding for federal health programs also is provided by other Subcommittees, including Defense (military health research) and State and Foreign Operations (global health), among others
House Budget Committee	Along with the Senate committee of the same name, the House Budget Committee, through a budget resolution, makes annual recommendations about the federal budget and health-care spending. While budget resolutions serve as a road map for the appropriations process, it does not have the force of law
House Education and Labor Committee	While this committee primarily is concerned with measures involving labor and education, it does have some jurisdiction over commercial/private sector health insurance plans and programs. In addition, the committee is involved in issues related to worker safety
House Energy and Commerce Committee	Holds legislative power over measures related to commerce, public health, energy, and technology. The Energy and Commerce Committee shares jurisdiction over some portions of the Medicare and Medicaid programs with the House Ways and Means Committee. Additionally, its Health Subcommittee holds responsibility over a wide range of health-related topics including measures related to biomedical research, mental health services, pharmaceuticals/prescription drugs, and medical devices
House Homeland Security Committee	The House Homeland Security Committee, as in the Senate, oversees the Department of Homeland Security. The Emergency Preparedness and Response Subcommittee enacts measures involving biosecurity and prevention and response to terrorism or natural disaster that may have implications on national health
House Judiciary Committee	Similar in jurisdiction to the Senate committee of the same name, the House Judiciary Committee has authority in health-related measures such as medical malpractice, tort liability, and health product liability
House Ways and Means Committee	Has similar jurisdiction to the Senate Finance Committee in that it holds jurisdiction over taxation and revenue measures. The Health Subcommittee has oversight related to the Social Security Act and therefore jurisdiction over Medicare, Medicaid, and other health measures included in the act

Source: Data from [5]; About the Budget Committee. House of Representatives Committee on the Budget. http://budget.house.gov/About/ Accessed May 11, 2012; About the Committee. House Energy and Commerce Committee. http://energycommerce.house.gov/about/about.shtml Accessed May 11,2012; About the Committee. Committee on Homeland Security. http://homeland.house.gov/about/history-jurisdiction Accessed March 11, 2012; Subcommittee on Emergency Preparedness, Response, and Communications. Committee on Homeland Security. http://homeland.house.gov/subcommittee-emergency-preparedness-response-communications Accessed March 11, 2012; Subcommittee on Emergency Preparedness, Response, and Communications. Committee on Homeland Security. http://homeland.house.gov/subcommittee-emergency-preparedness-response-communications Accessed March 11, 2012

many ways. An example of how physician-legislators can lead on health-care issues is the 2009 creation of the Republican Doctors Caucus, a group of various medical providers (and some other health professionals) from the House, organized to provide a unified voice in opposition to the PPACA [10]. This group successfully has used its collective standing as physicians to advocate in

Table 16.4 Physicians in the 113th Senate and Committee Membership

John Barrasso (R-Wyoming/Orthopaedic Surgeon)	Senate Energy and Natural Resources Committee, Senate Environment and Public Works Committee, Senate Indian Affairs Committee, Senate Foreign Relations Committee
Tom Coburn (R-Oklahoma/Family Physician)	Senate Banking, Housing, and Urban Affairs Committee; Senate Homeland Security and Governmental Affairs Committee; Senate Select Intelligence Committee
Rand Paul (R-Kentucky/Ophthalmologist)	Senate Foreign Relations Committee; Senate Health, Education, Labor, and Pensions Committee; Senate Homeland Security and Governmental Affairs Committee; Senate Small Business and Entrepreneurship Committee

Source: Data from Congressional Committees. GovTrack. http://www.govtrack.us/congress/committees/#. Accessed May 20, 2012

favor of repealing specific provisions of the PPACA, including the Independent Payment Advisory Board and the Community Living Assistance Services and Support Program (CLASS ACT) [11, 12]. The House of Representatives voted to repeal both of these PPACA provisions in the 112th Congress [13, 14].[5]

Getting Involved: Why and How

While running for Congress is the most intense and hands-on manner by which health-care providers can influence national health policy, it is not the only way physicians can have their voices heard. The demands of practice, lack of political or policy knowledge, indifference to the policy process, and concerns about taking time away from patient care and family obligations are all very valid reasons physicians may not seek to become active in the policymaking process. From where most physicians sit, it also may seem an impossible task to actually impact the deliberations that occur on Capitol Hill. However, individuals and organizations can have a strong influence in the genesis of public policy. Moreover, if physicians

do not take an active role in advocating for the best interest of his or her patients or specialty, policies impacting the health-care delivery system and the practice of medicine will be made without the input of physicians or those that know firsthand the strengths and weaknesses of the health-care delivery system. Therefore, it is extremely important that health-care providers become engaged and weigh in with their elected officials on issues of priority to them.

Because Systemic Changes Affect Physicians and Patients

As a result of rising US debt (which is now close to $16 trillion) and rising national health expenditures (a projected $2.8 trillion in 2012 and $4.6 trillion by 2020), the current health-care system is on an unsustainable path. Now more than ever the health-care system will need to be changed [15, 16]. Even with the 2010 passage of the PPACA, the process of health-care reform is far from over. Congress will continue to consider policies and changes (e.g., cuts to Medicare, changes to entitlement programs) that will impact the health-care delivery system for many years. These policies will directly and indirectly influence the way in which physicians practice and can deliver quality medical care to their patients, and, therefore, physician involvement in the process is more vital now than ever before.

---

[5] These measures repealing provisions of the PPACA were not been considered in the Senate, which in the 112th Congress is under democratic control, as it was when the PPACA passed the chamber in 2010 and as it is in the 113th Congress.

Table 16.5 Physicians in the 113th House of Representatives and Committee Membership

Dan Benishek (R-Michigan/General Surgeon)	House Agriculture Committee, House Natural Resources Committee, House Veterans' Affairs Committee
Ami Bera (D-California/General Practice)	House Foreign Affairs Committee; House Science, Space, and Technology Committee
Charles Boustany (R-Louisiana/Cardiovascular Surgeon)	House Ways and Means Committee
Paul Broun (R-Georgia/Family Physician)	House Homeland Security Committee; House Science, Space, and Technology Committee; House Natural Resources Committee
Larry Bucshon (R-Indiana/Thoracic Surgeon)	House Education and the Workforce Committee; House Transportation and Infrastructure Committee; House Science, Space, and Technology Committee
Michael Burgess (R-Texas/Ob-Gyn)	House Energy and Commerce Committee, House Rules Committee
Bill Cassidy (R-Louisiana/Gastroenterologist)	House Energy and Commerce Committee
Donna Christensen (D-US Virgin Islands/Physician)	House Energy and Commerce Committee
Scott DesJarlais (R-Tennessee/Family Physician)	House Agriculture Committee, House Education and the Workforce Committee, House Oversight and Government Reform Committee
John Fleming (R-Louisiana/Family Physician)	House Armed Services Committee, House Natural Resources Committee
John "Phil" Gingrey (R-Georgia/Ob-Gyn)	House Administration Committee, House Energy and Commerce Committee
Andy Harris (R-MD/Anesthesiologist)	House Natural Resources Committee; House Science, Space, and Technology Committee; House Transportation and Infrastructure Committee
Joe Heck (R-Nevada/Emergency Room Physician)	House Armed Services Committee, House Education and the Workforce Committee
Jim McDermott (D-Washington/Psychiatrist)	House Budget Committee, House Ways and Means Committee
Tom Price (R-Georgia/Orthopaedic Surgeon)	House Education and Workforce Committee, House Ways and Means Committee
David "Phil" Roe (R-Tennessee/Ob-Gyn)	House Education and the Workforce Committee, House Veterans' Affairs Committee
Raul Ruiz (D-California/Emergency Medicine)	House Natural Resources Committee, House Veterans' Affairs Committee
Brad Wenstrup (R-Ohio/Podiatric Surgeon, US Army Reserves Combat Surgeon)	House Armed Services Committee, House Veterans' Affairs Committee

Source: Data from Congressional Committees. GovTrack. http://www.govtrack.us/congress/committees/#. Accessed May 20, 2012

Because Physician Voices Matter

Who better to fuel legislative change in the health policy arena than the physicians on the frontline, those who take care of America's population on a daily basis? Physicians understand the shortcomings of the current health-care model and have the empirical evidence and experiences necessary to offer effective solutions to these systemic flaws. Not only do physicians have experience with – and an understanding of – the health-care system, but physicians also have the respect and support of the public. A recent survey conducted by Gallup found 73 % of Americans had confidence that physicians would recommend the right thing for reforming the US health-care system, while only 34 % of those surveyed trusted that Members of Congress would do the right thing [17]. This support and trust from the public should give physicians a sense of duty and responsibility to give input into policy decisions regarding the nation's health-care system.

Because If Not Us, Who?

Most Members of Congress and many other players in Washington do not have the firsthand knowledge about the delivery of health-care that physicians possess. Other organizations that do not share the physician community's concerns or viewpoints are likely meeting and communicating directly with Members of Congress on various issues that will impact the health-care delivery system. When it comes time to make a decision, Members of Congress only consider the viewpoints that they have heard, and you cannot assume that your view of a situation is widely shared or being advocated for on Capitol Hill. The point is clear: if physicians do not participate actively in affecting health-care policy, other players outside of the physician community will inevitably wield more power, in pursuit of their own legislative interests and desires, which could be in direct conflict with those of physicians.

How to Get Involved

While the public policy arena can seem intimidating and overwhelming, there are many easy ways for medical students and physicians to get involved. Advocacy does not just mean traveling to Washington, DC, to meet with your elected officials; it can be as quick and simple as sending an email or making a phone call. Your personal advocacy commitment can involve as much or as little time as you have and would like to dedicate to work toward affecting policy change.

Know Who Represents You

The first, easy step in getting involved is knowing who represents you in Congress. Using public websites – www.house.gov and www.senate.gov – you can find the names and contact information for your US Representative and two US Senators. You can then visit their websites and learn more about them by reading their bios, reviewing the issues they indicate are their priorities, and noting on which committees they serve. Keep in mind that due to redistricting, a number of representation changes occurred in 2012 so be sure you are using the most up-to-date information for the current session of Congress. You can contact the local or Washington, DC, offices of all three of your election officials to learn the name of the staff person who handles health-care issues. The websites provide the phone numbers, mailing addresses, fax numbers, etc., for your elected officials. Members' websites usually have an e-mail form that you may use to send a quick message and typically have an option to sign up for their newsletters and local meeting information; be sure to get connected to them through this easy mechanism. Keep the local and Washington, DC, contact information handy, and take the time to introduce yourself and offer your expertise and assistance (see the section in this chapter on "Get to Know Your Elected Officials and Their Staff").

Join a Medical Organization

Physicians and medical students can join a number of professional medical organizations that participate in organized lobbying; many of these organizations have a strong voice on the national health policy landscape. There are a variety of organizations that represent the many ideas, specialties, and political affiliations that belong to our heterogeneous medical community. These entities tackle a variety of different health policy issues, often through grassroots efforts. For example, the American Medical Association gives physicians the opportunity to lobby against cuts on Medicare reimbursements, while getting involved in the American Medical Student Association allows medical students the opportunity to collectively bring their voices forward against the discontinuation of subsidized Stafford loans for graduate and professional students [18, 19]. If you do not already know the group that best represents your issues of concern, general and specialty groups can be found through an internet search.

Most national health provider organizations have grassroots networks and other initiatives that involve unified "calls to action" or "action alerts" through which the organization urges its Members to communicate with their Members of Congress on a particular issue of interest. Such calls to action typically include a key message to convey and provide basic background and context to the policy issue. These organizations often prepare template messages that can be sent via e-mails, letters, and calls, and you can choose which method of communication fits your time and comfort level best. While such communications may seem generic, they can be very effective, as Members of Congress and their staff read, tally, and generally respond to each message [20]. Members of Congress routinely ask their staff Members "who are we hearing from" on a particular issue; unless physicians take advantage of opportunities to have their voices heard, these elected officials will be left with the impression that the physicians in their communities do not care about the issues at hand. With the number of professional organizations available for health-care professionals to join, it should not be hard to find a group that fits your professional interests and personal beliefs; Membership in such a group will provide you information and a conduit through which you can advocate on your primary policy issues of concern.

Get to Know Your Elected Officials and Their Staff

Members of Congress and their staff welcome physician advice and input on a number of health-related issues [21]; how you reach out is not as important as the fact that you do reach out. Beyond responding to calls to action from your professional societies, it is relatively easy to develop a relationship with elected officials and their staff. One terrific way to get started is to seek a meeting with your Members of Congress or his/her staff, either in Washington, DC, or "at home" in the state for Senators and in the district for House Members. To schedule a meeting, check the websites of the Member(s) you wish to meet with to see if there are any specific scheduling instructions posted. Sometimes offices will have a webform you can fill out to request a meeting.

Alternatively, you can call the Member's office and ask for the scheduler. When you talk to the receptionist, be sure to get the name of the scheduler and write it down, in case you need to call back to follow up later. Also be sure to iden-

tify yourself as a constituent when you call. You may need to leave a voice mail with the scheduler. Whether you speak to the scheduler or leave a message, remember to provide your name, identify yourself as a constituent, briefly explain the issue or issues you would like to meet with the Member about, and specify whether you would like to meet in DC or at home and when. If you do not hear a response from the scheduler within a week or two, politely call back and ask if the scheduler has a response to your request. You may have to follow up a number of times or submit your request in writing. The Congressional schedule can be very hectic, and it can be difficult to schedule appointments too far in advance. Throughout the process, remember to be persistent yet polite.

If the Member is unable to meet with you due to scheduling conflicts, he or she may refer you to a Member of the legislative staff. It is important to recognize the importance of Congressional staff, as these individuals assist the legislators in a wide variety of areas, including the drafting of legislation, deciding what stances to take on legislative issues, holding meetings, and communicating with constituents. Between committee hearings, dealings on the House or Senate floor, and various meetings, it is often not possible for Members to meet with every person who requests a meeting, even if they are a constituent: it is nothing personal against you or your issue. Staff are bright and competent and advise Members on many issues, so these meetings are just as beneficial to you, the office, and your cause. Tables 16.6, 16.7, and 16.8 provide more information on the common staff positions in an elected official's office and give recommendations for how to be effective in your communications with them.

It is helpful to learn as much as possible about your Members' voting history, bill cosponsorships, and committee Membership prior to meeting with them or their staff: be sure to do your homework. In preparation for meetings, it is important to educate yourself on the topics you wish to discuss in the meeting. Rather than trying to learn the intricacies of the legislative process, learn the basics, have a good idea of your Members' stance on policies important to

Table 16.6 Who works in a Congressional Office

As we mentioned earlier in the chapter, Members of Congress maintain busy schedules – Committee hearings, markups, constituent and lobbyist meetings, events, and travel to and from Washington, DC. The demands on legislators elevate the importance of their staff – often 20 and 30 year olds who devote their time and energy to the public policy process. Below is a brief overview of the different positions in a typical Congressional office.

Administrative Staff	Legislative Staff	State/District Staff	Committee Staff
Chief of Staff (CoS): Second highest ranking person in the office after the Member; responsible for overall office operations and evaluating political outcome of various legislative actions.	**Legislative Director:** Monitors the legislative schedule, work swith the CoS to develop priorities, advises on legislation, develops legislation, and oversees the legislative staff.	**State/District Director:** The State or District Director often serves as the Member's proxy at home - attending events, coordinating events while the Member is home, and acting as a liaison to the community.	Each Committee also has staff that specialize in issues related to the Committee's specific jurisidiction. These staff members may work generally for the Committee or may be assigned to a specific Committee member's office. For example, Senator Tom Harkin (D-IA), the HELP Committee Chairman's health LA is from the staff of the HELP Committee.
Scheduler: Responsible for apportioning the Member's time between hearings, meetings, events, and other activities and making any necessary travel arrangements.	**Legislative Assistant:** Offices have multiple LAs who each handle a portfolio of issues; LAs take meetings, draft legislation, and work with the LD to advise the Member on legislation.	**Community Representative:** Some offices may also have mid-level staff in the distric toffice that work with the state or district director in representing the Member back at home.	
Staff Assistant: Junior staff member usually responsible for answering the phones. Keep in mind that today's staff assistant can be tomorrow's Chief of Staff.	**Legislative Correspondent (LC):** LCs read and draft responses to constituent mail; LCs may also assist LAs with meetings, when necessary.	**Caseworker:** Staff, often in the state, but sometimes in DC, that act as a liaison between constituents and federal agencies and to assist with resolving constituent problems (passports, Veteran benefits, etc.)	

you, and focus on knowing your argument. Congressional websites, online biographies, and newspapers are useful in finding out this information. As noted earlier, a great reference is the Library of Congress website, THOMAS (www.thomas.loc.gov), which is an online database of bills and voting histories. THOMAS allows you to search for legislation by bill number, keyword, or legislator name. Prior to going to the meeting, make sure you have developed clear and focused talking points (plan on having between 15 and 30 min for the entire meeting), be cordial, and

Table 16.7 Becoming an Advocate and Trusted Resource

Research	Connect	Take Action
• Know who represents you at the federal, state, and local levels.	• Sign up for alerts from professional organizations of which you are a member.	• Contact your elected officials via phone, email, or letter to voice your opinion.
• Visit your elected officials' websites to find out their contact information, biographical information, and their stances on various policy issues.	• Subscribe to your elected officials' email newsletters.	• Seek local meetings by contacting the Members' schedulers or district staff.
• Call the offices to find out which staff member handles healthcare.	• Sign up for health-related organizations' newsletters to stay up to date on what is happening in the health policy field.	• Offer yourself as a resource and ask how you may be of assistance to the office.
• Anytime you contact an office, do your homework so you reference the correct bill and have some basic background information, if needed.	• Think about your existing connections to policy in your community - whether you know someone serving in public office or know of someone who may be able to introduce you to someone who does.	• After the meeting, follow up with a thank you and any information you said you would provide.
• Read national and local news sources and health policy blogs to stay abreast of key issues and developments.	• "Like the Facebook pages for your Members of Congress.	• Check in with the staffer with relevant information, when appropriate. This will keep you in the forefront of their mind, should they need a resource on your area of concern.
	• Follow your Members of Congress on Twitter.	• Continue to call and write the office - you never know when your issue may be relevant or resonate.
	• Attend a town hall meeting or other local event where you can meet your Member of Congress.	

leave behind materials after the meetings as reminders of the key points from your discussion.[6] If you are meeting as an individual citizen and not on behalf of – or with permission from – your employer, be sure to provide your personal contact information and not information from your work. Most importantly, offer your assistance and make clear you are happy to be a resource on health-care issues. You might consider inviting the staffer and/or Member to visit your practice, but be sure to get authorization first. After the meeting, follow up with the office:

thank the staffer and/or Member for the meeting, reiterate your main points, and provide any information you promised during the discussion.

In addition to meeting with and developing a relationship with your Senators and Representative and their staff, make an effort to participate in public meetings (e.g., town hall meetings), and offer or submit testimony regarding issues about which you are passionate. Physicians and medical students have been called upon by Congressional committees or outside groups to share their valued and respected opinions on health-related legislation. Finally, if there is a specific health issue that you feel strongly about that is currently not being addressed, consider bringing it to the attention of your elected officials and their staff, and you may find yourself working with them to draft legislation in response.

---

[6] Your health professional organization likely has a government relations and advocacy department that can assist you with scheduling meetings, developing talking points, and putting together a packet of supporting materials for your meeting. Do not hesitate to reach out for their assistance.

Table 16.8 How to ensure you and your messages have an impact

Keep your written or oral comments brief and easy to understand. Remember policymakers and their staff are like your patients – they did not go to medical school, they are not physicians. Do not use clinical terminology or technical terms – explain the issue in layperson's language

While you may have many issues that concern you – or make you crazy – do not try to tackle them all at once. Pick the most important (e.g., funding for graduate medical education) and reach out or write about that one first. Once you have success in weighing in on your top priority, you can have your voice heard on the other issues later

Include an example or illustration of the problem you are writing to address. Being mindful of HIPAA regulations, consider including a specific example from your practice that explains the issue in a way that is compelling. You can include statistics – but not too many – and keep in mind that a personalized story is more memorable

Keep a copy of your letter or e-mail – or make a record of any calls or meetings – so you can follow up later to ensure that you receive a response from the policymaker's office

If you have colleagues or coworkers who share your concerns or views, ask them to join you in your outreach. Bring someone from your practice with you and/or ask others to send in letters or make calls following up on your own communication. While one voice makes a difference, more voices have an even greater impact

Register to vote and exercise your right to vote in each and every election. If you do not like the direction things are going, do not just complain – take action through influencing the process and determining who represents you at all levels of government

Utilize the Media: Traditional and Social

The media can be a useful tool in the health policy process. Members of Congress and their staff monitor what is written in local newspapers and what is said on local television and radio stations, especially when it concerns public policy issues or mentions the elected officials themselves. In addition, technology has been transforming the way that Members of Congress interact with their constituents. Members of Congress increasingly are using social media tools, such as Facebook, Twitter, and YouTube, to get their message out [22]. Following your Members on Facebook and Twitter can provide you information about their activities in Washington as well as offer an additional forum through which you can interact with the Member and their staff.

All forms of media can be a valuable tool for delivering clear, direct messages, such as providing opinions on new legislation, communicating policy goals, and, if necessary, holding policymakers accountable in a public forum. Writing letters to editors of the local newspapers, showing up to local news conferences, connecting to your Members via social media, and offering yourself to local media outlets as a resource on health issues are all powerful ways to increase your visibility and have your voice heard in the health policy arena. Congressional offices take notice of these actions, which will keep you on their radar; generally, it is best to use the media in a positive way rather than punitive. For example, a quick thank you on Twitter following a meeting often generates a response and may start a positive dialogue with a Congressional office. By stepping out to show policymakers you appreciate their work, you raise your profile within their office and throughout the health-care policy field.

Take State, Local, and Community Action

Although this chapter has focused on the health policy players in Washington, the importance of local and state government should not be understated. A number of health-related activities fall under the jurisdiction of state and local government including public health, the financing and delivery of personal health services (including Medicaid), mental health services, direct delivery through public hospitals and health departments, environmental protection, and the regulation of the providers of medical care [18]. Perhaps of greatest significance is that the states are tasked with designing and operating the state health exchanges created under the PPACA, which are scheduled for implementation in 2014.

Therefore, taking advocacy action in health-care policy at the state and local levels can be beneficial as well. Through similar means such as becoming involved in state and local medical professional organizations (e.g., California Medical Association, Tennessee Orthopaedic Society) and seeking out meetings with state and local elected officials, you can pursue health policies that could have a profound difference for the communities in which you live and practice medicine.

Political Action Committees (PACs) and Super PACs

No discussion of Capitol Hill and Washington, DC, would be complete without a mention of Political Action Committees (PACs). PACs are created for the purpose of collecting finances to be donated to political candidates. A PAC can be affiliated with an entity, such as a labor, business, or trade organization, or a PAC may be created and funded by a group that exists primarily or solely for the purpose of giving money to specific candidates [23].[7] PACs collect and donate funds to political campaigns without having an active role in the campaign process. PACs can be formed by anyone but have been utilized mostly by labor groups, business corporations, and trade associations [23]. Today, PACs are subjected to multiple regulations, including restrictions on the total amount they can give to an individual candidate per election ($5,000 per election), the amount they can give to another PAC ($5,000), the amount they can receive from an individual ($5,000), and the amount they can give to a national party committee ($15,000) [24]. Multicandidate PACs are PACs that receive contributions from more than 50 Members and contribute to more than 5 political candidates [23]. Leadership PACs are formed by politicians to finance and support the campaigns of other politicians [24]. Health professionals, insurance companies, pharmaceutical companies, and hospitals all have developed PACs that make contributions to federal candidates. In 2010, a total of more than $54 million in campaign contributions were donated by 378 PACs from the health-care sector [25]. The Center for Responsive Politics operates a website – OpenSecrets.org – that reports the money spent on elections and lobbying and seeks to shed light on the role that money plays in politics and policymaking; the website provides detailed information where you can learn more about the specific political giving by a particular PAC, organization, individual, or sector.

Recently the process of making campaign contributions has undergone significant changes, with the advent of the "Super PAC," stemming from the Supreme Court's 2010 Citizens United ruling in which the court held that the First Amendment of the constitution does not allow the federal government to limit independent political expenditures by unions or corporations [26]. "Super PACs" are largely unregulated entities and can receive unlimited funds from individuals, corporations, unions, health organizations, etc. and can donate unlimited funds to support or oppose a politician [27]. This allows wealthy individuals, corporations, and others who create Super PACs to tap their own economic resources without relying on collecting money from PACs, either to aid the campaigns of politicians that share their political ideals or to speak out against the campaigns of politicians that do not support or comport to their interests. Unlike PACs, Super PACs are not able to directly donate funds to a politician's campaign [27]. For example, a Super PAC can run an unlimited number of television and magazine ads voicing support for Candidate X, but cannot contribute money directly to Candidate X's campaign funds. The November 2012 election was the first presidential election to be impacted by Super PACs. Conventional wisdom is that it is likely that Super PACs will have a major impact on the political process for years to come.

Conclusion

All levels of government – federal, state, and local – influence the practice of medicine directly and indirectly. With less than 2 % of

---

[7] Connected PACs are PACs associated with and governed by the labor, trade, or corporate association that originally created them. Non-connected PACs have no parent labor group or corporate organization [7].

the current Members of Congress as physicians, it is imperative that medical students and physicians bring their perspective and expertise to the nation's policymakers to ensure that the decisions they make are in the interest of doctors and patients. Unless physicians take the time to understand the policymaking process, get acquainted with elected officials and their staff, and weigh in on debates over Medicare, Medicaid, health-care reform, funding for biomedical research, etc., the policies, programs, and budgets that come out of Washington, DC, will be devoid of physician expertise and likely will be counter to what physicians and patients need in the twenty-first century. By reading this chapter and taking the recommended steps, you will help ensure that the next generation of physicians will have an even greater impact on our nation's health-care policies and programs.

References

1. US House of Representatives. How our laws are made. http://www.senate.gov/reference/resources/pdf/howourlawsaremade.pdf. Revised 30 June 2003. Accessed 11 May 2012.
2. US Senate. Enactment of a law. http://thomas.loc.gov/home/enactment/enactlaw.pdf. Revised 1997. Accessed 11 May 2012.
3. Committee FAQs. US house of representatives office of the clerk. http://clerk.house.gov/committee_info/commfaq.aspx. Accessed 5 May 2012.
4. Committees and Health Jurisdictions in Congress. In: Mann TE, Ornstein NJ, editors. Intensive care: how Congress shapes health policy. Washington, DC: American Enterprise Institute; Brookings Institute; 1995. http://www.questia.com/PM.qst?a=o&d=65451687. Accessed 5 May 2012.
5. Committees and subcommittees with jurisdiction over health legislation 112th Congress. American Hospital Association. www.aha.org/content/00-10/09congresshealthcommittees.pdf. Updated May 2011. Accessed 6 May 2012.
6. Jameson MG. Physicians and American political leadership. JAMA. 1983;249(7):929–30.
7. Kraus CK, Suarez TA. Is there a doctor in the house?...or the Senate? Physicians in US Congress, 1960–2004. JAMA. 2004;292(17):2125–9.
8. Reece R. Doctors in Congress. The health care blog. 2011 Jan 13. http://thehealthcareblog.com/blog/2011/01/13/doctors-in-congress/. Accessed 7 June 2012.
9. Suran M. The doctors in the house – but not all are on duty when it comes to reform. Washington: Medill Reports; 2009 July 23. http://news.medill.northwestern.edu/washington/news.aspx?id=136307. Accessed 19 May 2012.
10. Welcome message from Co Chairs. GOP doctors Caucus. http://doctorscaucus.gingrey.house.gov/WhoWeAre/WelcomeMessage.htm. Accessed 19 May 2012.
11. Repeal of insolvent, disastrous CLASS act vital first step. GOP doctors Caucus. http://doctorscaucus.gingrey.house.gov/News/DocumentSingle.aspx?DocumentID=277784. Accessed 19 May 2012.
12. House GOP doctors Caucus criticize IPAB in letter to President. American Society of clinical oncology in action. http://ascoaction.asco.org/Home/tabid/41/articleType/ArticleView/articleId/17/House-GOP-Doctors-Caucus-Criticize-IPAB-in-Letter-to-President.aspx. Accessed 19 May 2011.
13. Abraham J. House votes to repeal CLASS act, part of 2010 Obama health care law. HuffPost politics. 2012 Feb 1. http://www.huffingtonpost.com/2012/02/01/class-act-repeal_n_1248430.html. Accessed 18 May 2012.
14. Alonso-Zaldivar R. IPAB repeal: house votes to eliminate medicare cost-control board. HuffPost politics. 2012 Mar 22. http://www.huffingtonpost.com/2012/03/22/ipab-repeal-house-vote_n_1372879.html. Accessed 20 May 2012.
15. U.S. debt clock.org. http://www.usdebtclock.org/. Accessed 19 May 2012.
16. Centers for Medicare and Medicaid Services. National health expenditure projections 2010–2020. http://www.cms.gov/Research-Statistics-Data-and-Systems/Statistics-Trends-and-Reports/NationalHealthExpendData/Downloads/proj2010.pdf. Accessed 19 May 2012.
17. Saad L. On healthcare, Americans trust physicians over politicians. Gallup politics. 2009 June 17. http://www.gallup.com/poll/120890/healthcare-americans-trust-physicians-politicians.aspx. Accessed 13 June 2012.
18. Get involved. American Medical Association. http://www.ama-assn.org/ama/pub/advocacy/get-involved.page. Accessed 19 May 2012.
19. Current actions. American Medical Student Association. http://action.amsa.org/o/2083/p/dia/action/public/. Accessed 19 May 2012.
20. Congressional Management Foundation. Communicating with Congress: perceptions of citizen advocacy on Capitol hill. 2011. Accessed 17 Aug 2012.
21. Landers SH, Sehgal AR. How do physicians lobby their members of Congress? Arch Intern Med. 2000;160:3248–51.
22. Congressional Management Foundation. #Social Congress: perceptions and use of social media on Capitol hill. 2011. Accessed 17 Aug 2011.
23. Sabato LJ. The growth of political action committee. PAC POWER: inside the world of political action committees. New York: W.W. Norton & Co; 1994.

24. What is a PAC? Opensecrets.org. http://www.opensecrets.org/pacs/pacfaq.php. Accessed 4 May 2012.
25. Health: PAC contributions to federal candidates. Opensecrets.org. http://www.opensecrets.org/pacs/sector.php?cycle=2010&txt=H01. Accessed 4 May 2012.
26. SCOTUS for law students: a campaign finance face-off. SCOTUS Blog. http://www.scotusblog.com/?p=144987. Accessed 20 Aug 2012.
27. Super PACs. Opensecrets.org. http://www.opensecrets.org/pacs/superpacs.php?cycle=2012. Accessed 5 May 2012.

Government and State Agencies: Who Administrates Healthcare on Federal and State Levels?

17

Rishin J. Kadakia and Hassan R. Mir

Learning Objectives

After completing this chapter, the reader should be able to answer the following questions:

- Who administrates healthcare on the federal level?
- Who administrates healthcare on the state level?
- How do federal and state governments interact in Medicaid Administration?
- How do federal and state governments regulate the private health insurance sector?
- How are physicians and hospitals regulated by the federal and state governments?

Introduction

The "American healthcare system" is an amalgamation of many unique agencies that offer services to varying subpopulations of the American people. The specific regulations and policies of programs such as the federally regulated Medicare program or the state-based Medicaid programs

R.J. Kadakia, BS
Vanderbilt University School of Medicine,
Vanderbilt University Medical Center, Nashville,
TN 37232, USA
e-mail: rishin.j.kadakia@vanderbilt.edu

H.R. Mir, M.D. (✉)
Department of Orthopedic Surgery,
Vanderbilt University Medical Center, Nashville,
TN 37232, USA
e-mail: hassan.mir@vanderbilt.edu

have been described in great detail in previous chapters (see Chap. 2 and Chap. 3). This chapter delves into the various federal and state government agencies that regulate healthcare. How are these agencies organized into their respective government systems, and what are their responsibilities? The Medicaid program is unique in that it is regulated by both federal and state governments. How do federal and state agencies interact during the administration of Medicaid? The majority of American citizens receive healthcare through private health insurance plans. Although these private insurance programs may not be administered by a government agency, there are a multitude of federal and state guidelines that regulate the private health insurance sector that will also be touched upon in this chapter. Finally, this chapter will discuss how hospitals and physicians are regulated by state and federal governments.

M.K. Sethi and W.H. Frist (eds.), *An Introduction to Health Policy: A Primer for Physicians and Medical Students*,
DOI 10.1007/978-1-4614-7735-8_17, © Springer Science+Business Media New York 2013

Fig. 17.1 Organizational chart highlighting the various operating divisions and staff divisions with the Department of Health and Human Services (Reproduced from [2])

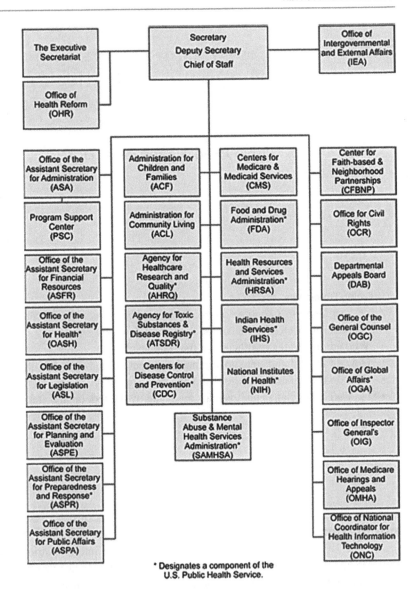

* Designates a component of the U.S. Public Health Service.

Healthcare Administration at the Federal Level

Department of Health and Human Services (HHS)

The Department of HHS is a cabinet-level member of the executive branch of the United States government that was established in 1980 via the Department of Education Organization Act, which split the Department of Health, Education, and Welfare (HEW) into the Department of Education and the Department of HHS [1]. This government department oversees an assortment of operating divisions that offer specific medical services and staff divisions, which help coordinate department functioning and provide leadership. See Fig. 17.1 and Table 17.1 for an organizational chart and table highlighting the various agencies under the Department of HHS and their respective functions.

In addition to providing healthcare for the American people, the Department of HHS also

Table 17.1 Mission statements and purpose of the primary agencies within the United States Department of Health and Human Services

United States Department of Health and Human Services	
Office of the Secretary	*Official Mission Statement*
Executive Secretariat	To serve as the primary consultant to the Secretary and Deputy Secretary
Office of Health Reform (OHR)	To provide leadership in establishing policies, priorities, and objectives for the Federal Government's comprehensive effort to improve access to health care, the quality of such care, and the sustainability of the healthcare system
Office of the Deputy Secretary	*Official Mission Statement*
Office of Intergovernmental and External Affairs (IEA)	To facilitate communication regarding HHS initiatives as they relate to State, local, tribal, and U.S. territorial governments
Operating Division	*Official Mission Statement*
Administration for Children and Families (ACF)	To promote the economic and social well-being of families, children, individuals, and communities
Agency for Healthcare Research and Quality (AHRQ)	To support, conduct, and disseminate research that improves access to care and the outcomes, quality, cost, and utilization of healthcare services
Administration for Community Living (ACL)	To promote the dignity and independence of people with disabilities and older adults and to help them to live at home with the supports they need while participating in communities that value their contributions
Agency for Toxic Substances and Disease Registry (ATSDR)	To serve the public by using the best science, taking responsive public health actions, and providing trusted health information to prevent harmful exposures and disease-related exposures to toxic substances
Centers for Disease Control and Prevention (CDC)	To promote health and quality of life by preventing and controlling disease, injury, and disability
Centers for Medicare & Medicaid Services (CMS)	To ensure effective, up-to-date healthcare coverage and to promote quality care for beneficiaries
Food and Drug Administration (FDA)	To rigorously assure the safety, efficacy, and security of human and veterinary drugs, biological products, and medical devices, and the safety and security of our Nation's food supply, cosmetics, and products that emit radiation
Health Resources and Services Administration (HRSA)	To improve health and achieve health equity through access to quality services, a skilled health workforce, and innovative programs
Indian Health Service (IHS)	To raise the physical, mental, social, and spiritual health of American Indians and Alaska Natives (AI/ANs) to the highest level
National Institutes of Health (NIH)	To employ science in pursuit of fundamental knowledge about the nature and behavior of living systems and the application of that knowledge to extend healthy life and reduce the burdens of illness and disability
Substance Abuse/ Mental Health Services Administration (SAMHSA)	To reduce the impact of substance abuse and mental illness on America's communities
Staff Division	*Official Mission Statement*
Assistant Secretary for Administration (ASA)	To help bring about improvements and effectiveness that can be achieved by structuring HHS as a united department, in support of the Secretary's goals
Program Support Center (PSC) – branch of ASA	To provide a full range of support services to HHS and other Federal agencies, allowing them to focus on their core mission
Assistant Secretary for Financial Resources (ASFR)	To provide advice and guidance to the Secretary on budget and financial management, and to provide for the direction and coordination of these activities throughout the Department

(continued)

Table 17.1 (continued)

United States Department of Health and Human Services	
Assistant Secretary for Health (ASH)	To provide senior professional leadership across HHS on cross-cutting public health and science initiatives and on population-based public health and clinical preventive services
Assistant Secretary for Legislation (ASL)	To advise the Secretary and the Department on congressional legislation and to facilitate communication between the Department and the Congress
Assistant Secretary for Planning and Evaluation (ASPE)	To provide advice and support to the Secretary on the development and analysis of cross-cutting, population-based health and human services policies
Assistant Secretary for Public Affairs (ASPA)	To serve as the Secretary's principal counsel on public affairs matters and to provide centralized leadership and guidance for public affairs activities within HHS
Assistant Secretary for Preparedness and Response (ASPR)	To serve as the Secretary's principal advisory staff on matters related to bioterrorism and other public health emergencies
Center for Faith-based and Neighborhood Partnerships (CFBNP)	To create an environment within HHS that welcomes the participation of faith-based and community-based organizations as valued, essential partners assisting Americans in need
Departmental Appeals Board (DAB)	To provide the best possible dispute resolution services for the people who appear before the board, those who rely on the decisions, and the public
Office for Civil Rights (OCR)	To ensure that all Americans have equal access to, and opportunity to participate in and receive services from, all HHS programs without facing unlawful discrimination, and that the privacy of their health information is protected while ensuring access to care
Office of the General Counsel (OGC)	To advance the Department's goal of protecting the health of all Americans and of providing essential human services, especially for those who are least able to help themselves
Office of Global Health Affairs (OGHA)	To promote the health of the world's population by advancing HHS global strategies and partnerships, thus serving the health of the people of the United States
Office of Inspector General (OIG)	To protect the integrity of HHS programs as well as the health and welfare of the beneficiaries of those programs
Office of Medicare Hearings and Appeals (OMHA)	To administer the nationwide hearings and appeals for the Medicare program, and to ensure that the American people have equal access and opportunity to appeal and can exercise their rights for healthcare quality and access
Office of the National Coordinator for Health Information Technology (ONC)	To provide leadership for the development and nationwide implementation of an interoperable health information technology infrastructure

Source: Data from [2]

governs other healthcare-related agencies such as the Food and Drug Administration (FDA), Centers for Disease Control (CDC), and the National Institutes of Health (NIH). As depicted by Fig. 17.1, the leadership of this department falls under the responsibility of the Secretary of the Department of HHS and the Deputy Secretary. The Secretary, appointed by the President of the United States, serves as the primary leader of the department and works closely with the White House, while the Deputy Secretary's primary function is to direct all department operations [2].

Center for Medicaid and Medicare Services (CMS)

CMS is an integral operating division within the Department of HHS. Established in 1977 and originally termed the Health Care Financing Administration, CMS administers the Medicare program and works with individual state governments to administer the Medicaid program and the State Children's Health Insurance Program (SCHIP) [3]. CMS is further subdivided into various administrative offices and subcenters, each

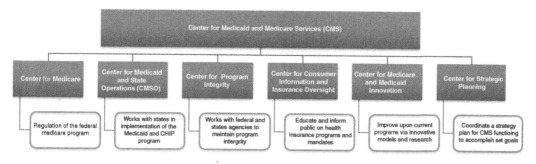

Fig. 17.2 Chart depicts the six centers within the Center for Medicaid and Medicare Services and a brief description of their functions

with unique functions. Figure 17.2 highlights the six subcenters within CMS and their respective functions. Center for Medicaid and State Operations (CMSO) is an integral part of CMS responsible for the administration of the Medicaid program at the federal level. A more thorough list of CMSO's responsibilities can be found in Table 17.3.

Indian Health Services (IHS)

Like CMS discussed earlier, the IHS is an operating division within the Department of HHS. The administration of healthcare for Native Americans was originally a responsibility of the Bureau of Indian Affairs (BIA); however, in 1955, this responsibility was transferred to the Department of HHS, specifically the IHS operating division [4]. IHS is responsible for the administration of healthcare to 562 federally recognized tribes, over 1.9 million Native Americans on or near reservations, and over 600,000 Native Americans in urban settings [5]. These individuals receive healthcare services through IHS clinics and healthcare centers, operated by their tribe, that receive IHS funding and support [5].

Veteran's Health Administration (VHA)

An important aspect of federal-based healthcare involves the services offered to American military veterans. Unlike the Medicare/Medicaid

programs, the healthcare programs offered to veterans are not administered by the Department of HHS. These alternative programs are provided by the Department of Veteran Affairs (VA), which is also a cabinet-level member of the executive branch of the government. The VHA, one of the three major administrations within the Department of VA, provides healthcare services to veterans. Although the practice of providing benefits and services for military veterans has existed since the early colonial era, the Department of VA and its tertiary organization were not officially established until 1988 [6]. The VHA administers healthcare to veterans via 152 hospitals, 1,400 outpatient clinics, and other medical facilities such as skilled nursing homes [7]. The Under Secretary for Health is the highest leadership position within the VHA and is responsible for overseeing all administrative functions [7].

Military Health System (MHS) and TRICARE

The MHS consists of a group of agencies that administer healthcare to individuals in active duty, veterans, and, in many cases, their dependents. The MHS is a member of the Department of Defense, another cabinet-level member of the executive branch of the government. Although MHS originally covered only active duty personal, Congress passed legislation in 1966 that created a healthcare plan offering coverage for active duty dependents and veterans and their dependents: the Civilian Health and Medical

Program of the Uniformed Services (currently called TRICARE) [8]. Other agencies within MHS include the Army, Navy, and Air Force Medicine Departments and specialized components such as the Hearing Center and Vision Center of Excellence.

Healthcare Administration at the State Level

State Health Departments

Much like the Department of HHS and its responsibilities with regard to healthcare for the entire nation, each state government contains a state health agency that is responsible for regulating and monitoring the public health within that respective state. The federal government has a limited role in the development and management of these state health departments. Therefore, the responsibilities and infrastructure of these state-based health agencies vary significantly. In the majority of states, the state health department is an independent government agency, while in

other states it is a component of a larger agency with broader roles [9]. In addition, some public health-related functions, such as medical facility inspections, can often be administered by state agencies outside of the state health department. Another level of complexity in state-based healthcare administration involves the regulation of local health departments that are often county or city based. The interaction between state and local health departments also varies by state: some states have local health departments that are run by the state health department, while some states have independently functioning local health departments [9]. Although there is immense interstate variability in the responsibilities of the state and local health departments, there are some general functions that are consistent for most departments, which have been summarized in Table 17.2. Finally, the majority of state health departments in the USA are run by the State Health Official (SHO). In most states, this is an appointed position by the state governor, and some responsibilities of the SHO include overseeing the daily functions of the department, setting policy, and maintaining standards of performance [10].

Table 17.2 State and local health department responsibilities

State and Local Health Departments Responsibilities	
Function	Description
Data collection for epidemiology study and surveillance	Collect information regarding incidence of infectious diseases, chronic conditions, and even cancers. Often report information back to CDC which compiles information across states. Also collects other health-related information such as immunization, birth, and death records
Laboratory testing	State labs perform much of the testing with regards to public health such as newborn screening, testing food products for infectious contaminants, and influenza virus typing
Responding to public health emergencies	Extremely vital in creating a strategy for handling any local health crisis. State agencies work with both local health departments and the CDC to ensure proper plans exist and can be implemented if the situation arises
Promoting good health and disease prevention/ control	Both state and local health departments create marketing campaigns and programs aimed at preventing disease and educating the public on specific health topics such as HIV/ AIDs, smoking risks, and other chronic conditions. Local health departments also contribute to disease prevention and control by offering immunization and screening services for infections and chronic medical conditions
Provide healthcare	In most cases, the state health department does not directly offer healthcare services to individuals. It is usually the local health departments that provide healthcare services such as immunizations, nutrition counseling services, and screenings for sexually transmitted diseases and other infections
Regulatory functions	In some states, the state health agency conducts inspections of health facilities and is responsible for licensing healthcare providers

Source: Data from [9]

Table 17.3 Responsibilities of the state and federal governments in the administration of the Medicaid program

Medicaid Administrational Responsibilities	
Federal Government (CMSO)	State Governments
Administer matching funds to states for appropriate expenses	Educate public regarding eligibility and assist with enrollment
Approving state Medicaid plans and amendments to existing plans	Determine which services will be covered and the reimbursement rates for these services
Provide explanations of federal requirements to state agencies and providers	Receive and process claims for services rendered to program participants
Ensuring states follow all federal guidelines for the Medicaid program	Prevent improper or fraudulent use of federal and state Medicaid funds
Enforce proper program administration in order to optimize efficiency	Employ programs to monitor quality of healthcare services provided to participants
Reduce improper expenditures and monitor for fraud	Collect relevant data regarding program functioning in order to increase effectiveness
Collecting data regarding expenditures and enforcing information collection from states	Settle arguments that may arise during administration between any parties involved in the program

Source: Data from [11]

In addition to the responsibilities summarized in Table 17.2, it is important to note that some state health agencies are also responsible for the administration of the state-based Medicaid program, while other states have independent Medicaid agencies [10]. The Medicaid program is an eligibility-based healthcare insurance program that offers coverage to the American people. Unlike Medicare, which is administered and funded solely by the federal government, the Medicaid program is regulated by both federal and state governments. Table 17.3 compares some of the major federal and state responsibilities with regard to the administration of the Medicaid program. While states are given flexibility regarding their unique Medicaid programs, CMSO provides basic framework and guidelines within which each state must operate their respective program.

The Interplay Between Federal and State Governments in the Administration of the Medicaid Program

The Role of CMSO in the Administration of Medicaid

A vital function of CMSO is providing matching federal funds to states for Medicaid-related expenses. States provide quarterly reports to CMSO regarding expenditures and receive quarterly reimbursements for approved expenditures. There is a possibility that CMSO and state Medicaid agency may disagree on whether a certain service is acceptable, and these disputes are handled by the Departmental Appeals Board, a staff division within the Department of HHS (Fig. 17.1) [11].

Although CMSO sets certain criteria for all Medicaid plans, states are given the option to alter their plan within the set guidelines via State Plan Amendments (discussed in the next section). CMSO is responsible for reviewing all plan amendments and determining if the change is acceptable. These decisions can have a significant financial impact, and in most cases, the Office of Management and Budget – a cabinet-level office within the executive branch of the federal government – is also involved in this decision-making process [11].

The federal government must also make certain that state agencies understand the federal Medicaid guidelines and must educate them on any new mandates; this process ensures that state-based programs are run correctly without any violations. The federal government retains the authority to punish states that do not comply with the federally set criteria for Medicaid, and this punishment often involves withholding payments to states until the noncompliance is resolved [11].

CMSO has a variety of roles in the administration of Medicaid that help prevent unnecessary expenditures. Medicaid is an extremely complex insurance program with multiple levels of administration, and CMSO enforces efficient administration at both the state and federal levels with the goal of reducing the administrative budget. The prevention of improper and fraudulent expenditures is primarily regulated by the Office of Inspector General (OIG), a staff division with the Department of HHS (Fig. 17.1). The OIG monitors all states and Medicaid providers for fraudulent activity, which can be punished by monetary penalties and sometimes expulsion from the program [11]. Individual states also have an OIG-like agency, the Medicaid Fraud Control Unit (MFCU), which will be discussed later. The OIG is responsible for the certification of each state's MFCU and ensures that each agency meets federal guidelines [11].

CMSO is also responsible for presenting expenditure and programming reports to Congress, and it must gather all the necessary information from state agencies and providers. In order to ensure that information is collected and reported in an efficient manner, the federal government has set guidelines to regulate data collection regarding the Medicaid program that must be followed by each state, including the implementation of a Medicaid Management Information System (MMIS) [11].

The Role of State Governments in Medicaid Administration

In order to receive federal funding for Medicaid, states must create a Medicaid program that meets the criteria set by CMSO, administer their program according to federal administrative guidelines, and create a single state agency that administers their Medicaid program. However, in practice, this last requirement is not always followed, as many state Medicaid offices work with other state and private agencies in the administration of their respective Medicaid program [11].

States are required to provide the opportunity for eligible individuals to enroll in their Medicaid program, and they must assist individuals during the application process. The process of determining eligibility must be unbiased and fair. After receiving an application for Medicaid, states must reach a decision and respond in a timely manner; federal guidelines generally require a response between 45 and 90 days after an application is received [11]. In order to ensure that funding is utilized in an appropriate manner, states must be very careful and thorough during their review of an application in order to ensure that only eligible individuals are accepted. The federal government can penalize states whose expenditures for ineligible individuals are greater than 3 % of their Medicaid benefit expenses [11]. While states must follow guidelines discussed herewith in regard to the enrollment/eligibility process, there is some flexibility for the enrollment process and marketing of programs to eligible candidates. For example, some states choose to market their Medicaid program together with SCHIP, while others choose to market them as separate entities [11].

CMSO sets minimal requirements with regard to the types of benefits that each state Medicaid program must cover, but states are given the option to expand upon these guidelines and given flexibility with regard to the extent of these benefits (e.g., setting a maximum length of hospital stay that will be covered by Medicaid [11]). Any modification to the state's program must be outlined in a State Plan Amendment (SPA) that is submitted to CMSO for review and approval.

It is important to note that any service rendered must be considered medically pertinent to the health of the recipient in order to be funded; eligibility of the recipient and coverage of the benefit do not matter if the service is deemed medically unnecessary. In most scenarios, states are given significant leeway in the process of determining which services are medically necessary. Sample exceptions to this policy include the administration of prescription drugs and the placement of individuals with mental illnesses into nursing homes. Most states are required to create "Drug Use Review" programs that will conduct reviews and set forth guidelines regarding the medical necessity and effectiveness of certain drug therapies [11]. The Preadmission Screening and Resident Review (PASRR) requires states to implement screening programs in order to ensure that individuals with mental illnesses are placed in nursing homes only if it is absolutely necessary [11].

States have some authority in determining reimbursement rates for services, but their policy must be thoroughly outlined in their state Medicaid plan. However, there are some federal restrictions with regard to reimbursements. For example, CMSO imposes an Upper Payment Limit on reimbursements for aggregate services in certain services [11]. States are also required to make the process by which they determine reimbursement rates for hospitals and nursing facilities completely open to the public [11]. While there are federal guidelines for certain services such as nursing homes, determining if a provider is qualified to participate in the Medicaid program is also a responsibility of the state.

In addition to regulating reimbursement rates, states are responsible for making payments to providers for approved services, and there are federal guidelines for this process. States are further required to have a formal claims review process before and after a payment has been made, and these payments must be made in a timely manner to ensure efficiency. There must also be a consideration of other sources of health insurance that may be applicable, such as Medicare or private health insurance [11]. These options must be exhausted before turning to the Medicaid program.

States have some authority in how they monitor the services offered to Medicaid recipients, but a monitoring plan must be approved by CMSO. The two exceptions in this case involve the monitoring of nursing facilities and clinical laboratories. States are required to conduct thorough reviews and inspections of nursing homes using federally set guidelines, and only laboratories that meet guidelines set by CMSO are eligible for participation in the Medicaid program [11].

All states are required to have a Medicaid Fraud and Abuse Control Unit (MFCU), which functions to monitor the Medicaid program for any fraudulent activity. This unit is considered a separate entity from the agency that administers Medicaid and is often run from the State Attorney General's office [11].

States are given less flexibility with regard to the management and collection of data pertaining to Medicaid, and there are multiple federal regulations that guide this important state responsibility. States are required to implement a Medical Management and Information System (MMIS), which must meet federally set requirements [11]. The federal regulation of MMIS ensures that all state-based programs have information systems that are nationally consistent and can be shared between states. In addition, states must make reports to the Secretary of HHS regarding the functioning of their Medicaid program; timely expenditure reports, projected expenditures, and annual enrollment information are just a few examples.

The Regulation of Private Health Insurance Plans

According to a report published by the United States Census Bureau on American healthcare from 2010, approximately 195.9 million Americans – 64.0 % of the population – are covered by private health insurance plans. Although this number has been decreasing annually since 2001, the private health insurance sector still provides insurance for the majority of the United States [12]. While these private health insurance companies have significant administrative freedoms, there are many federal and state regulations in place to ensure fair business practices among the insurers and protection for the consumers.

Regulation at the Federal Level

While private health insurance programs are significantly state-regulated, there are many federally implemented regulations as well. The Employee Retirement Income Security Act (ERISA) of 1974 marked one of the first major initiatives by the federal government to regulate private health insurance [13]. One of ERISA's provisions stipulated that self-insured employers who provided healthcare to their employees were free from most state regulations. A little over a decade later, the Consolidated Omnibus Budget Reconciliation Act (COBRA) of 1985 enhanced the benefits for employer-based health insurance by requiring certain employers to provide extended coverage – anywhere from 18 to 36 months – for employees who lose their employment for qualified reasons [13]. The Health Insurance Portability and Accountability Act (HIPAA) of 1996 is a relatively recent federal initiative that also regulates the private health insurance sector. One of the primary goals of HIPAA is to protect the consumer from discrimination based on preexisting medical conditions and health status. For example, the act redefined the term "preexisting condition" to guarantee that employment-based insurance plans were not unfairly labeling individuals and denying them coverage [13]. In addition, HIPAA also required private health insurance companies to guarantee a renewal of coverage for individuals in nearly all circumstances. These federal regulations apply to nearly all types of private insurance including employer- and individual-based plans. Many other federal regulations are in place for private insurance companies with regard to specific services that must be provided. For example, the Newborns' and Mothers' Health Protection Act of 1996 required all plans to cover hospital stays of 48h following delivery and 96h following Caesarean section [13].

Regulation at the State Level

The regulation of private insurance at the state level is predominantly a responsibility of the state insurance department and the state health insurance commissioner. Similar to the administration of Medicaid, there is great variability between individual states with regard to the regulation of private health insurance. However, the National Association of Insurance Commissioners (NAIC) which was originally formed in 1871 serves to unite state regulatory efforts. The NAIC consists of the insurance commissioners from each state and functions to conduct research, discuss policy and standards, and provide a unified national model for private insurance regulation that indi-

vidual states can base their policy upon [13]. Despite these efforts, significant differences still exist in private health insurance regulation between individual states.

Like federal regulation, states look to ensure that consumers of private insurance are protected from unfair practices. States often hire private firms to perform external reviews of private health insurance companies and have requirements for internal reviews of company functioning [13]. Private health insurance companies must be financially capable to cover all of the individuals they insure and conduct their business in a proper manner. For example, states require companies to be timely with their responses to insurance claims, and they must make all rates and policies open to the public for review.

States also impose a variety of coverage mandates with regard to the specific health services that must be included in most private health insurance plans and which individuals must be covered by these plans. There is certainly variability with regard to coverage between states, but nearly all states have multiple coverage mandates. In fact, only 2 states have less than 20 coverage mandates for private health insurance companies [13]. Since these mandates can have a significant economic impact for private companies, states have policies to ensure that only mandates deemed necessary and beneficial are implemented. States perform analyses on the economic benefits of certain mandates and also conduct retrospective studies. In terms of private health insurance and individual-based insurance plans, states also function to protect the consumer by preventing discrimination based on health insurance, limiting rate variation within communities, discouraging significant rises in premiums by companies, and, in most cases, requiring companies to provide insurance renewal [13].

The Regulation of Health Institutions and Providers

In addition to the regulation of health insurance, federal and state governments also influence American healthcare via regulation of institutions and providers. Although different agencies and processes regulate hospitals and physicians, the general concepts are similar for both: they must satisfy certain standards and be licensed in order to provide healthcare services. While the federal government sets certain guidelines and mandates for practicing medicine, the regulation of providers and institutions is primarily a state responsibility.

Regulation of Healthcare Institutions

States typically set certain guidelines that must be met in order for the healthcare facility to be licensed for practice in that state. There are a multitude of private organizations that inspect and offer accreditation to healthcare facilities, and most states adapt the guidelines set by an accrediting organization for their own licensing process. The Joint Commission (JTC) is the most well-known accreditation organization in the United States. Created in 1951, the JTC consists of representatives from a variety of healthcare associations such as the American College of Physicians and the American Hospital Association [14]. On a federal level, institutions must meet the Conditions for Coverage (CfCs) and Conditions of Participations (CoPs) set forth by CMS in order to participate in the Medicare and Medicaid program [15].

Regulation of Healthcare Professionals

The licensing of healthcare professionals is a responsibility of individual states. Each State Medical Board is comprised of healthcare professionals and is responsible for licensing providers within that state. The Federation of State Medical Boards (FSMB) is an organization consisting of all of the state medical boards that functions to unify all of the states. It conducts research on possible policy improvements and works to maintain consistency across state lines with regard to provider regulation [16]. Despite this attempt to maintain national consistency, there are still problems that can arise due to the

immense variability in regulation between individual states. For example, a provider who loses his or her license for improper conduct in one state may be able to receive a license in another state if there is no communication between state medical boards. For this reason, the federal government created the National Practitioner Data Bank (NPDB) in 1986 [17]. Individual states report conduct issues to this data bank, and the information is easily accessible to all states. This tool allows states to communicate with each other regarding regulation of healthcare providers.

Conclusion

The American healthcare system is comprised of many different private and public insurance programs. The multitude of available options greatly complicates the regulation of healthcare at both the federal and state levels. There are programs such as Medicare that are regulated solely by the federal government, while Medicaid is administered jointly by the federal and state governments. In addition, there are state-based healthcare services such as state health departments that are mostly run by the local state governments. Thus, the administration of healthcare in America is a complex process with responsibilities at both the state and federal governments, and it often includes varying magnitudes of responsibility at each level depending upon the specific program. It is important to note that many changes to healthcare in the United States will take place over the upcoming years. The Patient Protection and Affordable Care Act (PPACA) will drastically impact nearly every aspect of the American healthcare system, including the administration of healthcare [18, 19]. The PPACA and its implications will be discussed in Chap. 19.

References

1. U.S. Department of Health and Human Services. Historical highlights [Internet]. Washington, DC: Department of Health and Human Services (US); [cited 2012 Aug 21]. http://www.hhs.gov/about/hhsh-ist.html

2. U.S. Department of Health and Human Services. Strategic plan 2010–2015 appendix A: organizational chart for U.S. Department of Health and Human Services Operating and Staff Divisions [Internet]. Washington, DC: Department of Health and Human Services (US); [cited 2012 Aug 21]. http://www.hhs.gov/secretary/about/appendixa.html

3. Centers for Medicare and Medicaid services: history [Internet]. Baltimore, MD: Center for Medicare and Medicaid Services. Key milestones in CMS programs; [Updated 2012 Mar 27; cited 2012 Aug 21]; [PDF document on site]. http://www.cms.gov/About-CMS/Agency-Information/History/

4. Indian Health Service: contract health services [Internet]. Rockville, MD: Indian Health Service. [cited 2013 May 30]. http://www.ihs.gov/chs/index.cfm?module=chs_history

5. Indian Health service: the federal health program for American Indians and Alaska Natives [Internet]. Rockville, MD: Indian Health Service. IHS fact sheets: year 2008 profile; [updated 2008 Jan; cited 2012 Aug 21: [1 page]. http://www.ihs.gov/PublicAffairs/IHSBrochure/Profile08.asp

6. United States Department of Veteran Affairs [Internet]. Washington, DC: Department of Veteran Affairs (US). Publications: Books: VA history in brief; [updated 2012 May 15, cited 2012 Aug 21]: [PDF document on site – 36 pages]. http://www.va.gov/opa/publications/archives/docs/history_in_brief.pdf

7. United States Department of Veteran Affairs [Internet]. Washington, DC: Department of Veteran Affairs (US). About VHA; [updated 2011 Oct 5, cited 2012 Aug 21]: [2 pages]. http://www.va.gov/health/aboutVHA.asp#datasource

8. Best RA Jr. Military Medical Care Services: questions and answers. Foreign Affairs and National Defense Division, Congressional Research Service. Library of Congress. Washington, DC. Updated 2005 May 5.

9. Salinsky E. Governmental Public Health: an overview of state and local public health agencies. National Health Policy Forum [internet]. 2010 Aug 18 [cited 2012 Aug 21];77:5–15. http://www.nhpf.org/library/background-papers/BP77_GovPublicHealth_08-18-2010.pdf

10. Beitsch LM, Brooks RG, Grigg M, Menachemi N. Structure and functions of state public health agencies. Am J Public Health. 2006;96(1):167–72.

11. Schneider A et al. The Medicaid resource book [Internet]. Washington, DC: The Kaiser Commission on Medicaid and the Uninsured; c July 2002. Chapter 4: Medicaid Administration; [cited 2012 Aug 21]; pp. 129–164. http://www.kff.org/medicaid/loader.cfm?url=/commonspot/security/getfile.cfm&PageID=14262

12. DeNavas-Walt C, Proctor BD, Smith JC. U.S. Census Bureau Current population reports: income, poverty, and health insurance coverage in the United States: 2010. Washington, DC: U.S. Government Printing Office; 2011. pp. 60–239.

13. Jost TS. The regulation of private health insurance. National Academy of Social Insurance: Washington, DC, National Academy of Public Administration: Princeton: Robert Wood Johnson Foundation [Internet]. 2009 Jan [cited 2012 Aug 21]. http://www.rwjf.org/files/research/jost.pdf

14. The Joint Commission [Internet]. Oakbrook Terrace, IL: The Joint Commission; c2012. History of The Joint Commission [cited 2012 Aug 21]. http://www.jointcommission.org/about_us/history.aspx

15. Centers for Medicare and Medicaid Services [Internet]. Baltimore, MD: Center for Medicare and Medicaid Services. Conditions for Coverage (CfCs) & Conditions of Participations (CoPs); [Updated 2012 May 11; cited 2012 Aug 21]. http://www.cms.gov/Regulations-and-Guidance/Legislation/CFCsAndCoPs/index.html

16. Federation of State Medical Boards [Internet]. Euless, TX: Federation of State Medical Boards; c2010. FSMB Mission & Goals; [cited 2012 Aug 21]. http://www.fsmb.org/mission.html

17. The Data Bank: National practitioner, healthcare integrity & protection. Chantilly: The Data Bank. About us: NPDB; [cited 2012 Aug 21]. http://www.npdb-hipdb.hrsa.gov/topNavigation/aboutUs.jsp

18. Healthcare.gov: the health care law & you [Internet]. Washington, DC: United States Department of Health and Human Services. Initial guidance to states on exchanges; [cited 2012 Sept 9]. http://www.healthcare.gov/law/resources/regulations/guidance-to-states-on-exchanges.html

19. The Henry J. Kaiser Family Foundation [Internet]. Menlo Park, CA: The Henry J. Kaiser Family Foundation; c2012. Summary of new health reform law; 2011 Apr 19 [cited 2012Sept 9]; [summary.pdf]. http://www.kff.org/healthreform/8061.cfm

The 2006 Massachusetts Health Care Reform

Vasanth Sathiyakumar, Jordan C. Apfeld, Cesar S. Molina, Daniel J. Stinner, Andrew Han, and Manish K. Sethi

Learning Objectives

After completing this chapter, the reader should be able to answer the following questions:

- What are the origins of the 2006 Massachusetts Health Care Reform?
- What were the main changes made by the Massachusetts Health Care Reform?
- How has health-care reform progressed since the first set of reforms in 2006?
- What were the projections and what have been the effects of the health-care reform on health insurance coverage and costs?
- What are the prospects and major challenges going forward for health-care reform in Massachusetts?
- How did the 2006 Massachusetts Health Care Reform set the stage for the 2010 Federal Patient Protection and Affordable Care Act (PPACA)?

V. Sathiyakumar, B.A. • C.S. Molina, M.D. • A. Han
Department of Orthopedic Trauma, Vanderbilt University Medical Center, Nashville, TN 37232, USA
e-mail: vasanth.sathiyakumar@vanderbilt.edu;
cesar.molina@vanderbilt.edu;
andrew.m.han@vanderbilt.edu

J.C. Apfeld, B.A.
Vanderbilt Orthopedic Institute, Vanderbilt University Medical School, Nashville, TN 37232, USA
e-mail: jordan.c.apfeld@vanderbilt.edu

D.J. Stinner, M.D.
Vanderbilt Orthopedic Institute, Vanderbilt University Medical Center, Nashville, TN 37232, USA
e-mail: daniel.j.stinner@vanderbilt.edu

M.K. Sethi, M.D. (✉)
Director of the Vanderbilt Orthopaedic Institute Center for Health Policy, Assistant Professor of Orthopaedic Trauma Surgery, Department of Orthopaedic Surgery and Rehabilitation, Vanderbilt University School of Medicine, Nashville, TN 37232, USA
e-mail: manish.sethi@vanderbilt.edu

M.K. Sethi and W.H. Frist (eds.), *An Introduction to Health Policy: A Primer for Physicians and Medical Students*, DOI 10.1007/978-1-4614-7735-8_18, © Springer Science+Business Media New York 2013

Introduction

This chapter focuses on the pillars of the 2006 Massachusetts Health Care Reform. The factors and circumstances that made Massachusetts ripe for health-care policy change will first be addressed. Next, the specific aspects of reform will be discussed including the following: the individual mandate requiring health insurance coverage; the employer mandate requiring businesses to make a "fair contribution" towards health care for their employees; the creation of a health insurance exchange termed the "Health Connector" to facilitate the purchasing of insurance along with a new variety of health insurance programs known as "Commonwealth Choice" and "Commonwealth Care" programs; the expansion of public safety programs, particularly Massachusetts's Medicaid program termed "MassHealth"; the merging of the individual and small-group insurance markets; and the remodeling of the Uncompensated Care Pool into a new Health Safety Net Fund to finance medical treatment for uninsured residents. The chapter will conclude with an analysis of the development, reception, and amendments of the original reform over the past few years, as well as a glance towards the future of this law and the challenges that still need to be addressed.

Conditions for Reform

Many of the provisions included in the Massachusetts Health Care Reform – legally titled "Ch. 58 of the Acts of 2006" – were influenced by the political conditions of Massachusetts's policy scene. Prior to 2006, Massachusetts faced similar health-care problems compared to other states. One main issue included financial stresses resulting from treating uninsured patients [1]. After Congress passed the Emergency Medical Treatment and Active Labor Act (EMTALA) in 1986, hospitals were required to provide care to any person requiring emergency treatment. However, state governments were ultimately responsible for funding this

treatment [2]. Massachusetts already had a historically low rate of uninsured patients compared to other states [3]. However, then-Massachusetts Governor Mitt Romney, in collaboration with two former governors, initiated discussions to restructure health care and address coverage for uninsured citizens who were unable to pay for their treatment (termed "uncompensated care"). These discussions led to minor reforms and cost shifts that were designed to expand Massachusetts's contributions towards addressing uncompensated care [2–7]. These minor changes to some degree relieved the problems of uncompensated care for the state's budget. What is more important, however, is that Governor Romney and preceding governors established a culture of addressing health-care costs for the uninsured prior to sweeping reforms enacted in 2006 [2–8].

Furthermore, Massachusetts already had an expansive Medicaid program termed "MassHealth" under Section 1115 of the Social Security Act [8]. Using Section 1115 allows the Secretary of Health and Human Services to approve experimental programs in states wishing to implement programs with goals that coincide with those of Medicaid but do not fall within the strict regulations set forth by the federal government. In Massachusetts, the establishment of "MassHealth" under Section 1115 allowed for broader coverage and eligibility for low-income residents, while helping to shift costs in a more effective manner for the state to manage [8, 9]. The use of Section 1115 has allowed Massachusetts to easily switch financing between programs based on need, such as transferring funds from "MassHealth" to subsidizing new insurance coverage options for low-income residents established by the reform [8–10]. In addition to an established Medicaid program, Massachusetts had key insurance market reforms in place by 2006 that created an impressive network of health-care outreach programs and training missions for physicians and nurses that were funded by state- and insurance-sponsored grants [3–8]. Although the 2006 Reform in Massachusetts set the stage for the state to experience the most expensive health-care expenditures in the United States after 2006, focusing on a "coverage first" mentality had already been a manageable goal for the state.

These goals were manifested by a high rate of employer-sponsored coverage and Medicaid requirements with low restrictions [3–6]. By already enacting programs such as MassHealth that would reduce the burden of uninsured residents prior to reform, the state was prepared to absorb additional health-care reform costs as a result of the 2006 Reform.

The Individual Mandate

The individual mandate is a cornerstone of the Massachusetts Health Care Reform designed to increase health insurance coverage for state residents. Under this mandate, individuals over the age of 17 years who are considered "able to afford" health insurance were required to purchase a minimum coverage plan beginning on July 1, 2007 [9]. Individuals who are not covered face an annual tax penalty based on income level. At the time the reform was passed, the definition of "affordability" and specifics about penalties for noncompliance were determined by a new state-based health insurance exchange termed the Massachusetts "Health Connector" [7–9]. The Connector also set forth minimum coverage requirements for health insurance plans, such as emergency room and primary care services [5–9].

The institution of the individual mandate was the first of its kind in the United States, and the 2010 Federal Patient Protection and Affordable Care Act (PPACA) passed under President Obama has been the most notable law to follow with a similar provision [11]. Since implementation of the reform, the Health Connector specifically determined that the mandate applies to all residents over the age of 17 years whose annual income levels are 150 % above the Federal Poverty Line (FPL) [9, 10]. The Federal Poverty Line is a national threshold assessed by the Department of Health and Human Services every February specifying the annual costs that must be spent in order to meet food, clothing, shelter, and other basic needs. FPL is dependent on family size and is adjusted for inflation [12]. For example, in 2012 the FPL was $19,090 for a family of three [12]. Public programs such as Medicare or Medicaid often use the FPL to determine eligibility requirements. Using the 2012 FPL of $11,170 for an individual, all individuals whose annual incomes are at least $16,755 (150 % times the FPL) and are over the age of 17 years must have health insurance under the individual mandate in Massachusetts [9, 12].

Massachusetts's residents are required to demonstrate coverage of health insurance through annual income tax filings [4–10]. However, residents with incomes that are below 150 % of the Federal Poverty Line or residents who have religious obligations preventing the coverage of health insurance are not mandated to have insurance [4–10]. Nevertheless, these exempted residents still may be eligible for coverage under MassHealth, Massachusetts's Medicaid plan. Furthermore, if a citizen is able to demonstrate a lack of available "affordable" coverage, waivers may be obtained from the Health Connector that will help fully or partially cover the costs of premiums and facilitate the purchasing of insurance [13].

In order to help citizens purchase health insurance under the individual mandate, the state government reallocated funds that were used to reimburse hospitals for the treatment of uninsured patients [1, 3, 5]. These funds are now used to subsidize health insurance premiums based on income-sliding scales. In addition, certain individuals have access to the state's "Commonwealth Care Health Insurance Program," a series of privately subsidized health insurance options for low-income residents (discussed later in this chapter). Individuals who are eligible for Commonwealth Care must be over 19 years of age, not qualify for Medicaid, have employers who do not offer insurance, and have income levels less than 300 % of the Federal Poverty Line [9, 14].

Individual Mandate Penalties

In spring 2007, the Health Connector defined "affordability" as a certain maximum amount that individuals or families must pay for mandatory health insurance [15]. If insurance providers cannot offer insurance below this ceiling level, the individual mandate is waived for those who are

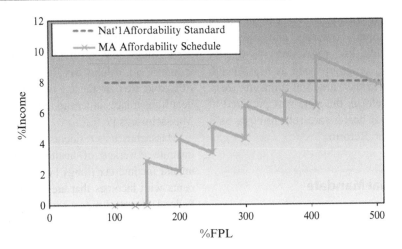

Fig. 18.1 National affordability standards vs. Massachusetts affordability standards. At about 500 % FPL, the Massachusetts Affordability Schedule defines coverage at affordable (Data from Ref. [11])

deemed incapable of affording health insurance. The Connector determined that the maximum individual contribution for residents who have income levels 150 % above the Federal Poverty Line (FPL) should be an "affordable" 2 % of individual income [6–9, 15]. In contrast, wealthier citizens with income levels that are 500 % above the FPL should contribute a maximum "affordable" amount equal to 9 % of individual income towards health insurance (Fig. 18.1). Other income contributory rates are tiered for individuals who have incomes between 150 % and 500 % over the FPL at 50 % increments of the FPL [10]. On the other side of the spectrum, individuals with annual incomes under 150 % of the FPL are not required to contribute any portion of income towards mandatory health insurance. The individual mandate is subsequently waived for these individuals. The Health Connector reexamines this affordability schedule annually to adjust levels of income contribution towards health insurance [10]. In order to determine whether a person can access "affordable" care, the Health Connector checks premium rates from Commonwealth Choice, an unsubsidized health insurance program available for uninsured citizens who are not eligible for MassHealth or Commonwealth Care (discussed later in this chapter), and compares the lowest premium rate option in these programs with affordability estimates [15].

Residents who do not prove health insurance coverage through tax filings originally lost personal tax exemptions worth $219 per individual annually. An additional cash penalty was included in a 2008 amendment, with maximum penalties at $76 per month ($912 per year) for those who are over 27 years old and have incomes that are 300 % over the Federal Poverty Level [9, 13].

Revenue from these penalties feeds into a newly created Commonwealth Care Trust Fund [16]. The Trust Fund is used to help fund Commonwealth Care – the Health Connector's lowest insurance options for uninsured adults who meet certain requirements – and a few other programs created under the 2006 Reform changes (discussed later in this chapter).

The Employer Mandate

Employer-provided health care covers more Massachusetts residents (65.1 % of residents in 2007–2008) than any other form of insurance [17]. This trend has persisted following passage of the health-care reform law, with nearly 76 % of residents covered through employer-sponsored plans in 2011 [18]. In addition to an individual mandate provision, the reform also contains an employer-mandated statute for providing health insurance options.

Under the reform, businesses with over 11 employees are mandated to either provide coverage for their employees or pay a penalty assessment that feeds into the newly established Health Safety Net Fund, a pool of revenue allocated by the state to pay for medically required services at community health centers and hospitals for uninsured and underinsured citizens in Massachusetts [6–9]. As long as an employee is sufficiently covered – by their own personal employer, their spouse's employer, or through a mixed contribution of the two – no such assessment will be charged to employers.

Employer Mandate Penalties

Employers are expected to provide "fair and reasonable contributions" to their employees' health insurance premiums [19]. In 2009, the Health Connector specifically set a "fair and reasonable contribution" benchmark with two main components. The first component is that if a business has over 50 full-time employees, then a quarter of that company's full-time workers must be enrolled in the company's health insurance plan [9]. The second component is that businesses with over 50 full-time employees must contribute 33 % of their employees' health insurance premium costs in order to pass "fair and reasonable" assessments [9, 19]. Only one of these two provisions needs to be met for companies that have between 11 and 50 full-time employees to pass the "fair and reasonable contribution" benchmark [19].

However, a company may resort to paying a penalty per employee if the penalties are overall less costly rather than covering insurance for their employees. These penalties are in place to assure compensation from every employer is being contributed to the health-care system [10–19]. This compensation is either through employers supplying health-care insurance for their employees, or through an employer "fair share contribution" penalty that feeds into the Health Safety Net Fund [9]. For businesses with ten or more employees that do not fulfill their "fair share," the Health Connector has chosen a maximum penalty of $295 per full-time employee that

businesses must pay [8]. Furthermore, to encourage businesses to offer health insurance and to deter Massachusetts workers from incorrectly using Health Safety Net Funds for medical treatment when these workers are able to afford insurance, the employer mandate also contains a "free rider" penalty. This penalty must be paid by businesses that have a large proportion of employees using Health Safe Net Fund dollars for medical treatment. Finally, the reform mandates that companies with more than 11 employees must offer federal "Section 125" insurance plans, which allow employees to purchase health insurance using their income prior to income tax withdrawals [4]. Allowing employees to purchase insurance plans using pre-income tax dollars reduces insurance costs for both employees and employers.

Creation of the Massachusetts Health Connector

The 2006 Health Care Reform created the Commonwealth Health Insurance Connector Authority [9]. Also known as the "Health Connector," this entity oversees the implementation of the health reform and also assists individuals, families, and employers in the purchase of mandatory insurance. The Connector is meant to function as an insurance broker and provides a centralized enterprise for purchasing affordable private or public insurance plans of sufficient quality and cost [4–10]. It serves as a forum where insurers submit bids to the Connector in order to be allowed into the exchange based on meeting minimum coverage and cost requirements. Buyers can then readily access and compare these plans to make the most knowledgeable and personally suited health insurance purchase on a yearly basis [4–12].

The Connector is aimed at increasing competition amongst insurance plans. This competition benefits consumers by increasing types of coverage provided by insurance plans while reducing premium prices as insurance companies vie for consumers [4–10]. Furthermore, the Connector mandates that insurance companies provide information on qualified plans to first-time insurance buyers. During the annual enrollment period, potential insurance consumers have the option to compare insurance plans side by side and receive real-time premium quotes to choose whichever plan is the best suited. By being accessible through a variety of sources – such as the Internet, health insurance agents, or in person – the Connector helps improve transparency of insurance companies and their available plans to help consumers make the most knowledgeable decision possible [3–10].

Commonwealth Choice Health Insurance Plans

Each participating health insurance plan in the Connector is considered a "Commonwealth Choice" plan [17, 18]. A "Choice" plan means that the plan has met minimum credible coverage services, such as ambulatory services, emergency services, preventive care services, and prescription drug coverage for acceptance into the Connector. In a sense, the Connector serves as a screening mechanism to ensure that accepted plans are of sufficient quality and reasonable cost to consumers. Furthermore, all qualified plans must follow marketing, quality improvement, and administrative guidelines to increase transparency and provide access for potential buyers to a network of providers [20]. These Commonwealth Choice plans are tiered at four separate levels – gold, silver, bronze, and young adult – depending on additional coverage benefits provided [20]. Individuals may purchase plans at the gold or silver level if they seek more types of specialized medical services that are not offered at the bronze level. Gold insurance plans typically have the highest monthly premium costs but have the lowest out-of-pocket costs when medical services are required. In contrast, bronze insurance plans have the lowest monthly insurance costs yet have the highest out-of-pocket costs when medical services are provided. The young adult plans are only available to residents who are between 18 and 26 years old and traditionally have low monthly insurance costs but higher out-of-pocket costs [9]. Young adult plans

also have prescription plan coverage options. All insurance companies that are part of the Connector – such as Blue Cross Blue Shield of Massachusetts, Fallon Community Health Plan, Tufts Health Plan, and Harvard Pilgrim Health Care – offer plans at each of these four levels [20]. Depending on the plan selected, age, and geographic location, premiums in Massachusetts can currently range from $100 to over $900 per month. Choice plans with smaller premiums usually come with slightly higher co-payments and deductibles, whereas plans with larger premiums have lower co-payments and deductibles.

Commonwealth Care Health Insurance Programs

Citizens who are 19 years or older, do not qualify for Massachusetts's Medicaid program, and are not provided an option to purchase insurance though their employers have other specialized insurance plans available for purchase through the Connector [9, 14]. Termed "Commonwealth Care," this program comprises five subsidized insurance plans contracted with the Massachusetts government to serve eligible residents. Then-Governor Romney specifically announced that the average uninsured Massachusetts resident should be able to purchase insurance for $175 each month [4–7, 9]. The five insurance plans that are currently contracted with Massachusetts to serve the Commonwealth Care population typically have premiums lower than $150 per month.

Commonwealth Care explicitly covers residents who have incomes that are at the Federal Poverty Level or up to 300 % of the Federal Poverty Line [8, 9]. Residents who are below 100 % of the Federal Poverty Line are eligible to apply for Massachusetts's Medicaid program ("MassHealth") and are only responsible to cover prescription co-payment costs. However, residents with incomes between 100 % and 150 % of the Federal Poverty Line will similarly only be responsible for co-payments for prescription drugs and medical services and will not be responsible for paying monthly premiums for their Commonwealth Care plan [4–6, 9].

Individuals with incomes greater than 150 % of the Federal Poverty Line (FPL) are categorized into groups at progressive 50 % FPL intervals, with wealthier citizens paying higher monthly premiums for their Commonwealth Care plans. For example, a citizen who has an income that is 250–300 % over the Federal Poverty Line pays on average $140 per month on Commonwealth Care premiums, whereas a resident who has an income that is 150–200 % over the FPL pays on average only $50 for monthly Commonwealth Care insurance premiums [9]. These premium estimates have been traditionally set to be "affordable" and "low" due to a decision in July 2008 by the Health Connector to only sponsor Commonwealth Care plans that have low premiums with subsequent high co-payments.

Expansion of Massachusetts's Medicaid: "MassHealth"

The 2006 Health Care Reform included a provision to expand coverage and funding for the Massachusetts Medicaid program – "MassHealth" – which is available to low-income residents who have annual incomes below 100 % of the Federal Poverty Line. MassHealth both contributes to and implements Medicaid funds received from the federal government [21]. It is also bundled with the state's Children's Health Insurance Program (CHIP) that provides matching funds for uninsured families with children.

As part of the reforms, the Centers for Medicare and Medicaid Services extended the Massachusetts's Medicaid program, allowing 10,500 people previously on the wait list to enroll in the MassHealth "Essential" program [9, 21]. The "Essential" program covers long-term unemployed adults who had incomes below 100 % of the Federal Poverty Level [9, 21]. Additionally, the 2006 Reform dedicated $3 million for community outreach programs to encourage the state's 100,000 uninsured, Medicaid-eligible citizens to enroll within MassHealth [9, 11]. For children, MassHealth eligibility was expanded from family income levels below 200 % of the Federal Poverty Line to family income levels below 300 % of the Federal Poverty Line.

The reform also restored certain benefits, such as expanded prescription drug coverage, that were cut during the 2002–2003 recession.

Changes in the State's Safety Net

Significant alterations were made to the former Uncompensated Care Pool [9]. The pool was originally created as a safety net in 1985 to reimburse hospitals and community care clinics for services provided to uninsured or underinsured residents who had incomes up to 200 % of the Federal Poverty Line. Furthermore, residents with incomes between 200 % and 400 % of the Federal Poverty Line received some subsidized care from the pool [22]. During times of medical hardships, the pool also covered individuals whose medical costs exceeded 30 % of family income [22]. The premise behind the creation of the pool was to not deny high-quality coverage for any resident based upon inability to pay. Both the private and public sectors primarily funded the Uncompensated Care Pool. Private sector contributions included payments from hospitals, insurers, health maintenance organizations, and individuals. The public sector contribution is derived from the Massachusetts's legislature appropriating funds to the pool on an annual basis [22]. Prior to health-care reform, the pool's annual budget wavered around $450 million per year. Due to expenditures from the pool exceeding annual budgets and hospitals inappropriately using portions of the pool to reimburse Medicaid-related services, the reform replaced the Uncompensated Care Pool with the Health Safety Net Fund (HSNF) to better regulate expenditures associated with uninsured residents [9, 22].

The new Health Safety Net Fund still pays hospitals for treatments provided to the uninsured, but at different rates. Instead of paying lump sums to compensate for free care, the HSNF anticipates and funds rises in new health-care insurance coverage resulting from the individual mandate and the expansion of Commonwealth Care [8, 10, 22]. Funding for the HSNF comes from employer mandate penalties; employers who do not offer employee health benefits are required to pay $295 to the HSNF for every full-time employee [6, 8, 10, 22].

Between 2006 and 2008, total funding for the HSN was $1.3 billion annually. Prior to health-care reform, the majority of the Uncompensated Pool went towards supplementing managed care organizations, but, after reform, funds were spent more on designated state health programs and the newly established Commonwealth Care.

Other Insurance Market Reforms

Merging of Non-Group and Small-Group Insurance Markets

Concurrent with the implementation of Commonwealth Care by the Health Connector, the reform merges the private individual market – termed the non-group market – with the private 'small-group market,' which offers insurance plans for companies with 50 or fewer employees [23]. Advocates claim that this merger provides individuals with greater access to health plans, such as those that are typically only available in the small-group market that do not require waiting periods or contain preexisting condition limitations. Furthermore, by grouping together all individual and small-group insurance plans into one pool, premium rates are now determined by competition amongst all these plans [9, 23]. Pooling together health risks over a larger population helps to lower costs by lowering premiums as a result of increased competition. Before reform, residents who purchased insurance in the non-group market were typically older and sicker than the average resident. This resulted in claims costs that were 40 % higher on average than for insurance claims in the small-group market. After the merger, however, premiums in the merged market were on average 33 % lower than the premiums in the non-group market prior to reform [6–8, 10, 22, 23]. Insurance plans in the combined pool, therefore, have been more affordable post-reform.

Massachusetts also implemented an additional law in 2011 affecting the structure of the combined non-group and small-group market by establishing an annual enrollment period when citizens can enroll in a plan [4–10]. Prior to this law, individuals had the option to enroll into insurance when expensive medical coverage was required. These individuals could subsequently drop coverage once insurance plans covered their bills. However, under the new law, residents are prohibited from engaging in this behavior because they only have one period each year to enroll. Citizens are exempt from this law if they prove a "good faith effort" towards purchasing health insurance but have merely missed the open enrollment period or if residents have lost insurance due to job loss after the enrollment period has closed [24].

Underage/At-Risk Groups

The reform includes a provision that changed the definition of "dependent." After July 2007, young adults up to the age of 26 years who did not have access to employer-based coverage had access to similar plans through the Health Connector [6–9]. "Dependents" were further defined to also have access to parents' health insurance plans until the age of 25 years, or for an additional 2 years after the designation of "dependent" status is revoked (whichever comes first). Furthermore, due to the young adult tiered plans in the Health Connector, many young adults currently have access to some of the least costly premium plans and the most specifically designed insurance products [8].

Health Maintenance Organization (HMO) Plans

Under health-care reform, health management organizations (HMOs) can offer coverage plans that are linked to health savings accounts as long as participants have incomes that are above 300 % of the Federal Poverty Line [1, 6]. Combining an HMO with a health savings account allows individuals access to cost-saving measures inherent in HMO plans – such as low premiums, low or no deductibles, and low or no co-payments – with the tax savings inherent in a health savings account. Furthermore, individuals will have access to a large network of providers that are part of the particular HMO plan [1, 6].

Financing Health-Care Reform

In 2006, prior to reform, Massachusetts allocated a substantial amount to its Uncompensated Care Pool for its uninsured and underinsured citizens. Beginning in 2007 as a result of the reform, the state now had new fiscal responsibilities including covering children whose family incomes are 300 % above the Federal Poverty Level; supporting the "MassHealth" benefits for the newly qualified uninsured residents; financing new increases in Medicaid reimbursements to primary care physician services and hospital services; providing subsidies for Commonwealth Care plans; and funding of new administrative work and overhead costs as a result of the reforms, especially the implementation and functioning of the newly established Health Connector (Table 18.1) [2–10]. The reform also has provisions to balance both

new spending and existing obligations by shifting money out of older programs and into newer ones.

Financing for the health reform relies on the principle of "shared responsibility." Under this principle, the expansion of publicly funded state programs such as "MassHealth" will help cover costs for the low-income uninsured [25]. Private sector contributions that once paid for "free care" will shift towards subsidizing insurance plans for uninsured individuals who can afford private health insurance plans. Employers will cover additional costs associated with providing employer-sponsored plans for uninsured workers due to the "employer mandate." Finally, individuals themselves will be responsible for covering health insurance costs associated with state-determined levels due to the "individual mandate" [25]. Both federal contributions to health-care reform and state funds are projected to increase every year to

Table 18.1   Revenues and expenditures for Massachusetts Health Care

Massachusetts Health Care reform bill spending projections (in millions)[a]

Sources	FY07	FY08	FY09
Federal Safety Net Revenue	605.0	610.5	610.5
New Federal Medicaid Match	184.6	242.1	299.6
Hospital Assessment	160.0	160.0	160.0
Payor Assessment	160.0	160.0	160.0
Free Rider Surcharge	50.0	40.0	25.0
Fair Share Assessment	45.0	36.0	22.5
General Fund	125.0	125.0	125.0
Total revenues	1,329.6	1,373.6	1,402.6
Uses			
Existing Obligations			
MCO Supplemental Funding	287.0	180.0	160.0
Free Care Pool/Safety New Fund	610.0	500.0	320.0
Subtotal	897.0	680.0	480.0
New Spending			
Children to 300 %	18.2	27.4	37.4
Restored MassHealth Benefits	48.0	53.0	58.0
Medicaid Provider Rate Increases	100.0	180.0	270.0
Commonwealth Care Subsidies	160.0	400.0	725.0
Subtotal	346.2	660.0	1090.4
Total spending	1,243.2	1,340.4	1,570.4
Net balance	+106.4	+33.2	−167.9

Source: Reproduced with permission from Blue Cross MA Foundation. Massachusetts Health Care Reform Bill Summary Book. 2010

[a]Funding for other MassHealth expansions (e.g., Essential, enrollment cap increases) will be included in the state fiscal year 2007 budget and are not included in the table above

help cover costs of reform. For example, from 2007 to 2008, federal contributions towards health-care costs in Massachusetts increased nearly $6 million to $981 million total, and state funds increased $75 million to $338 million total [2–10, 22, 25].

Amendments to the Original Reform

In 2008, a series of amendments to the 2006 Reform were included to improve cost containment, transparency, and efficiency in the state's health-care system [8, 10, 25]. The amendments specifically created a program to provide physicians and prescribers greater transparency on the therapeutic effectiveness and cost-containment measures of different prescription drugs. Furthermore, the amendments set forth regulations and incentives to establish a statewide electronic health record system by 2015 [8–10, 25]. The final major amendment in 2008 included new methods for recruitment and training of primary care providers while establishing new guidelines for streamlining billing and coding by insurers.

In 2010, an amendment was added to the original reform that required insurance providers to have mandatory biannual open enrollment periods during which individuals have options to switch insurance plans. These individuals also have options to sometimes switch plans regardless of corporate preexisting condition exclusions or waiting periods [8, 10, 25]. Furthermore, individuals who have demonstrated coverage of health insurance but subsequently have lost health insurance due to unemployment can enter a special enrollment period. This enrollment period is determined as needed to help consumers enroll in new insurance plans still required by the individual mandate.

In 2012, further amendments were made to the reform to help contain rising health-care costs. The state specifically set a goal of reducing $200 billion in health-care costs [4–6, 8–10, 25]. To accomplish this, the state decided to set increases to health-care costs equal to increases in the gross state product of Massachusetts.

The gross state product measures the economic output of Massachusetts and is analogous to the gross domestic product that represents the economic output of the entire country. By indexing rises in health-care costs to rises in gross state product, the reform ensures that Massachusetts will pay the same percentage in health-care costs each year. The amendment also created new boards and appointees to oversee insurance provider performance improvements and transparency efforts and to enforce compliance of cost-cutting compliance through spending caps. Further minor amendments included employers paying "fair share" contributions if they employ 21 or more workers (previously 11) and a restructuring of premium contribution standards for employers.

Measurable Results of the Reform

As a result of the reform, 401,000 citizens have gained health insurance coverage from 2006 to 2010. By 2010, 98.1 % of adult citizens and 99.8 % of state children carried health insurance that fulfilled coverage requirements set forth by the individual mandate and the Connector [8–10, 25]. Compared to the national average of 83.7 % of citizens having health insurance, Massachusetts currently has the highest rate of health insurance coverage out of any state. As of 2011, 40 % of newly insured residents are now covered through Commonwealth Care, 16 % are covered through individual private insurance, and 43 % are covered through MassHealth [8–10, 25]. Newly insured residents by type of insurance for the first 6 years of reform are shown in Fig. 18.2. Non-elderly adults make up the largest proportion of the newly insured but still constitute the largest proportion (95 %) of uninsured citizens. Furthermore, residents of Hispanic backgrounds, those with low annual incomes that are under 300 % of the Federal Poverty Line, and young males are currently the most likely to not have health insurance [8–10, 25]. In 2009, the national average of uninsured residents was 16.7 % of all Americans, which is markedly higher than the 2.7 % uninsured rate seen in Massachusetts.

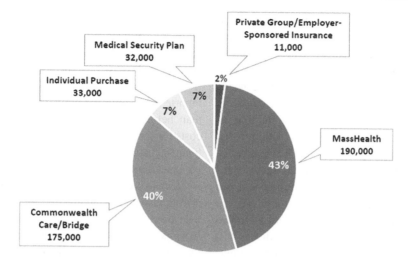

Fig. 18.2 Insurance sources for the newly insured after reform (numbers may not add up due to rounding) (Reprinted with permission from Massachusetts Division of Health Care Finance and Policy. Key Indicators. May 2011 and June 2011)

When considering all insured citizens in Massachusetts as a group, private group and employer-sponsored coverage continues to cover the majority of residents (79 %), compared to MassHealth which covers 16 % of citizens in comparison [8–10, 21–25].

By 2010, Commonwealth Care beneficiaries had not "crowded out" or outgained the market share of employer-sponsored insurance as some economic analysts had projected [8, 26]. As of 2009, employer-sponsored plans covered nearly 68 % of residents in the state who had insurance. This is a nearly 2 % increase in insurance market share when compared to 2007–2008, and employer-sponsored plans constitute the largest source of insurance compared to any other option [8–10, 25, 26]. As a comparison, public and other coverage options comprised 27 % of the insurance market in 2009. Although only 12 % of businesses in Massachusetts are required to follow "Fair Share" requirements because they have greater than 11 employees, nearly 95 % of these companies passed "Fair Share" benchmarks as described earlier. Furthermore, more companies were willing to offer insurance and meet "Fair Share" requirements in lieu of facing penalties [8–10, 25, 26]. As a result of reform, businesses are more likely to use federal tax provisions that allow employees to purchase health insurance

prior to income tax withdrawals, thereby saving employers potential costs. Employees are also more likely after reform to carry insurance offered through their employers. However, employers currently contribute fewer dollars towards covering their employees' premiums, as premium costs have steadily risen due to medical inflation over the past few years.

Reception of Health-Care Reform

There has been notable acceptance and praise by the Massachusetts population towards the 2006 Reform. Of the 4.2 million in the state who are required to file taxes annually, 97 % comply with the individual mandate that required these citizens to prove their health insurance status on tax forms. Furthermore, 95 % of these individuals carried health insurance year-round [8–10]. Exemptions from tax filings were mostly due to low incomes, inability to afford coverage, or religious exceptions. Although 17 % of the state's uninsured were subject to a penalty under the individual mandate, only 1.2 % of these residents were actually assessed a penalty in 2008 due to individual mandate exemptions [2–5, 8–10].

With respect to accessibility and quality of care, Massachusetts continues to have the greatest number of physicians and specialists per capita in the United States. Patients in 2009 recorded fewer out-of-pocket expenses and faced fewer unmet needs due to costs or for any other reason compared to in 2006. Cost and coverage needs were met especially for those in middle- and low-income brackets, as well as for those in minority or chronically ill population groups. Additionally, more adults currently have established sources of care such as primary care physicians, take advantage of more preventative care visits, and see improvements in health-care access and use as a result of reform across all population groups including income, race, and ethnic disparities. Adults in Massachusetts currently face fewer out-of-pocket costs after reform. Those who are still uninsured have greater access to health-care resources.

In 2006 after passage of the reform, public support was 69 % for the law and was consistent across most demographic groups including sex, race, and income. By 2009, support dipped slightly to 67 %. As a whole, 52 % of Massachusetts citizens currently believe health reform has been positive for their state [8]. Nearly 88 % of medical doctors believe the reform either improved or did not affect care or quality of care provided for residents. Almost 79 % of the state's population believes reform helped those people previously uninsured. Finally, 75 % of state residents believe health-care reform in Massachusetts should continue [8, 25].

Current Challenges

Although proponents of the health-care reform cite encouraging trends, extrapolations, and predictions in terms of greater access to health care and fewer health disparities amongst different segments of the population, reform in Massachusetts still faces many challenges. Financially, it is projected that total state spending on health care will nearly double from 2010 to 2020 [8–15]. Massachusetts currently spends the most on health care compared to any other state. Massachusetts spends nearly 15 % more on per capita health-care expenditures compared to expenditure for the average American. Nearly

37 % of this spending is from Medicaid and Medicare services, with remaining expenditures from private market plans. All these components are expected to rise over the next 10 years as well [8–15]. Furthermore, in 2009 more insured adults reported difficulties paying their medical bills than before the reforms due to rising medical costs for services and treatments. Addressing the financial aspects of the reform will be a continuing challenge for the state.

Health-care costs account for most increases in private insurance spending and more than half of the increases in outpatient services spending. Hospital costs in Massachusetts currently constitute 38 % of per capita spending [27]. Along with nursing home care costs, these provider-related expenditures comprise a majority of the difference in health-care spending when comparing Massachusetts to the United States as a whole [27]. To address these rising health-care costs, employers are passing more of the premium costs onto employees. Unfortunately, these increasing costs are outstripping stagnant income trends. Therefore, a current climate exists in Massachusetts whereby citizens are spending larger proportions of their annual household budgets on health care without experiencing any increases in income [8–10, 21, 25]. On the state level, rising government expenditures towards health care will continue to squeeze other public spending priorities such as infrastructure and education.

Furthermore, although Massachusetts has the nation's smallest uninsured pool, there are still nearly 5.6 % of residents in the state who do not have health insurance [8]. There are a variety of reasons why there still remain some uninsured residents. It may be difficult to convince these residents to purchase insurance, they might be exempt from the individual mandate due to income restrictions or religious obligations, or they may not qualify for government subsidies or employer-sponsored insurance due to their annual incomes. Most of the remaining uninsured residents after health-care reform cannot afford insurance even after government subsidies and aids. Furthermore, many of the uninsured are young adults or male adults in good health, and 75 % of them have incomes that fall within 300 % of the Federal Poverty Line [8, 25].

One final challenge that must be taken into account is the lack of widespread preventative care in the state. In 2010, overall access to health care increased due to more residents having health insurance. However, one in five non-elderly adults in Massachusetts had difficulty with finding an available primary care physician as a result of an expanded insured pool that placed increasing strains on primary care services [2–5, 8]. Those with chronic diseases, especially diabetes, received less than ideal preventative care due to longer wait times. Finally, nearly half of the emergency department visits in 2010 were potentially preventable. These emergency room visits cost the health-care system over $510 million in unnecessary expenditures [1–5]. These costs are unfortunately increasing with no provisions or amendments in the current structure of the reform to further reduce these expenditures. While there have been indisputable improvements in health-care access and coverage, these cost concerns are a legitimate threat to the sustainability of health care in Massachusetts. The major discussions in the state today deal with how to reverse this rise in costs.

Conclusion

The 2006 Massachusetts Health Care Reform was the first of its kind in the nation to require insurance carriage through specific mandates. Although the reform is still relatively new and trends are still being analyzed in terms of impact of the reform, Massachusetts nevertheless has the highest rate of insured citizens out of any state. A well-established understanding of the changes that occurred in the 2006 Reform serves as a platform for understanding wide-sweeping health-care reform and the challenges that such dramatic change presents.

References

1. An employers' guide to the 2006 Massachusetts Health Care Reform Act. Mintz. 2008 Jan 21. http://www.mintz.com/newsletter/2007/EBEC-Alert-MHCRA-Guide-02-07/MHCRA-Emp-Guide.pdf. Accessed 21 Aug 2012.
2. Symonds WC. In Massachusetts, health care for all? Bloomberg Businessweek. 2006 Apr 3. http://www.businessweek.com/stories/2006-04-03/in-massachusetts-health-care-for-all-businessweek-business-news-stock-market-and-financial-advice. Accessed 21 Aug 2012.
3. Massachusetts Health Reform of 2006. Families USA. 2007 Aug. http://www.familiesusa.org/assets/pdfs/state-expansions-ma.pdf. Accessed 21 Aug 2012.
4. Holahan J, Blumberg L. Massachusetts health reform: solving the long-run cost problem. Urban. 2009 Jan. http://www.urban.org/UploadedPDF/411820_mass_health_reform.pdf. Accessed 21 Aug 2012.
5. Massachusetts Health Care Reform bill summary. BlueCross BlueShield. http://69.30.54.70/sites/default/files/060700MHRLawSummary_0.pdf. Accessed 21 Aug 2012.
6. Raymond AG. The 2006 Massachusetts Health Care Reform Law; Progress and challenges after one year of implementation. BlueCross BlueShield. 2007 May. http://masshealthpolicyforum.brandeis.edu/publications/pdfs/31-May07/MassHealthCareReformProgess%20Report.pdf. Accessed 21 Aug 2012.
7. Consumers' experience in Massachusetts: lessons for national health reform. Kaiser. 2009 Sept. http://kaiserfamilyfoundation.files.wordpress.com/2013/01/7976.pdf. Accessed 14 Mar 2013.
8. Health reform in Massachusetts: assessing the results. BlueCross BlueShield. https://www.mahealthconnector.org/portal/binary/com.epicentric.contentmanagement.servlet.ContentDeliveryServlet/Health%2520Care%2520Reform/Overview/HealthReformAssessingtheResults.pdf. Accessed 21 Aug 2012.
9. Session Laws: Chapter 58: An act providing access to affordable, quality, accountable health care. The Commonwealth of Massachusetts. https://malegislature.gov/Laws/SessionLaws/Acts/2006/Chapter58. Accessed 21 Aug 2012.
10. Massachusetts Health Care Reform: six years later. Kaiser. 2012 May. http://kaiserfamilyfoundation.files.wordpress.com/2013/01/8311.pdf. Accessed 21 Aug 2012.
11. Feller M. Health care home run: Massachusetts' new universal health care law has everyone watching. National conference of states legislatures. 2006 June. http://www.ncbi.nlm.nih.gov/pubmed/16791975. Accessed 21 Aug 2012.
12. 2012 HHS Poverty Guidelines. US Department of Health and Human Services. http://aspe.hhs.gov/poverty/12poverty.shtml. Accessed 15 Nov 2012.
13. Massachusetts Health Insurance Requirements. Mass Resources. http://www.massresources.org/health-reform.html. Accessed 21 Aug 2012.
14. Commonwealth Care. Health Connector. https://www.mahealthconnector.org/portal/site/connector/template.MAXIMIZE/menuitem.3ef8fb03b7fa1ae4a7ca7738e6468a0c/?javax.portlet.tpst=2fdfb140904d489c8781176033468a0c_ws_MX&javax.portlet.prp_2fdfb140904d489c8781176033468a0c_viewID=content&javax.portlet.prp_2fdfb140904d489c878117

6033468a0c_docName=CommCareOverview& javax.portlet.prp_2fdfb140904d489c8781176033468 a0c_folderPath=/About%20Us/CommonwealthCare/. Accessed 21 Aug 2012.

15. Mcdonough JE. Massachusetts health reform implementation: major progress and future challenges. Health Aff. 2008;27(4):w285–97.

16. Commonwealth Care Trust Fund. BlueCross BlueShield. http://bluecrossmafoundation.org/tag/chapter-58/commonwealth-care-trust-fund. Accessed 21 Aug 2012.

17. Urban Institute. Health care reform in Massachusetts. http://www.urban.org/projects/massahusetts.cfm. Accessed 21 Aug 2012.

18. Massachusetts household and employer insurance surveys: results from 2011. Commonwealth of Massachusetts. 2013 Jan. http://www.mass.gov/chia/docs/r/pubs/13/mhisreport-1-29-13.pdf. Accessed 15 Mar 2013.

19. Employers. HealthConnector. https://www.mahealthconnector.org/portal/site/connector/template. MAXIMIZE/menuitem.3ef8fb03b7fa1ae4a7ca7738e 6468a0c/?javax.portlet.tpst=2fdfb140904d489c8781 176033468a0c_ws_MX&javax.portlet.prp_2fdfb140 904d489c8781176033468a0c_viewID=content &javax.portlet.prp_2fdfb140904d489c87811760334 68a0c_docName=content&javax.portlet.prp_2fdfb14 0904d489c8781176033468a0c_folderPath=/ FindInsurance/Employer/Obligations/Fair%20 Share%20Contribution/&javax.portlet.begCache Tok=com.vignette.cachetoken&javax.portlet. endCacheTok=co. Accessed 21 Aug 2012.

20. Commonwealth Choice Overview. HealthConenctor. https://www.mahealthconnector.org/portal/site/connector/template.MAXIMIZE/menuitem.3ef8fb03b7f a1ae4a7ca7738e6468a0c/?javax.portlet.tpst=2fdfb14 0904d489c8781176033468a0c_ws_MX&javax.portlet.prp_2fdfb140904d489c8781176033468a0c_viewID=content&javax.portlet.prp_2fdfb140904d48 9c8781176033468a0c_docName=Commchoice%20

Overview&javax.portlet.prp_2fdfb140904d489c8781 176033468a0c_folderPath=/About%20Us/Commonwealth%20Choice/&javax.portlet.begCache Tok=com.vignette.cachetoken&javax.portlet. endCacheTok=com.vignette.cachetoken. Accessed 21 Aug 2012.

21. MassHealth: An Overview. MassResources. http://www.massresources.org/masshealth.html. Accessed 21 Aug 2012.

22. The uncompensated care pool: saving the safety net. Massachusetts Health Policy Forum. 2002 Oct 23. http://masshealthpolicyforum.brandeis.edu/publications/pdfs/16-Oct02/IB%20UncompCarePool%2016. pdf. Accessed 21 Aug 2012.

23. Impact of Merging the Massachusetts Non-Group and Small Group Health Insurance Markets. 2006 Dec 26. http://www.mass.gov/ocabr/docs/doi/legal-hearings/nongrp-smallgrp/finalreport-12-26.pdf. Accessed 19 Aug 2012.

24. Gooch JJ. Massachusetts ties healthcare cost increases to the state's gross state product. Managed Healthcare Executive. 2012 Aug 15. http://managedhealthcareexecutive.modernmedicine.com/managed-healthcare-executive/news/massachusetts-ties-healthcare-cost-increases-states-gross-state-pr. Accessed 21 Aug 2012.

25. Raymond AG. Massachusetts health care reform: a five-year progress report. BlueCross BlueShield. 2011 Nov. https://www.mahealthconnector.org/portal/binary/com.epicentric.contentmanagement.servlet.ContentDeliveryServlet/Health%2520Care%2520Reform/Overview/BlueCrossFoundation 5YearRpt.pdf. Accessed 21 Aug 2012.

26. Expanding access to affordable, quality health care. Governor's Budget. http://www.mass.gov/bb/h1/fy14h1/exec_14/hbudbrief3.htm. Accessed May 2013.

27. Hospital costs in context: a transparent view of the cost of care. Massachusetts Hospital Association. http://www.mhalink.org/AM/Template.cfm?Section=Home&CONTENTID=11241&TEMPLATE=/CM/ContentDisplay.cfm. Accessed 21 Aug 2012.

The 2010 Patient Protection and Affordable Care Act: What Is It and How Will It Change Health Care?

19

Richard Latuska, Alexandra Obremskey, and Manish K. Sethi

Learning Objectives

The main objective for this chapter is to highlight key provisions of the Patient Protection and Affordable Care Act (PPACA), signed into legislation by President Barack Obama on March 23, 2010.

After completing this chapter, the reader should be able to answer the following questions:

- The history of and rationale for how the PPACA came into legislation.
- The various ways in which the PPACA hopes to expand accessible and affordable health insurance coverage to a greater number of Americans such as the Individual Mandate, expansion of Medicaid/SCHIPs, creation of the exchanges, and implementing several changes in employer-sponsored health plans and private insurance plans.
- Changes to health insurance taxes intended to help fund this reform and attempt to contain costs in the future.
- How the PPACA seeks to improve the quality of care that is delivered by placing a greater emphasis on preventive care, primary care, and long-term care.

R. Latuska, B.S.
Vanderbilt University School of Medicine, Nashville,
TN 37232, USA
e-mail: richard.f.latuska@vanderbilt.edu

A. Obremskey
University of Southern California, Los Angeles,
CA 90089, USA
e-mail: obremske@usc.edu

M.K. Sethi, M.D. (✉)
Director of the Vanderbilt Orthopaedic Institute Center
for Health Policy, Assistant Professor of Orthopaedic
Trauma Surgery, Department of Orthopaedic Surgery
and Rehabilitation, Vanderbilt University School of
Medicine, Nashville, TN 37232, USA
e-mail: manish.sethi@vanderbilt.edu

The Problem

The issue of health-care reform has been discussed in presidential elections dating back to the early 1900s when the idea of creating federally funded programs to provide health insurance for certain populations unable to obtain private insurance first surfaced [1]. For a detailed discussion of the history of medicine in the United States, please see Chap. 1. It was not until 1965 however, under Former President Lyndon B. Johnson's administration, that Medicare and Medicaid were created to provide health insurance for the elderly

M.K. Sethi and W.H. Frist (eds.), *An Introduction to Health Policy: A Primer for Physicians and Medical Students*, 235
DOI 10.1007/978-1-4614-7735-8_19, © Springer Science+Business Media New York 2013

over the age of 65 and for individuals or families with low incomes who were unable to purchase health insurance, respectively [1]. While the idea of health-care reform has been discussed in previous presidential elections, it has never been as dominating of an issue or platform as it was in the 2008 election between Democrat Barack Obama and Republican John McCain or as it was in the 2012 presidential election between President Obama and Republican Mitt Romney.

With the induction of President Obama into office following the 2008 election, Americans knew it was only a matter of time before some form of health-care reform legislation was proposed. In 2009, addressing the topic of health-care reform plans, President Obama stated, "what is truly scary—truly risky—is the prospect of doing nothing. If we maintain the status quo, we will continue to see 14,000 Americans lose their health insurance every day. Premiums will continue to skyrocket. Our deficit will continue to grow and insurance companies will continue to profit by discriminating against sick people" [2]. One year later, on March 23, 2010, President Obama signed into law the Patient Protection and Affordable Care Act (PPACA), commonly referred to as "Obamacare" [3].

The primary rationale behind this statute is the need to expand health-care insurance coverage to cover more Americans. According to the National Bureau's report on Income, Poverty, and Health Insurance Coverage in the United States, 16.3 % of Americans were uninsured in 2010, which translates to 49.9 million Americans without some form of health-care insurance [4]. While there is a large variety of reasons behind this number (i.e., inability to purchase insurance, transitioning between jobs, or choosing not to purchase), it is still a staggering number of uninsured Americans that the PPACA hopes to reduce.

Another important rationale behind the PPACA is that it hopes to tame the current out-of-control high costs of health care in America. In 2009, costs of health care in the United States were 17.6 % of the gross domestic product (GDP) [5], and these costs are expected to rise to 25 % of GDP by 2015 [6]. In 2010, health-care costs reached approximately $2.6 trillion [7]. As a

comparison, the UK spent only 9.6 % of its GDP on health care in 2010 [7].

Given these rising costs, private insurance plans, premiums, and deductibles have followed similar patterns, and consumers now in turn bear the burden. Since 2000, employer-sponsored health insurance premiums have doubled, which is three times faster than increases in employee wages [8]. In 2008, if a family purchased their health insurance plan through an employer, it cost approximately $12,680, which is the average amount someone working a full-time job in the United States earns in a year [8]. Therefore, while the PPACA seeks to expand coverage to a greater number of Americans, it also aims to control costs in the long run, with the main goal of reducing the overall national deficit over the next 10 years [9].

While the USA spends more on health care than any other nation, the quality of health care that Americans are receiving does not seem to match up. When compared to other developed countries, the United States ranks in the lower third for life expectancy [10]. Another study examined preventable mortality between 19 countries and found that the United States had the highest rate of deaths from preventable or treatable conditions [11]. Furthermore, when comparing the United States to ten European countries, it was found that the United States had a much higher prevalence of cancer, heart disease, and stroke in its population over age 50 [12].

In the current health-care system, there are also many problems that exist even for those Americans who are financially able to afford health insurance. One of the more pressing problems is that in 45 out of the 50 states in America, insurance companies are able to refuse insurance to an individual due to a preexisting health condition [13]. Such "preexisting" conditions may range from serious illnesses like cancer to mild conditions such as asthma [13].

Issues such as these provide the framework for many of the main goals of the PPACA which aim to expand access to care. Provisions that seek to expand access to care include implementing the Individual Mandate, increasing federally funded programs such as Medicaid and SCHIPs, creating health insurance exchanges, expanding employer-based coverage, and placing certain regulations and limitations on current insurance company policies. Advocates of the PPACA also believe that the introduction of certain tax changes related to health insurance and the implementation of other programs and policies can help control the skyrocketing costs without sacrificing quality of care. This chapter will provide an overview and summary of these provisions while also demonstrating how they will affect the patient, the physician, the state, insurance companies, and employers/employees.

The Individual Mandate

One of the most controversial provisions in the PPACA is the Individual Mandate which requires US citizens and legal residents to purchase qualifying health-care coverage for themselves and for their tax dependents each month by 2014 [14]. The "minimum qualifying policy" would cover 60 % of costs, and any remaining costs would be paid by those enrolled in the form of deductibles, co-payments, or coinsurance [15]. Individuals would still retain their freedom to choose where and from whom they obtain health insurance, whether that be through their employer, a privately purchased insurance plan, a new health insurance exchange (discussed later in this chapter), a grandfathered plan (allowing people who already have individual or employer coverage to continue that coverage even though it might not meet the new benefit standards), or a government-sponsored plan such as Medicaid or Medicare [14].

Those who do not obtain coverage and are without coverage for longer than 3 months will have to pay a penalty in the form of a tax, known as the "shared responsibility payment" [15]. The penalty will ultimately reach a level of 2.5 % of their income beginning in 2016, but until then it will be phased in, beginning with 1 % of income in 2014 and 2 % in 2015 [16]. Therefore, in 2016, if an individual's income is $50,000, he/she would be required to pay a penalty of $1,016 [16]. Furthermore, for families with children who are uninsured, parents would be required to pay

half of the imposed penalty for each member of the house that is uninsured [15]. There are limitations to this penalty as well: the penalty cannot exceed the average premium amount that would be required in the insurance exchange, and a family would not be required to pay more than three times the amount of the individual penalty (which would be $2,250 in 2016) [15].

The legislation does allow certain groups to be exempt from the mandate and thus the tax penalty as well. These groups include those with religious objections, undocumented immigrants, individuals in prison, American Indians, those who are uninsured for a short period of time (3 months or less, such as individuals who may be switching jobs), and, finally, those who meet the criteria of financial hardship [14]. The issue of religious exemption, specifically details as to which religious groups would be exempt, has not been fully discussed. As it stands now, groups would need to file for exemption, and those likely to be exempt must have a history of belief that discourages accepting benefits of any private or public insurance. An example of one religious group that would be exempted from this mandate would be Muslims since the Islamic faith believes insurance to be a form of "risk taking" and is thus banned [17].

The criteria set for "financial hardship" is for those with an annual income 100 % of the federal poverty line, those whose incomes are below the tax filing threshold (which was $9,350 for single taxpayer under the age of 65 and $18,700 for couples in 2009) [16], and individuals for whom the required amount to purchase basic coverage would be more than 8 % of their annual income [15, 16].

Clearly, many families may not meet this set of criteria for financial hardship exemption, yet this does not mean the requirement to purchase coverage will not be a significant burden for a large percentage of low-income families. In order to address this concern and not only increase coverage but increase *affordable* coverage, the PPACA proposes the expansion of federally funded public programs such as Medicaid and SCHIPs, premium and cost-sharing subsidies to individuals, an increase in employer-sponsored coverage, creation of health insurance exchanges to offer more affordable qualified health plans, and cost-sharing assistance/tax credits for individuals or families with low incomes of certain levels of the federal poverty level [16]. Each of these provisions seeks to expand affordable health-care coverage to Americans, and each will be discussed in further detail in this chapter.

Expansion of Public Programs (Medicaid and SCHIPs)

Medicaid is a federally funded public program designed to provide health insurance coverage for individuals with low incomes. Every one of the 50 states currently participates in the Medicaid program, but, in doing so, it must follow certain guidelines the government establishes as to who is eligible to be a part of the program and how costs are distributed and handled [14]. Presently, Medicaid offers coverage for pregnant women, children less than 6 years of age who belong to families with incomes below 133 % of the federal poverty line (FPL), children between the ages of 6–18 who belong to families with incomes at or below 100 % of the FPL, any adult who was financially eligible for the former cash assistance program (AFDC), and those who are able to receive Supplemental Security Income benefits due to their low income or disability status [14].

To start, the PPACA called for an expansion of Medicaid to include all individuals under the age of 65 who are not eligible for Medicare (which would thus include young adults and adults without children) with incomes up to 133 % FPL [16]. Furthermore, each state would maintain the option of additionally expanding coverage beyond the 133 % FPL requirement [9]. Expansion would also increase coverage to Puerto Rico and the surrounding territories [9]. It is estimated that this expansion would help provide coverage to approximately 32 million previously uninsured Americans [18]. All who are newly eligible would be guaranteed a baseline benefit package that offers the same health benefits that are available to individuals who obtain insurance through the exchanges [16].

In order to execute this expansion, the federal government claims it will cover 100 % of the costs of this expansion from 2014 through 2016 and then steadily decrease to 90 % funding in 2020 and so on [16]. Similarly, states that have already expanded coverage to adults with income at or below 100 % FPL will receive a similar steady increased federal funding until it is even with the other states by 2019 [16]. The state will be responsible for enrolling these newly eligible individuals into Medicaid no later than January 2014 but have the option of beginning enrollment any time after 2011 [16].

Furthermore, these expansions are not limited to increasing solely health insurance coverage but will also increase several services available through newly acquired Medicaid coverage. Such services include freestanding birth centers, Medicaid hospice services for children, family planning services, and community-based attendant services to those who otherwise would need a nursing home or some other form of intermediate care [9].

Another federally funded program, the State Children's Health Insurance Program (SCHIP), known as "Children's Medicaid," began in 1997 and provides health coverage to approximately eight million children in families that have high enough incomes that prevent qualification for Medicaid, but low enough that they cannot afford private coverage [19].

The PPACA will maintain the same SCHIP eligibility standards that are already in place from the time of its enactment until 2019 [19]. What it will change, however, is the federal funding to the program by increasing payments by 23 % points (up to a maximum of 100 % funding through 2019) [19]. For children that still may be affected by this cap, the PPACA will allow these children to be eligible for exchange credits in order to obtain coverage [9]. Another barrier for many low-income families that are eligible to obtain Medicaid or SCHIPs, however, is actually enrolling in these programs, as it may be a difficult process for families unfamiliar with such programs. In order to overcome this problem, the PPACA also provided an additional $40 million in federal funding in order to increase enrollment in SCHIP and Medicaid [19]. An example of this effort is the creation of state-run benefit application websites that requires states and programs to coordinate enrollment and application procedures in order to aid families in the enrollment process for Medicaid and SCHIP [9]. Each state now has the option to choose whether to participate in these expansions or not, following the Supreme Court ruling in June 2012 (discussed later in this chapter).

Health Insurance Exchanges

One of the other critical provisions of the PPACA that intends to expand access to health insurance coverage is the creation and enactment of health insurance exchanges. These exchanges are "a new entity intended to create a more organized and competitive market for health insurance by offering a choice of plans, establishing common rules regarding the offering and pricing of insurance, and providing information to help consumers better understand the options available to them" [20]. These exchanges, formally referred to as American Health Benefit Exchanges (beginning July 1, 2013) and Small Business Health Options Program (SHOP) Exchanges (beginning in 2017), will be available for uninsured individuals or small businesses with up to 100 employees (restricted to US citizens and legal immigrants) to purchase qualifying coverage [16]. The main goal of the exchanges is offering multiple plans that provide similar benefits, subsequently increasing competition, lowering prices, and allowing individuals to compare between plans in an easier manner [20]. More than one exchange may exist in a state, but exchanges will not be allowed to overlap in the geographic regions that they serve [20].

In the "public plan option," which is a community health insurance option, these exchanges will make available at least two multistate plans to individuals, which differ as to what services are allowed to be offered [16]. There will also be the creation of a Consumer Operated and Oriented Plan (CO-OP) program which would be run by nonprofit members of health insurance

companies, would be offered in all 50 states, and would not be an existing health insurer company (or sponsored by state/local government) [16]. Similar to the other exchanges, the CO-OP also proposes to provide more affordable, qualifying health insurance coverage for uninsured individuals. The CO-OP would be allowed to purchase items and services at its discretion, but disallow the utilization of provider payment rates [9]. The PPACA states that any profits that CO-OP produces must be used to lower premiums, improve benefits for consumers, or improve quality of health care that is delivered [16]. The government will provide $4.8 billion in funds to launch the CO-OP program [16].

As previously mentioned, each plan offered in the exchange will be similar, but since a completely uniform benefit plan would prevent consumers from having the freedom to choose between plans and decrease innovative plan improvement/development, a four-tier benefit plan will be utilized (as well as an additional "catastrophic" plan). Each plan will provide the same essential health benefits and have the same out-of-pocket limits (set by the Health Savings Account (HSA) law) which are currently $5,950 for individuals and $11,900 for families [16]. The "essential health benefits" that all plans are required to provide include ambulatory services, emergency services, hospitalization, maternal and newborn care, mental health/substance use services, prescription drugs, rehabilitation services, laboratory services, preventative and wellness services, and pediatric services [9]. The four benefit plans will differ, however, in the percentage of the benefit costs it covers, known as the "actuarial value": the bronze plan would cover 60 % of costs, the silver plan 70 %, the gold plan 80 %, and the platinum plan 90 % of costs [16]. The catastrophic plan, which would only be available in the individual market, will be available for individuals under the age of 30 (or those exempt from the Individual Mandate pending its enactment) and provide "catastrophic coverage," i.e., the minimum amount of coverage level that the HSA law sets [16]. The exception to this minimum coverage is that preventative care and three primary care visits would be free from the deductible [16]. In another effort to expand *affordable* coverage, the out-of-pocket limits would also be reduced for low-income families: those with incomes 100–200 % FPL would have one-third of the limits, those with incomes 200–300 % FPL would have one-half of the limits, and those with incomes 300–400 % FPL would have two-thirds of the limits [16].

Another purpose of the exchanges is to make the purchasing of health insurance more transparent by providing the consumer with more information. Each exchange will be required to hire navigators to help with outreach and enrollment in the exchange and to use a uniform enrollment form and a standard format to present plan information [16]. Additionally, exchanges will be required to have a call center for customer service to help with enrollment and with communication of information about the plans [16]. By providing qualifying options in a single, easy-to-use marketplace, the exchanges also hope to increase competition, thereby lowering premiums. All of these requirements are intended to help catch those who fall through the cracks and do not obtain coverage because of the previous complications of enrolling in programs or choosing between plans.

States will be allowed to apply for a 5-year waiver in order to be exempt from some of these new health insurance requirements, as long as the state can prove that they are providing coverage to all residents that is equally as comprehensive as coverage offered through the exchange *and* prove that this plan does not significantly increase the federal budget deficit [16].

Premium and Cost-Sharing Subsidies to Individuals

In an attempt to provide further assistance for low-income US citizens and legal immigrants purchasing insurance through the exchanges, the PPACA proposes premium tax credits and cost-sharing subsidies, available beginning January 2014, that will lower premiums, deductibles, and out-of-pocket costs such as co-payments and coinsurance. These benefits will not be available, however, to those who obtain coverage through employer-sponsored plans unless that plan does not cover a minimum of 60 % of costs (which is the amount of costs covered in the lowest exchange category, the bronze plan) or if the individual's portion of the premium is greater than 9.5 % of their income [16].

The premium tax credits will be refundable and available to individuals or families with incomes between 133 % and 400 % FPL, and the percentage of tax credit they receive will be based on a sliding scale depending on their income [16]. The premium tax credits will also be associated with the silver plan category of the exchanges, and the value of the credits will also be adjusted each year to control for inflation and family size [16, 21].

For families with incomes 250 % FPL and lower, cost-sharing subsidies will further help decrease out-of-pocket costs, whether in the form of lower deductibles, lower coinsurance rates, or lower co-payments [22]. Once again, there is a scale determining the percentage of the subsidies provided to help cover these charges: those with incomes between 100 % and 150 % FPL will receive 94 % additional protection, incomes between 150 % and 200 % FPL will receive 87 %, and incomes between 200 % and 250 % FPL will receive 73 % [22].

Changes to Private Insurance

Some of the more widely accepted provisions in the ACA are the changes that will occur regarding new regulations on insurance policies. As previously mentioned in the introduction, there are currently no restrictions for increasing premiums, discriminating against preexisting health conditions (ranging from serious to mild conditions), or dropping individuals from a plan if coverage costs become too great.

Currently, the young adult population is significantly more vulnerable to losing health insurance than most others. The majority of adolescents in the USA are covered under their parent's insurance plans as dependents coverage, but, upon turning 19, many of these adolescents lose this coverage [23]. Along with this transition into young adulthood, many find themselves financially independent from their parents and struggling with school, finding a job, beginning a family, and so forth. Therefore, they are much less likely to obtain their own coverage. In 2008, it was reported that young adults aged 19–29 comprise approximately one-third of the uninsured, which constitutes the greatest uninsured rate compared to any other age group [23]. Clearly, young adults who are unemployed are at a greater risk for being uninsured, but even those who are employed struggle to obtain insurance, since young adults are more likely to begin work in small businesses or work part time (both of which might not offer health insurance as a benefit) [23]. With the ACA implementations, young adults will have the ability to remain on their parents' insurance policies until the age of 26, or if they choose not to remain on their parent's plan, young adults will have other options to choose from, including the exchanges (discussed previously) or the expanded employer-sponsored coverage (discussed later in this chapter) [23].

Another significant change to insurance policies is the restriction on discriminating against people with preexisting health conditions as well as prohibiting individual and group plans from implementing lifetime limits on the value of coverage beginning January 2014 [16]. Furthermore, restrictions will be set to deter insurance companies from increasing premiums and requirements will be made that force insurance companies to justify and report any planned increases [16]. Limitations will also be set for deductibles for plans that exist in the small group market: $2,000 for individuals and $4,000 for families [16]. In order to provide coverage for individuals with preexisting conditions, as well as those uninsured for longer than 6 months, a "national high-risk pool" will be created. In an effort to enhance affordability for entering this pool, the PPACA will offer subsidized premiums for eligible individuals. Currently, insurance companies can use a large number of variables to perform a "risk assessment" and calculate the premium ratings for a given individual. In this new pool, however, the only variables that may be taken into account are age, (which cannot increase a premium rating

by more than a factor of 4), geographic region, family size (which cannot increase a premium rating by more than a factor of 3), and tobacco use (which cannot increase a premium rating by more than a factor of 1.5) [16, 24]. The government will allocate $5 billion to launch and fund this high-risk pool for individuals with preexisting conditions [16]. For those who choose to remain on grandfathered plans, the same limitations and restrictions will also apply to these policies [16]. Additionally, a requirement will be set for private insurance companies to pay nearly $25 billion between 2014 and 2016 in order to fund a temporary, nonprofit reinsurance program that covers other high-risk individuals [16].

In addition to these changes, all insurance policies (through the individual market and through the exchanges) must comply with one of the four benefit categories (bronze, silver, gold, platinum) discussed earlier in this chapter; however, they will not be expected to comply with the same new set of benefit standards that the exchange policies set [16]. In 2006, insurance companies will be allowed to enter what is known as "interstate compacts" which allow plans to be purchased outside of the state in which an individual resides [9]. Opening up the insurance market in this way will, it is hoped, promote competition between insurance companies and improve benefits (such as lower premiums) for individuals to choose from [9].

Finally, the PPACA will help establish a website in order to help individuals to choose between different plans [16]. To further enhance the process of applying for coverage, a standardized format for applying and presenting information will also be utilized [16].

Role of the Employer

A common way many Americans obtain health insurance coverage is through their employers. While the PPACA will not necessarily *require* all employers to offer health insurance coverage to their employees, beginning January 2014 it will try to increase the incentive for employers to offer more affordable coverage to their employees by penalizing companies with fees depending on the number of uninsured employees they have [25]. For example, employers with more than 50 full-time employees who do not offer any type of coverage *and* have one or more employees receiving a premium tax credit through the exchange will have to pay $2,000 for every full-time employee (excluding the first 30 employees) [25]. According to the federal law, full-time employees are defined as those working 30 or more hours per week, except for "full-time" seasonal employees who work for less than 120 days of the year [26]. Employers with 50 or more employees who do offer coverage but still have at least one full-time employee receiving premium tax credits through the exchange (implicating that the offered coverage is either not affordable or does not provide the minimum value of coverage) will have to pay the lesser of either $3,000 for every employee that receives a premium tax credit or $2,000 for every full-time employee (again excluding the first 30 employees) [16]. According to the Congressional Budget Office (CBO), approximately one million individuals every year will enroll in an exchange plan and receive a premium tax credit because an employer's plan was considered unaffordable [25]. While these provisions and penalties are targeted at medium-sized businesses, larger businesses of more than 200 full-time employees *will* be required to automatically enroll all employees into the health insurance plan that they offer [16]. These plans must meet affordability and essential benefit standards since employees will not be given the option to opt out of this coverage [16].

Premium Subsidies to Employers

The previous section discussed penalties the PPACA has set in place for larger employers (50 or more full-time employees), but, for smaller business employers (no more than 25 employees with average annual wages of $50,000), the PPACA will offer tax credits in two phases to employers that offer health insurance coverage [16]. Phase I, which will take place between 2010 and 2013, will offer a tax credit up to 35 % of the

amount an employer contributes towards his/her employee's premiums, if and only if that amount is at least 50 % of the total premium or 50 % of a benchmark premium [16]. For even smaller businesses (with no more than ten employees and average annual wages of $25,000), a full tax credit will be available [16]. As indicated, the size of the tax credit for which a business is eligible will be inversely correlated to the size of the business and its employer's average annual wages [16]. In Phase II, which begins in 2014, up to a 50 % tax credit will be available for small businesses that obtain coverage through the exchanges [16]. The policy in Phase I for smaller businesses (up to ten employees) being eligible for full tax credits also applies in Phase II [16].

Employers of various business sizes and their employees have been discussed, but what about elderly individuals who no longer work but are still in need of obtaining health insurance because they are not yet eligible for Medicare? Beginning January 2014, the PPACA will create a temporary "reinsurance program" for employers who offer health insurance coverage for retirees over the age of 55 who are not eligible for Medicare [16]. If the employer or insurer makes insurance claims for these retired individuals between an amount of $15,000 and $90,000, the government will refund the employer 80 % of these costs [16]. The government has also decided to provide $5 billion in order to finance this program [16].

Tax Changes Related to Insurance

The previous sections of this chapter have focused on the numerous ways the PPACA intends to expand health insurance coverage to Americans by making it more accessible *and* more affordable. In order for these provisions and changes to be successful, however, there needs to be a way to finance them. Therefore, the PPACA has proposed several taxes in various sectors in order to help finance health-care reform. The pharmaceutical industry is one of the largest sectors to be hit with these new tax changes, which impose fees that will steadily increase over the next few years (Table 19.1) [16].

Table 19.1 Fees to be imposed on the pharmaceutical industry

Amount	Year
$2.8 billion	2012–2013
$3.0 billion	2014–2016
$4.0 billion	2017
$4.1 billion	2018
$2.8 billion	2019

Source: Data from [16]

Table 19.2 Tax increases to be imposed on the health insurance industry

Amount	Year
$8 billion	2014
$11.3 billion	2015–2016
$13.9 billion	2017
$14.3 billion	2018

Source: Data from [16]

Another large-scale sector that will be subject to tax increases is that of the health insurance industry, and these fees will also be phased in and steadily increased beginning in 2014 (Table 19.2) [16].

The fees mentioned here only apply to insurance companies that make a profit, as fees calculated for nonprofit insurers will only take into account 50 % of net premiums [16].

Other areas subject to taxation include indoor tanning services (10 % tax) which began in July 2010 and medical device sales (excise tax of 2.3 %) beginning December 2012 [16].

Additionally, to help fund this health-care reform, higher income individuals or couples/families (individuals with an income of $200,000 or couples with an income of $250,000) will experience a fairly significant .9 % increase in Medicare Hospital Insurance tax [27].

There are also several changes related to health-care flexible spending accounts and health-care savings accounts that employers often use for employees. For example, employees are now only allowed to contribute a maximum of $2,500 to a health-care flexible spending account (formerly, employees would contribute approximately $4,000–$5,000) [28]. Additionally, individuals are no longer allowed to use money in these accounts to pay for over-the-counter (OTC) medications

[28]. Finally, the penalty for nonqualified distributions of funds in these health savings accounts has been doubled to 20 % [28].

Other tax changes include the elimination of deductions employers are allowed to take for offering Medicare Part D prescription drug coverage for retired employees (beginning 2013), a tax increase on itemized deductions for medical expenses from 7.5 % to 10 % (beginning 2013), and the introduction of 40 % excise tax on high-cost plans (over $10,200 for individuals and $27,500 for families) beginning in 2018 [28].

Cost Containment

In a recent health report, it was noted that "78 % of senior citizens are worried that at some point, either they or someone they know might incur a health-care cost that wouldn't be covered by their health insurance and that, on average, an older couple may need to save $300,000 to pay for health-care costs not covered by Medicare alone" [29]. In addition to these concerns, many Americans fear that the proposed expansion of Medicare will simply force the program further into debt as it strives to provide health insurance coverage to a significantly larger number of individuals. In 2009, the Medicare Trustees Report estimated that the Medicare Part A Trust Fund would be exhausted by 2017 [29]. Therefore, the PPACA has implemented several provisions to contain the cost of expanding these public, federally funded programs. One of the methods to reduce costs is to change the means by which payments are made to Medicare Advantage (MA) plans by distributing higher payments to areas with lower fee-for-service rates and lower payments to areas with higher fee-for-service rates [16]. It is believed that reducing these excessive government payments to particular Medicare Advantage plans that are not in as great a need could save the government, taxpayers, and Medicare beneficiaries approximately $100 billion over the next 10 years [29]. Reform will also ensure that the money in the Medicare Trust Fund goes towards improving the quality of care for its seniors, rather than towards private insurance companies [16]. The PPACA also eliminated the 21 % physician payment cut in 2010 in order to promote and increase the number of physicians providing health care to the elderly covered through Medicare [29]. An "Innovation Center" within the Centers for Medicare and Medicaid Services will also be created to promote the development and evaluation of new, innovative payment structures to Medicare, Medicaid, and SCHIPs without compromising the quality of care that is delivered to patients [16]. In order to contain costs and promote better quality of care, Medicare payments will be reduced by 1 % for conditions that are acquired in hospitals [16].

To further help contain costs within the Medicaid program, drug rebates will be increased for brand-name drugs to 23.1 % [16], with the exceptions being clotting factor drugs and drugs that are approved exclusively for children, for which the drug rebate will increase to 17.1 % [16].

Fraud

Fraud and abuse are other significant causes that contribute to losses from Medicare spending, which ultimately lead to an increase in premiums. Recently, one of the largest fraud settlements in history was made when Pfizer, the well-known pharmaceutical company, agreed to pay $2.3 billion because of its illegal marketing practices [30]. Fortunately, due to this settlement, approximately $1 billion was returned to Medicare/Medicaid funds and other government-operated insurance companies [30]. Unfortunately, this instance of abuse is not isolated and many others have been getting away unpunished. When this happens, it is the elderly and the tax payers who suffer the consequences in the form of increased taxes and skyrocketing premiums. In an attempt to control fraud and abuse with the expansion of Medicare and therefore (it is hoped) control costs, the PPACA proposes several changes intended to help detect fraud/abuse as well as increase the penalties for those culpable. These include the proposal allowing suspected Medicare providers to be screened (with a $200 screening charge) to help detect cases of fraud/abuse [9], enhancing

oversight periods for new providers and suppliers (including an increased 90-day period of enhanced oversight for durable medical equipment suppliers), allowing possible suspension of enrollment into the Medicare program in areas at "high risk" for fraud/abuse, promoting greater communication and facilitation across states, and increasing penalties for submitting false claims (the exact increase has yet to be determined) [9, 16]. The Congressional Budget Office believes that these changes could save over $1 billion over the next 10 years [29].

Prescription Drugs

Finally, one of the most important fields in dire need of cost containment is that of the pharmaceutical industry. Prescription drug prices continue to increase, and, while Medicare helps cover drug costs for senior citizens, there is a catch known as the "donut hole," which refers to a price range of medications not covered by Medicare that many individuals fall into. With the way coverage currently works, an individual is required to pay monthly premiums for coverage and 100 % of out-of-pocket costs up until $310 of the deductible amount on drugs has been reached. After this point, one only needs to pay 25 % of the cost of drugs, while Medicare covers the rest—that is, until the total amount reaches $2,800. This point marks the beginning of the "donut hole," as an individual is once again required to pay 100 % of costs until the total reaches the other end of the spectrum (which is the yearly out-of-pocket limit of $4,450) before one is safely covered again. Therefore, it is the patients who need drugs costing between $2,800 and $4,450 that are most affected [31]. It has been reported that, in 2007, over eight million seniors were stuck in this "donut hole" [29]. One of the more concerning problems for those who find themselves in this donut hole is the issue of decreased medication compliance. Many patients caught in the donut hole end up not purchasing and taking the medications they require because they must put the money towards other living necessities (rent, groceries, etc.).

In an attempt to solve this critical issue, the PPACA will phase in changes that should slowly close the donut hole. Already, senior citizens entering the donut hole are eligible to receive a one-time $250 rebate check to help cover the cost of their medications [31]. In 2011, a 50 % discount for brand-name drugs was implemented, with efforts to further reduce generic drug prices beginning in 2013 [31]. The PPACA hopes to completely close the donut hole coverage gap by 2020, with individuals only having to pay 25 % of the cost of drugs until the out-of-pocket spending limit is reached (at which point Medicare would cover the rest) [31].

Quality of Care

While the previous sections of this chapter have focused on ways to expand health insurance coverage and finance these expansions, the following sections will focus on how the PPACA seeks to improve the quality of health care that is delivered despite the common belief that improving access to care and quality of care are mutually exclusive.

Several new programs and institutes are called for with an emphasis on improved coordination of care, patient-centered care, and quality improvement research and implementation strategies. Efforts aimed at improving the quality of care for Medicare beneficiaries include the creation of the Patient-Centered Outcomes Research Institute to compare the clinical effectiveness of different treatments; a Medicare pilot program to evaluate a bundled payment package for several different acute inpatient and outpatient services; an "Independence at Home Demonstration" program to provide primary care to high-need Medicare patients in their homes; and a hospital value-based purchasing program that rewards hospitals based on performance and quality of care [16, 29]. With Medicaid, a new plan will be created to allow individuals with two or more chronic conditions (or at a high risk for developing a second chronic condition) and those with chronic, serious mental health conditions to choose a specific provider as a "health home" [16]. A health home is a provider or team of providers specially trained to deliver integrated health care

[16]. Additionally, investments will be made to establish "patient-centered medical homes" and "accountable care organizations" that similarly utilize an interprofessional team of health-care professionals to more effectively coordinate a patient's care with the intention to improve the quality of care while reducing costs [9].

While all states will not be required to expand Medicaid as proposed given the Supreme Court ruling (discussed later in this chapter), they still have the option to expand it as they see fit, which will inevitably lead to a greater number of individuals insured under Medicare and thus requiring primary care services [32]. However, the American Academy of Family Physicians reported that the number of medical students entering primary care (which includes family medicine as well as general internal medicine, general pediatrics, and geriatrics) has dropped by 51.8 % since 1997, and it estimates a shortage of 40,000 family physicians by 2020 [33]. Given that primary care fields such as these are crucial for preventing emergency room visits and other hospital admissions, the PPACA aims to improve primary care reimbursement, training, and services. In 2011, primary care providers began receiving a 10 % bonus for claims made to Medicare for primary care services [9]. Beginning in 2013, the new law will require payments to physicians who provide primary care services to be at least 100 % of Medicare rates [26]. To increase incentives for medical students entering primary care, the PPACA intends to improve the Primary Care Student Loan program by making it easier for students to qualify for loans, shortening payback periods, reducing the maximum service obligation from 20 years to 10 years [9], and increasing funding to the National Health Service Corps scholarship and loan repayment program, so more students may be eligible for these loans/programs [16]. Grant programs have also been created to support the expansion of primary care residency programs and the filling of unused residency positions with primary care physicians (especially for areas that are in the greatest need) [9]. Finally, the PPACA will create a Primary Care Extension Program to educate and train primary care providers on evidence-based medicine, preventative medicine, chronic disease management, and mental health issues [9].

Prevention and Wellness

In addition to the emphasis that needs to be placed on increasing and enhancing primary care providers and services, there also needs to be a stronger focus on the delivery of high-quality preventative health services in order to effectively reduce future health-care costs and improve the overall health of Americans. According to the National Commission on Prevention Priorities, increasing the use of just five preventive services would save more than 100,000 lives annually in the USA [34]. In 2008, the CDC reported that 38 % of adults over the age of 50 have never had a colonoscopy or sigmoidoscopy [29] and an estimated 14,000 additional lives could be saved each year if this percentage was increased to 90 % [34]. In terms of cost, preventative measures such as educating at-risk adults about regular aspirin use, smoking cessation counseling, immunizations, alcohol abuse education/counseling, and vision screening have all been proven to save more money in the long run [34].

Under the PPACA health-care reform, seniors over the age of 50 would no longer need to pay out of pocket for a colonoscopy screening or any other preventative service [29], and Medicare will also cover annual wellness visits, providing its beneficiaries with a "Personalized Prevention Plan" that would include health risk assessments, BMI measurements, and other preventive screenings, without the requirement of any co-payments or deductibles [35]. Coinsurance requirements for a large portion of preventative services, including initial preventative physical exams, will be waived as Medicare will also cover 100 % of these costs [35]. States will also be eligible for special grants as incentives to promote Medicaid beneficiaries to participate in certain "healthy lifestyle programs" that aim to cease alcohol misuse/tobacco use, lower blood pressure and cholesterol levels, and better manage/control diabetes or other chronic medical conditions. There will also be funds and programs established to promote other preventive health programs, community health centers, and education centers; to increase the number of vaccinations for children and adults; and to ensure that chain restaurants (those with more than 20 establishments under the same name) have a standardized menu showing nutrition labels and information [16, 35].

Long-Term Care

Another area of care that tends to be neglected is that of long-term care for the elderly who wish to remain in their homes or communities but require certain health-care services that are often not provided. Approximately 65 % of seniors over the age of 65 live at home and require care that they do not receive [36].

The PPACA had hoped to address this problem with several grants and programs aimed at expanding coverage plans to include long-term care for in-home and community-based services. One of the main programs under this provision, known as the Community Living Assistance Services and Supports (CLASS), was a plan to offer an average of $50 cash benefits for those with certain medical limitations to receive nonmedical support and services in their community [27]. In September 2011, however, the Senate Appropriations Committee announced the deletion and abandonment of this program as members realized how unfeasible it would be to fund such a program, thus leaving the USA without a solution to the crucial problem of long-term care [37]. This is one example that highlights the key difference between politics and implementing policy—in other words, where the "rubber meets the road"—and thus calls into the question the practicality of the implementation of other provisions under the PPACA [37].

Supreme Court Decision

After the signing of the Patient Protection and Affordable Care Act in 2010, several states argued that certain provisions of the reform were unconstitutional [14]. In November 2011, the

Supreme Court elected to hear the debate on two key provisions included in the PPACA: the Individual Mandate and expansion of Medicaid, as well as the constitutionality of the ACA as a whole (all discussed earlier in this chapter) [14]. This section will highlight the arguments from both sides and discuss the final ruling from the Supreme Court [38].

Those filing claims against the constitutionality of the Individual Mandate included the National Federation of Independent Businesses (NFIB) and two individual plaintiffs without health insurance [14]. First and foremost, the Supreme Court had to decide if the Individual Mandate was constitutional or not (i.e., whether or not it is within Congress's power to regulate commerce and taxes), and, if found unconstitutional, it had to decide whether or not the entire provision must be dropped or if parts of it could remain [14]. Ultimately, the federal government argued that the Individual Mandate was constitutional based on three clauses of Congress: the Commerce Clause, the Necessary and Proper Clause, and Taxing Power [14]. The Commerce Clause states that Congress has the ability to "regulate Commerce with foreign Nations and among the several States, and within Indian tribes"; however, this clause does not differentiate between economic activity and inactivity [14]. Those against the ACA argue that not purchasing health insurance is a form of inactivity, which should not be covered under the Commerce Clause. The Necessary and Proper Clause asserts Congress's power to "enact all laws that are 'necessary and proper' for executing its enumerated powers, such as the Commerce Clause" [14], yet defendants argue that if the Individual Mandate is unconstitutional under the Commerce Clause, then this clause should not have the power to reverse that decision. Finally, the federal government states that the Individual Mandate falls under Congress's taxing ability since the consequence for not purchasing health insurance is the payment of a tax, while defendants argue that this is a penalty and thus not valid under this clause as well.

As for the Medicaid expansion, the federal government claimed it was constitutional under Congress's spending power, while the defendants argued that the expansion is coercive since states already depend so greatly on Medicaid funding such that choosing between adopting the expansion and foregoing all federal Medicaid payments essentially forces states to abide by the expansion [14]. The federal government, however, argued that it retains the rights to attach any conditions to federal funds it distributes to the states [14]. The idea that the expansion is coercive was unprecedented, but the federal government also argued that Medicaid has been expanded in the past and that they will cover a large majority of the costs of the expansion as well [14].

On June 28, 2012, the Supreme Court announced the final ruling concerning the ACA and these two provisions. Regarding the Individual Mandate, it determined that the mandate did exceed Congress's Commerce Clause by attempting to regulate inactivity; however, it also decided that the fee for not purchasing health insurance is in fact considered a tax and, therefore, ruled the Individual Mandate constitutional under Congress's Taxing Power [39]. Many other aspects associated with the Individual Mandate, which include insurance companies being prohibited from dropping individuals for preexisting conditions or individuals being allowed to remain on their dependent's plans until 26, were also upheld [39]. The Individual Mandate and its related provisions will be enacted starting in 2014 [14].

The conditions attached to the Medicaid expansion, however, were not upheld as the Supreme Court agreed with the defendants that the withholding of all Medicaid funds to states that choose not to participate in the expansion is considered coercive [39]. Therefore, states now have the option of choosing whether or not to participate in the expansion without losing any current funds they receive for Medicaid [39]. All other provisions of the Affordable Care Act were upheld.

Conclusion

In conclusion, with the exception of the Medicaid expansion and long-term care provisions, the majority of the health-care reform bill has been upheld. Over the next few years, millions of previously uninsured Americans will receive health insurance, and numerous changes will be made to the way in which this coverage is offered and received, as well as to how health care in general is delivered. There are plenty of advocates for this reform as well as opponents, with each claiming to have "evidence" in support of their views. As was seen with the long-term care provision, however, there will inevitably be more changes to come as we move forward, whether in legislation itself or in the provisions implemented.

References

1. Henry J. Kaiser Family Foundation. Timeline: history of health reform in the US [Internet]. 2011 [updated 2011]. http://healthreform.kff.org/flash/health-reform-new.html

2. Obama B. Why we need healthcare reform. The New York Times [Internet]. 2009 Aug 15 [cited 2012 Jun 11]. Opinion. http://www.nytimes.com/2009/08/16/opinion/16obama.html?_r=1&pagewanted=all

3. Stolberg S. Obama signs healthcare overhaul bill, with a flourish. The New York Times [Internet]. 2010 Mar 23 [cited 2012 Jun 11]. Money and Policy. http://www.nytimes.com/2010/03/24/health/policy/24health.html

4. DeNavas-Walt C, Proctor B, Smith J. Income, poverty, and health insurance coverage in the United States: 2010. Washington, DC: US Government Printing Office; 2011, 179p.

5. Henry J. Kaiser Family Foundation. Trends in healthcare costs and spending [Internet]. 2009 Mar [cited 2012 Jun 12]. http://www.kff.org/insurance/upload/7692_02.pdf

6. Orszag P. Growth in health care costs: statement before the committee on the budget, United States Senate. Washington, DC: Congressional Budget Office; 2008, 20p.

7. Centers for Medicare and Medicaid Services, Office of the Actuary. National health expenditures projections 2011–2012 [Electronic Report]. 2012 Jan [cited 2012 Jun 12]. 23p. http://www.cms.gov/Research-Statistics-Data-and-Systems/Statistics-Trends-and-Reports/NationalHealthExpendData/Downloads/Proj2011PDF.pdf

8. Henry J. Kaiser Family Foundation and Health Research Education Trust. Employer health benefits, 2011 annual survey [Internet]. 2011 Sep 27 [cited 2012 Jun 12]. 220p. http://ehbs.kff.org/pdf/2011/8225.pdf

9. American Academy of Family Physicians. Patient protection and affordable care act, Senate Health Care Bill [Internet]. 2009 Nov 30 [cited 2012 Jun 12]. http://www.aafp.org/online/en/home/policy/federal/issues/reform/ppaca.html

10. Docteur E, Berenson R. How does the quality of US HealthCare compare internationally? Timely analysis of immediate health policy issues [Internet]. 2009 Aug [cited 2012 Jun 12]. http://www.urban.org/uploadedpdf/411947_ushealthcare_quality.pdf

11. Nolte E, McKee CM. Measuring the health of nations: updating an earlier analysis [Internet]. Health Aff 2008; 27(1):58–71. http://www.commonwealthfund.org/usr_doc/1090_Nolte_measuring_hlt_of_nations_HA_01-2008_ITL(web).pdf?section=4039

12. Thorpe KE, Howard DH, Galactionova K. Differences in disease prevalence as a source of the U.S.-European health care spending [Internet]. Health Aff (Millwood) 2007; 26(6):678–86. http://ejournals.ebsco.com/Direct.asp?AccessToken=6VHLFLX89KCIZOVCFJN3MJFJX2LC8H9VVC&Show=Object&msid=941102954

13. Seshamani M. Coverage denied: how the current health insurance system leaves millions behind [internet]. 2012 Jun 8 [cited 2012 Jun 12]. http://www.healthreform.gov/reports/denied_coverage/index.html

14. Henry J. Kaiser Family Foundation. A guide to the Supreme Court's review of the 20120 healthcare reform law [Internet]. 2012 Jan [cited 2012 Jun 12]. http://www.kff.org/healthreform/upload/8270-2.pdf

15. Merlis M, Dentzer S. Health policy prief: individual mandate [Internet]. Health Aff. 2010; 31(6). http://www.healthaffairs.org/healthpolicybriefs/brief.php?brief_id=14

16. Henry J. Kaiser Family Foundation. Summary of the new health reform law [Internet]. 2011 Apr 15 [cited 2012 Jun 12]. http://www.kff.org/healthreform/8061.cfm

17. Mikkelson B, Mikkelson D. Health insurance exemptions. http://snopes.com/politics/medical/exemptions.asp. Accessed 12 Jun 2012

18. DeParle N. The affordable care act helps America's uninsured [Internet]. 2010 Sep 16 [cited 2012 Jun 12]. http://www.whitehouse.gov/blog/2010/09/16/affordable-care-act-helps-america-s-uninsured

19. Centers for Medicaid and Medicare Services. Children's Health Insurance Program (CHIP) [Internet]. Baltimore, MD. [cited 2012 Jun 12]. http://www.medicaid.gov/Medicaid-CHIP-Program-Information/By-Topics/Childrens-Health-Insurance-Program-CHIP/Childrens-Health-Insurance-Program-CHIP.html

20. Henry J. Kaiser Family Foundation. Explaining healthcare reform: what are health insurance exchanges? [Internet]. 2009 May [cited 2012 Jun 12]. http://www.kff.org/healthreform/upload/7908.pdf

21. American Cancer Society. Health reform premium and cost sharing subsidies [Internet]. [cited 2012 Jun 13]. http://www.acscan.org/pdf/healthcare/implementation/background/HealthReformPremiumCostSharingSubsidies.pdf

22. Henry J. Kaiser Family Foundation. Explaining health care reform: questions about health insurance subsidies [Internet]. 2010 Apr. [cited 2012 Jun 13]. http://www.kff.org/healthreform/upload/7962-02.pdf

23. Seshamani M. Young Americans and health insurance reform: giving young Americans the security and stability they need [Internet]. [cited 2012 Jun 12]. http://www.healthreform.gov/reports/youngadults/index.html.

24. American Cancer Society. Affordable Care Act: private insurance [Internet]. 2010 Apr 22 [cited 2012 Jun 12]. http://www.acscan.org/pdf/healthcare/implementation/factsheets/hcr-private-insurance.pdf

25. Chaikind H, Peterson C. Summary of potential employer under the Patient Protection and Affordable Care Act [Internet]. Congressional Research Service. 2010 May 14 [cited 2012 Jun 14]. http://www.shrm.org/hrdisciplines/benefits/Documents/Employer Penalties.pdf

26. Martin S, Bracht F, Jolivette G, Murawski L, Wurden M. The Patient Protection and Affordable Care Act: an overview of its potential impact on state health program. Sacramento, CA. Legislative Analyst's Office Report. 2010 May 13 [cited 2012 Jun 14]. 28p. http://www.lao.ca.gov/reports/2010/hlth/fed_healthcare/fed_healthcare_051310.pdf

27. Senate.gov. Responsible reform for the middle class – The Patient Protection and Affordable Care Act [Internet]. [cited 2012 Jun 14]. http://www.dpcc.senate.gov/?q=health+reform+bill&p=search&site=dpcc&num=10&filter=0&x=0&y=0

28. Pryde J, Senior Tax Editor. Health care reform: 13 tax changes on the way [Internet]. 2010 Oct 8. [cited 2012 Jun 12]. http://www.kiplinger.com/businessresource/forecast/archive/health-care-reform-tax-hikes-on-the-way.html

29. HealthReform.gov. Office of Health Reform, Department of Health and Human Services. Health insurance reform and Medicare: making Medicare stronger for America's seniors [Internet]. [cited 2012 Jun 15]. http://www.healthreform.gov/reports/medicare/index.html

30. HHS.gov. US Department of Health & Human Services. Justice Department announces largest health care fraud settlement in its history [Internet]. 2009 Sep 2 [cited 2012 Jun 15]. http://www.hhs.gov/news/press/2009pres/09/20090902a.html

31. Blum J, Deputy Administrator and Director for the Center of Medicare at the Centers for Medicare and Medicaid Services. What is the donut hole? [Internet]. 2010 Aug 9 [cited 2012 Jun 15]. http://www.healthcare.gov/blog/2010/08/donuthole.html

32. Mann S. Addressing the physician shortage under reform [Internet]. Association of American Medical Colleges. Washington, DC: 2011 Apr [cited 2012 Jun 16]. https://www.aamc.org/newsroom/reporter/april11/184178/addressing_the_physician_shortage_under_reform.html

33. Lloyd J. Doctor shortage looms as primary care loses its pull. USA Today [Internet]. 2009 Aug 17 [updated 2009 Aug 18; cited 2012 Jun 16]. Health and Behavior. http://www.usatoday.com/news/health/2009-08-17-doctor-gp-shortage_N.htm

34. Partnership for Prevention. Preventive care: a national profile on use, disparities, and health benefits [Internet]. C2007 Aug 7. [cited 2012 Jun 16]. http://www.prevent.org/data/files/initiatives/ncpppreventive carereport.pdf

35. HealthyAmericans.org. Patient Protection and Affordable Care Act (HR 3590). Selected Prevention, Public Health & Workforce Provisions [Internet]. [cited 2012 Jun 16]. http://healthyamericans.org/assets/files/Summary.pdf

36. Kemper P, Komisar H, Alecxih L. Long-term care over an uncertain future: what can current retirees expect? Inquiry [Internet]. 2005 [cited 2012 Jun 16]; 42(4):335–50. http://www.ncbi.nlm.nih.gov/pubmed/16568927

37. Issar N, Hassan M, Obremsky W, Jahangir A, Sethi M. The demise of the CLASS act: implications for the future of long term care. American Academy of Orthopaedic Surgeons [Internet]. Mar 2012 [cited 2012 Jul 27]. http://www.aaos.org/news/aaosnow/mar12/advocacy4.asp

38. Liptak A. Supreme Court upholds health care law, 5-4, in victory for Obama. The New York Times. [Internet]. 28 Jun 2012 [cited 2012 Jun 16]. http://www.nytimes.com/2012/06/29/us/supreme-court-lets-health-law-largely-stand.html?_r=2&hp

39. Buckley M. United States: Supreme Court rules on Affordable Care Act. [Internet] 28 Jun 2012 [cited 2012 Jul 2]. http://www.mondaq.com/unitedstates/x/185512/Healthcare/Supreme+Court+Rules+On+Affordable+Care+Act

Index